D1093038

Perinatal Psychiatry

Perinatal Psychiatry
The legacy of Channi Kumar

Edited by

Carmine M. Pariante

Sue Conroy

Paola Dazzan

Louise Howard

Susan Pawlby

Trudi Seneviratne

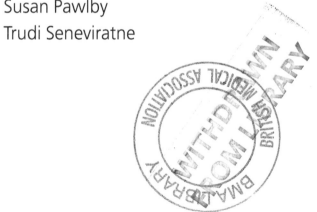

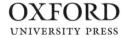

OXFORD
UNIVERSITY PRESS

OXFORD
UNIVERSITY PRESS

Great Clarendon Street, Oxford, OX2 6DP,
United Kingdom

Oxford University Press is a department of the University of Oxford.
It furthers the University's objective of excellence in research, scholarship,
and education by publishing worldwide. Oxford is a registered trade mark of
Oxford University Press in the UK and in certain other countries

© Oxford University Press 2014

The moral rights of the authors have been asserted

First Edition published in 2014

Impression: 1

Published in the United States of America by Oxford University Press
198 Madison Avenue, New York, NY 10016, United States of America

British Library Cataloguing in Publication Data
Data available

Library of Congress Control Number: 2013952762

ISBN 978-0-19-967685-9

Printed and bound by
CPI Group (UK) Ltd, Croydon, CR0 4YY

Oxford University Press makes no representation, express or implied, that the
drug dosages in this book are correct. Readers must therefore always check
the product information and clinical procedures with the most up-to-date
published product information and data sheets provided by the manufacturers
and the most recent codes of conduct and safety regulations. The authors and
the publishers do not accept responsibility or legal liability for any errors in the
text or for the misuse or misapplication of material in this work. Except where
otherwise stated, drug dosages and recommendations are for the non-pregnant
adult who is not breast-feeding

Links to third party websites are provided by Oxford in good faith and
for information only. Oxford disclaims any responsibility for the materials
contained in any third party website referenced in this work.

Foreword

Channi Kumar (Figure 1) was born in the Punjab, and came to England on his own at the age of 13, which perhaps caused him to have an independent mind. After qualifying in medicine he complemented his medical training with a doctorate in pharmacology. He trained in psychiatry at the Maudsley, and collaborated in the creation of the mother and baby unit in 1981—now re-named after him. From the beginning, he collaborated with others in carrying out a programme of research into puerperal illness, including research into which psychotropics pass into breast milk. Channi launched the Marcé Society, along-side Ian Brockington and James Hamilton, for research into mental illness associated with childbearing, and was its second president from 1986 to 1988. This has subsequently blossomed into a French Marcé society, and then an International Marcé society.

Many psychiatrists run good clinical services, other colleagues are good scientists and researchers, but it is rare to find both of these excellent qualities in the same person; however, Channi Kumar managed to do it. He did this by combining a genuine concern for others with a sharp enquiring mind. But he also combined warmth and gentleness with huge charm.

I read his papers long before I met him—that occurred when I started as the psychiatrist on the MRC's Small Grants Committee, and attended my first meeting as an observer, while Channi attended his last meeting in order to introduce me to my new task, and spoke to projects in both psychology and psychiatry. He advised me to see what was good in a project, and put my best foot forward in describing it to other members of the committee.

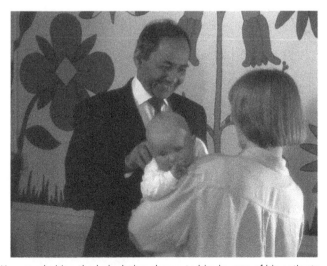

Fig. 1 Channi Kumar admiring the baby being shown to him by one of his patients.

Even at the Institute of Psychiatry he had no enemies, and managed to be friendly and helpful to all of us. In 1993 he offered to help to revise our postgraduate teaching. This meant potentially making enemies—but this seemed not to happen. His early death felt quite strange to us, the survivors—it seemed ironic that the nicest psychiatrist in the place was abruptly not there any more.

Channi was not just important to his psychiatric colleagues and his patients: he was also an important figure to both the nurses on his unit, and to midwives, both here at KCH, and more widely. The memorial service held by the midwives he had trained at KCH was a most moving occasion.

His contribution to science lives on—but my guess is that the memorial he would most have appreciated was the gratitude and respect that he inspired in his patients, as well as the better later adjustment experienced by the babies whose mothers were treated at his unit.

David Goldberg

Contents

Section 4 **Biological aspects of perinatal mental disorders**

Section 5 **Safeguarding mothers and children: the ongoing debate**

Contributors

Kathryn M. Abel
Professor
Centre for Women's Mental Health,
Institute of Brain Behaviour and Mental
Health,
University of Manchester

Ian Brockington
Professor Emeritus
University of Birmingham, UK

John Cox
Professor Emeritus, University of Keele, UK
Past President, Royal College of
Psychiatrists
Secretary General, World Psychiatric
Association (2002–2008)

Paola Dazzan MSc PhD FRCPsych
Reader in the Neurobiology
of Psychosis
Honorary Consultant Psychiatrist
Department of Psychosis Studies, Institute
of Psychiatry
De Crespigny Park
London, UK

Cindy-Lee Dennis, RN, PhD
Professor in Nursing and Medicine, Dept.
of Psychiatry
Shirley Brown Chair in Women's Mental
Health Research, Women's College
Research Institute
University of Toronto,
Toronto, Ontario
Canada

Therese Dowswell
Department of Women's and Children's
Health

The University of Liverpool, Liverpool
Women's NHS Foundation Trust
Crown Street
Liverpool, UK

Bárbara Figueiredo
Professora Associada com Agregação
Escola de Psicologia, Universidade do Minho
Braga, Portugal

Nine M.-C. Glangeaud-Freudenthal
PhD, Sci D
Senior researcher
CNRS at INSERM
Paris, France

Vivette Glover
Institute of Reproductive and
Developmental Biology
Imperial College London
Hammersmith Campus
London, UK

Sarah L. Halligan
Department of Psychology
University of Bath
Bath, UK

Louise M. Howard
Section of Women's Mental Health,
Health Services and Population Research
Department
Institute of Psychiatry
Kings College London
London, UK

Stephanie H. M. van Goozen
Professor of Psychology,
School of Psychology,
Cardiff University,
Cardiff, UK

Dale F. Hay
Professor of Psychology,
School of Psychology,
Cardiff University,
Cardiff, UK

Alison E. Hipwell, PhD., ClinPsyD
Associate Professor of Psychiatry
and Psychology
University of Pittsburgh Medical Center
Pittsburgh
PA, USA

Simonetta Agnello Hornby

Ian Jones
Professor of Psychiatry
Deputy Director
National Centre for Mental Health
Director of Clinical Training and
Public Engagement
MRC Centre for Neuropsychiatric
Genetics and Genomics
Cardiff University, UK

Shigenobu Kanba
Professor
Department of Neuropsychiatry
Graduate School of Medical Sciences
Kyushu University,
Fukuoka, Japan

Remi Kapo
c/o Quartet Books
London, UK

Michael W. O'Hara
Department of Psychology
University of Iowa
Iowa City, IA, USA

Lynne Murray
Stellenbosch University,
South Africa,
and University of Reading, UK

Margaret R. Oates
Clinical Director, East Midlands
Strategic Clinical Network
for Mental Health, Dementia
& Neurological Conditions,
NHS England and
Consultant Perinatal Psychiatrist,
Nottinghamshire Healthcare NHS Trust

Thomas G. O'Connor
University of Rochester Medical Center,
NY, USA

Kieran O'Donnell
Douglas Mental Health University
Institute
McGill University
Montreal, Canada

Carmine M. Pariante
Professor of Biological Psychiatry
and Head of the Sections of Perinatal
Psychiatry & Stress, Psychiatry
and Immunology
Institute of Psychiatry,
Kings College London,
Department of Psychological Medicine
London, UK

Susan Pawlby
Sections of Perinatal Psychiatry & Stress,
Psychiatry and Immunology
Institute of Psychiatry, Kings College
London, Department of Psychological
Medicine
London, UK

Atif Rahman
University of Liverpool, Institute of
Psychology, Health & Society, Child
Mental Health Unit
Alder Hey Children's NHS Foundation
Trust, Liverpool, UK

Lisa S. Segre
College of Nursing
University of Iowa
Iowa City
IA, USA

Deborah Sharp
Professor of Primary Health Care
Centre for Academic Primary Care, School
of Social and Community Medicine
University of Bristol, UK

Margaret Spinelli MD
Associate Professor of Clinical Psychiatry
Columbia University College of Physicians
and Surgeons
New York, NY, USA

Cerith S. Waters
Clinical Psychologist,
School of Psychology,
Cardiff University, Cardiff, UK

Hiroshi Yamashita
Senior Lecturer
Department of Child Psychiatry
Kyushu University Hospital
Fukuoka, Japan

Keiko Yoshida
Professor
The Department of Child Psychiatry
Kyushu University Hospital
Fukuoka, Japan

Section 1

Clinical and epidemiological aspects of perinatal mental disorders

Chapter 1

The obstetric outcome of pregnant women with psychotic disorders

Louise M. Howard

Introduction

In 1996, when I was working with Channi as a psychiatry trainee, we were both struck by how often we were seeing women with psychotic disorders in the outpatient clinic who were seeking advice on whether or not they should try to conceive and have a family. Although there was a small amount of literature on the parenting difficulties some of these women would experience, there was a very limited evidence base on their risk of adverse obstetric outcomes. We felt we needed to know more about the outcome of pregnancy for women with pre-existing psychotic disorders, and this led to my PhD, funded by a Wellcome Trust Clinical Training Fellowship, with Channi as my primary supervisor. Channi became too ill to continue working on this project, but our work together led to my perinatal mental health research programme, for which I will always be in his debt. This chapter describes this early PhD research, and the research it has led on to, over the subsequent years.

The fertility of women with psychotic disorders

We initially thought about collecting detailed clinical outcome data from the women we were seeing locally, who came from a large catchment area. However, to obtain a large enough sample size would take many years and it became clear we needed large epidemiological datasets in order to optimize statistical power and minimize bias. We therefore started to look for such data, with the first dataset available coming from colleagues at the Institute of Psychiatry—the PRiSM psychosis study (Thornicroft *et al.* 1998). The PRiSM psychosis study research team conducted the complete ascertainment of all prevalent cases of psychosis in the two study catchment areas in the index year (1991–1992) providing us with a representative population of mothers with psychotic disorders. We found that 63% of women with psychotic disorders (*n* = 155) were mothers, and that these women were more likely to be older and live in unsupported accommodation than women who had not had children, although they had similar levels of disability and health and social care needs (Howard *et al.* 2001). An Australian group of researchers reported a similar proportion of women (59%) with severe mental disorders in contact with community mental health teams in Australia to be mothers (McGrath *et al.* 1999), so we concluded that most women with chronic psychotic disorders do become mothers at some point in their lives. However, this does not in itself tell us much about how their fertility compares to the general population.

We therefore then investigated the fertility of women with psychotic disorders using the UK General Practice Research Database, a large dataset of around 5% of the UK population with electronic information on demographic, clinical, and drug prescription data on almost the whole population in the primary care catchment areas (as very few people are not registered with primary care in the UK). We found that the general fertility rate is considerably lower in women with psychotic disorders, particularly in women with a diagnosis of schizophrenia—these women had a general fertility rate (GFR) of 0.46 (95% CI 0.36–0.58), compared with age-matched women (Howard *et al.* 2002). Several studies published since our work have confirmed this decreased fertility in women with schizophrenia and bipolar disorder (and actually even more so in men), and GFRs of around 0.4 were found in a meta-analysis published in 2011 (Bundy *et al.* 2010).

There is evidence that the fertility of women with schizophrenia has increased in recent years, with a recent study reporting the GFR to be 1.16 times higher in 2007–2009 than in 1996–1998 (Vigod *et al.* 2012). This is likely to be due to the use of atypical antipsychotics, many of which do not have a sustained effect on prolactin and therefore do not impact on fertility; we also found that the traditional prolactin-raising neuroleptics had a particularly significant impact on fertility of women with affective psychosis (Howard *et al.* 2002).

We then investigated the outcome of these pregnancies including the psychosocial outcomes, using the General Practice Research Database and the UK Marcé Database. Our findings on the psychiatric and parenting outcomes are beyond the scope of this chapter. The rest of this chapter focuses on the obstetric and fetal outcomes of these pregnancies and reviews the growing literature, by our group and others, on the possible reasons for this increased risk.

Fetal outcomes

Using the General Practice Research Database I carried out a matched retrospective cohort study that compared the outcomes for women with a history of a psychotic disorder (and their infants), who gave birth in 1996–1998, with women matched for age and general practice (199 cases and 787 controls) and their infants. There was no significant difference between the cohorts in the risk of most individual obstetric complications, but we did not have reliable data on birth weight and prematurity and therefore could not investigate these outcomes. However, there were significantly more Caesarean sections among the women with psychotic disorders and, in the adjusted and unadjusted analyses, there was a significantly greater proportion of stillbirth and neonatal deaths in infants of women with psychotic disorders compared with the comparison cohort (Howard *et al.* 2003). Our data were included in a meta-analysis published in 2005 (Webb *et al.* 2005), which reported a twofold increase in the risk of stillbirths in women with psychotic disorders. This has been replicated in subsequent studies (e.g. Webb *et al.* 2006; MacCabe *et al.* 2007).

There is also a growing research literature, using Scandinavian and Australian registers, which consistently finds that schizophrenia (Bennedsen *et al.* 1999; Jablensky *et al.* 2005; King-Hele *et al.* 2007) and affective psychosis (MacCabe *et al.* 2007) are associated with around a twofold increased risk of low birth weight, prematurity, and small for gestational age babies. This is even after adjustments for confounders such as smoking, although the risks are attenuated in multivariate analyses (Nilsson *et al.* 2002, 2008; MacCabe *et al.* 2007). Obstetric complications also appear to be more common (Sacker *et al.* 1996) (Leight *et al.* 2010), with Jablensky highlighting the increased risk of placental abruption (Jablensky *et al.* 2005), and others reporting an increased risk of Caesarean section (Boden *et al.* 2012). There is therefore consistent evidence that women with psychotic disorders, both schizophrenia and affective psychotic disorders, have pregnancies that are at increased risk of low birth weight, prematurity, obstetric complications, stillbirths, and neonatal deaths and infant deaths. Moreover we and others have also reported an increased risk of neonatal deaths and sudden infant death syndrome (SIDS) in the infants of women with psychotic disorders (Bennedsen *et al.* 2001; Howard *et al.* 2003; King-Hele *et al.* 2007). These are therefore vulnerable babies who do not grow optimally in utero, and are at increased risk of death in infancy.

Mechanisms

There are a number of potential mechanisms that could account for these findings, but the first question to ask is whether these increased risks are specific to psychotic disorders, or whether they also extend to other mental disorders? Studies using Scandinavian registers report an increased risk for women with a history of a psychiatric admission, whatever the diagnosis, with particularly high rates of adverse outcomes in women admitted with alcohol or drug misuse disorders. The relative risks reported previously are comparable to those in the offspring of parents admitted for other mental disorders, such as affective disorder and alcohol/drug-related disorder (Webb *et al.* 2006). Rates of death by natural causes do not appear to be raised with any specific diagnosis (King-Hele *et al.* 2007; Nilsson *et al.* 2008; Webb, J.B. *et al.* 2008) but fatal birth defect risk is modestly elevated with maternal affective disorder, and to a greater degree with maternal schizophrenia (Webb, R. *et al.* 2008). Similarly SIDS rates are elevated with schizophrenia and other mental disorders, though the highest SIDS risk is with maternal alcohol/drug-related disorder (King-Hele *et al.* 2007), which is a well-established risk factor for SIDS.

However, it is not only pregnant women with a history of a psychiatric admission (a marker of severity of mental disorder) that have an increased risk of these adverse outcomes. A recent meta-analysis examining the relationship between maternal depression and birth outcomes also found an increased risk of low birth weight, prematurity, and small for gestational age babies, although the effect was only found for women experiencing socioeconomic deprivation (Grote *et al.* 2010). Other research groups have reported on an increased risk of pregnancy loss associated with a range of mental disorders (Gold *et al.* 2007), and, using a case–control study design, using data from the General Practice Research Database, we found depression in pregnancy was associated with SIDS in which no cases were admitted during pregnancy, or on psychotropic medication (Howard 2007).

There has been some inconsistency in the research literature on whether behavioural risk factors, such as smoking, explain these findings. In many studies, data on these covariates are not available; in others, the risk is attenuated by controlling for these confounders, and sometimes no independent association is found (Boden *et al.* 2012), but in some studies a significant risk remains (Nilsson *et al.* 2002). With all of these studies, miss-classification bias is likely to be a problem, as smoking and other risk factors are under-reported and under-recorded. What is clear is that much of the increased risk for adverse pregnancy outcomes is probably accounted for by covariates, as these potential confounders are particularly common in women with psychotic disorders, and more importantly perhaps are potentially modifiable. I am therefore going to discuss research on these comorbid factors in the following sections. However, there are other risk factors that are not covered here (although they are covered elsewhere in this book) and need to be borne in mind, which I will briefly discuss.

First, psychotropic medication, which is covered extensively in Chapter 5, will often be prescribed during pregnancy in women with severe mental illnesses. Even if women stop medication when they realize they are pregnant, exposure during major organ formation in the first trimester will have already occurred. Debate continues as to whether antipsychotic medication impacts on the risk of congenital anomalies and fetal outcomes such as birth weight, while it is already known that some mood stabilizers (particularly valproate) (Meador *et al.* 2008) are linked with a substantially increased risk of neural tube defects and other major malformations. However, many women with severe mental disorders will need to take medication during pregnancy to stay well, while minimizing risks by using the lowest effective dose and using drugs that have not been reported to be associated with significant increases in risk where possible.

Second, it is possible that some of the adverse outcomes reported are due to genetic factors. It is known that higher rates of minor physical anomalies have been found in people with schizophrenia and their close relatives (Ismail *et al.* 1998), and shared genetic factors between the mother and baby may explain some of these adverse outcomes. However, the increased risk of fatal birth defects was found only in maternal schizophrenia, not paternal schizophrenia, in the study discussed above (Webb, R. *et al.* 2008).

Third, the impact of the illness itself may explain some of the adverse outcomes, and this is rarely adequately controlled for in studies investigating outcomes for women with psychotic disorders. This is understandable as controls with the same disorders not on medication are difficult to detect in register studies and are rare. The literature on the impact of illness is covered in chapters XX and although most of this literature is not on psychotic disorders, the mechanisms discussed are also likely to be relevant to this population.

Finally, many of the risk factors discussed next are associated with socioeconomic deprivation, and most women with chronic psychotic disorders have financial difficulties and live in difficult circumstances (Howard *et al.* 2001), with unmet health and social care needs that are not detected by professionals but are likely to impact on health during pregnancy (Howard and Hunt 2008; Webb *et al.* 2010). Deprivation is a complex concept and a distal risk factor, which is difficult to measure in its entirety, but it undoubtedly contributes to the health inequalities described next.

Risk factors

Smoking

Smoking is the leading preventable cause of fetal morbidity and mortality in the UK and other high-income countries. Smoking is associated with an increased risk of miscarriage, congenital malformations, low birth weight, prematurity, stillbirths, SIDS, and physical and mental disorders in childhood (Royal College of Physicians 2010). Smoking prevalence in pregnancy varies from 3% to 30% across England, with an average of 13% still smoking at delivery (Health and Social Care Information 2012), and similar rates reported in other high-income countries. Women with mental disorders are more likely to be smoking at conception, at antenatal booking, and up until delivery (Shah and Howard, 2006; Goodwin *et al.* 2007), and to find it more difficult to stop smoking, even if they accept referral to smoking cessation services (Howard *et al.*, 2012). People with severe mental disorders are particularly likely to smoke heavily and be more addicted to nicotine (Aubin *et al.* 2012).

There is good evidence from a large Cochrane systematic review (72 randomized controlled trials (RCTs); $n > 25,000$) that smoking cessation programmes reduce the proportion of pregnant women continuing to smoke, and improve rates of low birth weight and prematurity (Lumley *et al.* 2004), but trials in pregnant women have failed to measure the impact of mental disorders on the effectiveness of smoking cessation interventions in pregnancy. Nevertheless in non-pregnant people with mental disorders (both severe psychotic disorders and depressive disorders), smoking cessation interventions are effective (Banham and Gilbody, 2010; Tsoi *et al.* 2010), though patients are likely to need more support. Uptake of smoking cessation services during pregnancy is low in general (Taylor and Hajek, 2001), and The American Congress of Obstetricians and Gynecologists (ACOG) in 2005 and the UK National Institute for Clinical Excellence (now known as the National Institute for Health and Care Excellence from 2013) in 2010 (NICE 2010a) emphasize that pregnant women who continue to smoke are often heavily addicted to nicotine and should be encouraged at every follow up visit to seek help to stop smoking. However, translation of this guidance into practice is far from complete, and a recent audit in a South London hospital found that smoking was rarely discussed after the initial antenatal booking visit (Howard *et al.* 2012).

There has been one RCT of a cognitive behavioural intervention in high-risk African-American women with comorbidities including depression, smoking, and partner violence, with modules directed at each risk factor provided; this led to improved maternal and fetal outcomes including very low birth weight and very premature birth (El-Mohandes *et al.* 2009; Joseph *et al.* 2009). There is also evidence that smoking cessation in pregnancy is associated with improvements in symptoms of depression (Munafò *et al.* 2008). In addition, public health campaigns, such as the SIDS reduction campaigns, can impact on antenatal smoking in women with severe mental disorders, although smoking rates in women with a history of a severe mental disorder remain high (Webb *et al.* 2010). Smoking cessation in pregnant women with psychotic disorders is therefore possible, without worsening of mental health.

However, data from the UK and the USA suggest that primary and maternity care staff are less likely to record antenatal smoking behaviour in pregnant women with major mental health problems (Kelly *et al.* 1999; Howard *et al.* 2012). Smoking cessation interventions for pregnant women are thus in urgent need of research and development. Tailoring of interventions to risk factors present in pregnant smokers seems important, since a randomized trial of an intensive depression-focused intervention for smoking cessation in pregnancy found that women with high levels of depressive symptoms receiving the depression-focused treatment achieved higher abstinence and improved depressive symptoms, whilst women with low levels of depressive symptoms had better outcomes if they received a control intervention (Cincirpini *et al.* 2010).

Although recent drivers such as the various NICE guidelines on perinatal care (NICE, 2007, 2010) have advocated routine screening by midwives for smoking (and antenatal mental health problems and domestic violence), one additional strategy would be to target women with mental disorders before pregnancy by providing preconception counselling via mental health services (Lewis 2011). This, and other innovations to improve uptake and efficacy of cessation support in pregnancy, are urgently needed.

Alcohol and substance misuse

Alcohol in pregnancy is associated with miscarriage, preterm birth, low birth weight, and developmental delays, including partial and full fetal alcohol syndrome (Makarechian *et al.* 1998; O'Leary *et al.* 2009). Alcohol use in pregnancy is predicted by pre-pregnancy alcohol consumption (i.e. quantity and frequency of typical drinking) and exposure to abuse or violence (Skagerstrom *et al.* 2011), with inconsistent evidence for an association between antenatal psychiatric disorders or symptoms and alcohol misuse (Lancaster *et al.* 2010; Skagerstrom *et al.* 2011). A Cochrane review (of only four RCTs) suggests that psychological and educational interventions may result in increased abstinence from alcohol, and a reduction in alcohol consumption among pregnant women (Stade *et al.* 2009), but there have been no trials on women with both mental disorders and alcohol abuse.

The prevalence of illicit drug use in pregnant women in the general population is also significant, with marijuana the most commonly used illegal drug, with more than 10% of UK inner city pregnant women screening positive for cannabis at booking (Sherwood *et al.* 1999). High rates of smoking (>80%) are often reported in substance-misusing women, which may be more harmful than other substances (and is commoner), but other substances have an independent effect on foetal outcomes (e.g. Lutiger *et al.* 1991; Kuhn *et al.* 2000)). Pregnant women with mental disorders are more likely to abuse alcohol and substances (Howard *et al.* 2012) but again there is very little evidence on how to help these women most effectively.

Obesity and nutrition

There has been a significant increase in first-trimester maternal obesity (BMI >30 kg/m^2) over the last two decades in the UK (7.6% in 1989; 15.6% in 2007) (Heslehurst *et al.* 2008; Heslehurst *et al.* 2010), with an impact on maternal deaths (Lewis 2011). There is a growing evidence base on the impact of obesity on adverse pregnancy outcomes, including congenital neurological defects, obstetric and fetal complications (e.g. gestational diabetes, shoulder dystocia, macrosomia) (Stothard *et al.* 2009; Lewis 2011). This is likely to be a particular issue for pregnant women with psychotic disorders. A recent study has reported overweight/obesity in pregnancy in around 50% of women with psychotic disorders prescribed antipsychotic medication (Boden *et al.* 2012) and there is some preliminary evidence of an association between obesity and other mental disorders (Howard and Croker 2012). Studies have also reported an increased risk of gestational diabetes in women with psychotic disorders, even after adjusting for maternal factors, with a similar risk increase for the more obesogenic and diabetogenic antipsychotics clozapine and olanzapine as for other antipsychotics, though this may reflect a lack of statistical power to detect differences (Reis and Källén 2008; Boden *et al.* 2012). We have also recently reported a case of resistant hyperinsulinaemia in an infant exposed to olanzapine, with no maternal obesity, which suggests adverse metabolic impacts on the infant of the medication itself (Rowe *et al.* 2012). Nutritional deficiencies in women with or without obesity are also more common in women with mental disorders, and a recent systematic review found a higher risk of folate and vitamin B12 deficiencies in childbearing age women with psychotic disorders (McColl *et al.*). Weight management/nutritional interventions are currently being developed and evaluated (e.g. the UPBEAT study; Poston *et al.* 2013), but there has been limited focus on how to help women with additional mental health problems. The nutrition of pregnant women with mental disorders is an area that undoubtedly needs research, but while data are awaited health care professionals need to support women with psychotic disorders to optimize BMI before conception, to help them with their nutritional needs in pregnancy, and to ensure gestational weight gain is optimal.

Domestic violence

Domestic violence is defined in the UK as any incident or pattern of incidents of controlling, coercive or threatening behaviour, violence, or abuse, between those aged 16 or over who are or have been intimate partners or family members, regardless of gender or sexuality. This can encompass, but is not limited to, psychological, physical, sexual, financial, or emotional abuse. It is associated with mental disorders across the diagnostic spectrum (Trevillion *et al.* 2012; Howard *et al.* 2013) and many of the comorbidities described above (e.g. antenatal smoking and alcohol abuse). There is a growing literature on its association with adverse pregnancy including low birth weight and prematurity (Feder *et al.* 2009). It may therefore also be an important confounder when evaluating the impact of medication on pregnancy outcome. In the majority of cases, antenatal violence continues into the postnatal period, and both antenatal and postnatal violence are associated with adverse child behavioural outcomes (Flach *et al.* 2011). A recent Cochrane review on interventions for domestic violence in pregnancy included nine trials ($n = 2391$ women) but for most outcomes very few studies contributed data (Jahanfar *et al.* 2011). There was evidence from one study that the total number of women reporting episodes of partner violence during pregnancy, and in the postpartum period, was reduced for women receiving a psychological therapy intervention but only one study reported findings for fetal outcomes such as preterm delivery and birth weight, and there were no clinically significant differences between groups. There is therefore insufficient evidence to assess the effectiveness of interventions for domestic violence on pregnancy outcomes, and no trials of women with psychotic disorders. However, good practice recommendations include referral and care pathways for women experiencing domestic violence with routine enquiry about domestic violence when seeing pregnant women with mental disorders (Howard 2012).

Implications and conclusions

It is clear that the pregnancies of women with psychotic disorders are high-risk pregnancies. The woman herself during pregnancy is at risk of relapse if she stops taking medication or postnatally due to the increased risk of illness in women with psychosis (Munk-Olsen *et al.* 2006), and there are clear risks also for the fetus and infant. This is not only due to the illness and possible medication effects; women with psychotic disorders are more likely to have comorbid risk factors for adverse fetal and neonatal outcomes compared with the general population of pregnant women. Maternity professionals need to be aware of this increased risk so that they can ensure optimal care is delivered.

When examining the effects of psychosis on pregnancy, fetal and infant outcomes, studies therefore need to ensure confounders are appropriately measured and taken into account in the analysis. Many confounders are comorbidities that are particularly common in pregnant women with mental disorders, including smoking, substance misuse, and nutritional deficiencies. Comorbidities are also important to bear in mind when considering the risks and benefits of medication in a particular woman as they can act as effect modifiers. For example, socioeconomic status interacts with antenatal depression so that in pregnant women of low socioeconomic status depression is associated with low birth weight, but no association is found between depression and low birth weight in pregnant women from less deprived backgrounds (Grote *et al.* 2010). These co-morbidities can also impact directly on the effectiveness of medication, for example by induction of CYP1A2 by smoking (Taylor *et al.* 2012).

There is still some debate as to the nature of comprehensive care for pregnant women with psychotic disorders, with little guidance for clinicians. However, some clinical guidelines now advocate screening for severe mental illness history (NICE 2007) and/or domestic violence (NICE 2008, 2010b), increased monitoring of glucose metabolism during pregnancy (SIGN 2012), and modification of maternal care pathways for women with substance misuse problems and other complex social factors (NICE 2010b). At present, as discussed earlier, there is a very limited evidence base on which to base clinical decision-making, both for medication and for interventions addressing comorbidities.

It is hoped that this book will facilitate further research into this important area, and help answer the questions Channi and I grappled with in his welcoming office at the Institute of Psychiatry in the 1990s.

References

American Congress of Obstetricians and Gynecologists (ACOG). Smoking cessation in pregnancy Technical Bulletin 316. Washington DC, ACOG.

Aubin, H.J., Rollema, H., Svesnsson, T.H., *et al.* (2012). Smoking, quitting, and psychiatric disease: a review. Neuroscience and Biobehavioral Reviews **36**(1): 271–284.

Banham, L. and Gilbody, S. (2010). Smoking cessation in severe mental illness: what works? Addiction **105**(7): 1176–89.

Bennedsen, B., Mortensen, P., *et al.* (1999). Preterm birth and intra-uterine growth retardation among children of women with schizophrenia. British Journal of Psychiatry **175**: 239–45.

Bennedsen, B., Mortensen, P., *et al.* (2001). Congenital malformations, stillbirths, and infant deaths among children of women with schizophrenia. Archives of General Psychiatry **58**(7): 674–79.

Boden, R., Lundgren, M., *et al.* (2012). Antipsychotics during pregnancy: relation to fetal and maternal metabolic effects. Archives of General Psychiatry **58**(7): 674–9.

Boden, R.L., Brandt, M.L., *et al.* (2012). Antipsychotics during pregnancy: relation to fetal and maternal metabolic effects. Archives of General Psychiatry **69**(7): 715–21.

Bundy, H., Stahl, D., *et al.* (2010). A systematic review and meta-analysis of the fertility of patients with schizophrenia and their unaffected relatives. Acta Psychiatrica Scandinavica **123**(2): 98–106.

Cincirpini, P., Blalock, J., Minnix, J.A., *et al.* (2010). Effects of an intensive depression-focused intervention for smoking cessation in pregnancy. Journal of Consulting Clinical Psychology **78**(1): 44–54.

El-Mohandes, A. A., Kiely, M., *et al.* (2009). Prediction of birth weight by cotinine levels during pregnancy in a population of black smokers. Pediatrics **124**(4): e671–80.

Feder, G., Ramsay, J., *et al.* (2009). How far does screening women for domestic (partner) violence in different health-care settings meet criteria for a screening programme? Systematic reviews of nine UK National Screening Committee criteria. Health Technology Assessment **13**(16): 1–113, 137–437.

Flach, C., Leese, M., *et al.* (2011). Antenatal domestic violence, maternal mental health and subsequent child behaviour: a cohort study. BJOG: An International Journal of Obstetrics and Gynaecology **118**(11): 1383–91.

Gold, K.J., Dalton, V.K., *et al.* (2007). What causes pregnancy loss? Preexisting mental illness as an independent risk factor. General Hospital Psychiatry **29**(3): 207–13.

Goodwin, R.D., Keyes, K., *et al.* (2007). Mental disorders and nicotine dependence among pregnant women in the United States. Obstetrics & Gynecology **109**(4): 875–83.

Grote, N. K., Bridge, J.A., *et al.* (2010). A meta-analysis of depression during pregnancy and the risk of preterm birth, low birth weight, and intrauterine growth restriction. Archives of General Psychiatry **67**(10): 1012–24.

Health and Social Care Information (2012). Statistics on women's smoking status at time of delivery. 2012. Available from http://www.hscic.gov.uk/catalogue/PUB11039 (accessed 24 September 2013).

Heslehurst, N., Rankin, J., Wilkinson, J.R., *et al.* (2010). A nationally representative study of maternal obesity in England, UK: trends in incidence and demographic inequalities in 619 323 births, 1989–2007. International Journal of Obesity **34**(3): 420–8.

Heslehurst, N., Simpson, H., Ells, L.J., *et al.* (2008). The impact of maternal BMI status on pregnancy outcomes with immediate short-term obstetric resource implications: a meta-analysis. Obesity Reviews **9**(6): 635–83.

Howard, L. (2007). Sudden infant death syndrome and maternal depression. Journal of Clinical Psychiatry **68**(8): 1279–83.

Howard, L. (2012). Domestic violence: its relevance to psychiatry. Advances in Psychiatric Treatment **18**: 129–36.

Howard, L. and Hunt, K. (2008). The needs of mothers with severe mental illness: a comparison of assessmentts of needs by staff and patients. Archives of Women's Mental Health **11**(2): 131–6.

Howard, L.M. and Croker, H. (2012). Obesity and mental health. In Obesity and pregnancy. M. Gillman and L. Poston, editors, Cambridge, Cambridge University Press 70–79.

Howard, L., Kumar, C., Thornicroft, G., *et al.* (2001). The psychosocial characteristics of mothers with psychotic disorders. British Journal of Psychiatry **178**: 427–32.

Howard, L., Kumar, C., Leese, M., *et al.* (2002). The general fertility rate in women with psychotic disorders. American Journal of Psychiatry **159**(6): 991–7.

Howard, L. M., Goss, C., Leese, M., *et al.* (2003). Medical outcome of pregnancy in women in psychotic disorders and their infants in the first year after birth. British Journal of Psychiatry **182**: 63–7.

Howard, L., Bekele, D., Rowe, M., *et al.* (2012). Smoking cessation in pregnant women with mental disorders: a cohort and nested qualitative study. An International Journal of Obstetrics and Gynaecology **20**(3): 362–70.

Howard, L.M., Oram, S., Galley, H., *et al.* (2013). Domestic violence and perinatal mental disorders: a systematic review and meta-analysis. PLoS Med. **10**(5): e1001452. doi: 10.1371/journal. pmed.1001452.

Ismail, B., Cantor-Graawe, E., McNeil, T.F., *et al.* (1998). Minor physical anomalies in schizophrenic patients and their siblings. American Journal of Psychiatry **155**(12): 1695–702.

Jablensky, A., Morgan, V., Zubrick, S.R., *et al.* (2005). Pregnancy, delivery, and neonatal complications in a population cohort of women with schizophrenia and major affective disorders. American Journal of Psychiatry **162**: 79–91.

Jahanfar, S., Janssen, P., Howard, L.M., *et al.* (2011). Interventions for preventing or reducing domestic violence against pregnant women Cochrane Database of Systematic Reviews (11): CD009414.

Joseph, J., EL-Mohandes, A., Kiely, M., *et al.* (2009). Reducing psychosocial and behavioral pregnancy risk factors: results of a randomized clinical trial among high-risk pregnant african american women. American Journal of Public Health **99**(6): 1053–61.

Kelly, R.H., Banielsen, B.H., Goulding, J.M., *et al.* (1999). Adequacy of prenatal care among women with psychiatric diagnoses giving birth in California in 1994 and 1995. Psychiatric Services **50**(12): 6.

King-Hele, S., Abel, K., Webb, R.T., *et al.* (2007). Risk of sudden infant death syndrome with parental mental illness. Archives of General Psychiatry **64**: 1323–30.

Kuhn, L., Kline, J., Ng, S., *et al.* (2000). Cocaine use during pregnancy and intrauterine growth retardation: new insights based on maternal hair tests. American Journal of Epidemiology **152**(2): 112–19.

Lancaster, C.A., Gold, K.J., Flynn, H.A., *et al.* (2010). Risk factors for depressive symptoms during pregnancy: a systematic review American Journal of Obstetrics & Gynecology **202**(1): 5–14.

Leight, K.L., Fitelson, E.M., Weston, C.A., *et al.* (2010). Childbirth and mental disorders. International Review of Psychiatry **22**(5): 453–71.

Lewis, G.B. (2011). Saving mothers' lives. Confidential enquiry into maternal deaths 2005–8. BJOG: An International Journal of Obstetrics and Gynaecology 118, Supplement 1.

Lumley, J., Oliver, S., Dowswell, T., *et al.* (2004). Interventions for promoting smoking cessation during pregnancy (Review). Cochrane Database Systematic Review Jul 8;(3):CD001055. doi: 10.1002/14651858.CD001055.pub3

Lutiger, B., Graham, K., Einarson, T.R., *et al.* (1991). Relationship between gestational cocaine use and pregnancy outcome: a meta-analysis. Teratology **44**: 405–11.

MacCabe, J., Martinsson, L., Lichtenstein, P., *et al.* (2007). Adverse pregnancy outcomes in mothers with affective psychosis. Bipolar Disorders **9**(3): 305–9.

Makarechian, N., Agro, K., Devlin, J., *et al.* (1998). Association between moderate alcohol consumption during pregnancy and spontaneous abortion, stillbirth and premature birth: a meta-analysis. The Canadian Journal of Clinical Pharmacology **5**: 169–76.

McColl, H., Dhillon, M., Howard, L.M., *et al.* A systematic review of the nutritional status of pregnant women with severe mental illness. Archives of Women's Mental Health **16**(1): 39–46.

McGrath, J., Hearle, J., Jenner, L., *et al.* (1999). The fertility and fecundity of patients with psychoses. Acta Psychiatrica Scandinavica **99**(6): 441–6.

Meador, K., Reynolds, M., Crean, S., *et al.* (2008). Pregnancy outcomes in women with epilepsy: a systematic review and meta-analysis of published pregnancy registries and cohorts. Epilepsy Research **81**(1): 1–13.

Munafò, M.R., Heron, J., Araya, R., *et al.* (2008). Smoking patterns during pregnancy and postnatal period and depressive symptoms. Nicotine & Tobacco Research **10**(11): 1602–9.

Munk-Olsen, T., Laursen, T.M., Pedersen, C.B., *et al.* (2006). New parents and mental disorders: a population-based register study. JAMA **296**(1): 2582–9.

NICE (2007). Antenatal and postnatal mental health: clinical management and service guidance. NICE. London.

NICE (2008). Antenatal care. NICE Clinical Guideline 62. London, NICE, National Institute for Health and Clinical Excellence.

NICE (2010a). Quitting smoking in pregnancy and following childbirth. NICE Public Health Guidance 26. London, NICE, National Institute for Health and Clinical Excellence.

NICE (2010b). Pregnancy and complex social factors. NICE Clinical Guideline 110. London, NICE, National Institute for Health and Clinical Excellence.

Nilsson, E., Lichtenstein, P., Cnattingius, S., *et al.* (2002). Women with schizophrenia: pregnancy outcome and infant death among their offspring. Schizophrenia Research **58**(2–3): 221–9.

Nilsson, E., Hultman, C., Cnattingius, S., *et al.* (2008). Schizophrenia and offspring's risk for adverse pregnancy outcomes and infant death. British Journal of Psychiatry **193**(4): 311–15.

O'Leary, C., Nassar, N., Kurinczuk, J.J., *et al.* (2009). The effect of maternal alcohol consumption on fetal growth and preterm birth. BJOG: An International Journal of Obstetrics and Gynaecology **116**: 390–400.

Poston, L., Holmes, B., Barr, S., *et al.* (2013). Developing a complex intervention for diet and activity behaviour change in obese pregnant women (the UPBEAT trial); assessment of behavioural change and process evaluation in a pilot randomised controlled trial. BMC Pregnancy Childbirth **13**(1): 148.

Reis, M. and Källén, B. (2008). Maternal use of antipsychotics in early pregnancy and delivery outcome. Journal of Clinical Psychopharmacology **28**(3): 279–288.

Rowe, M., Gowda, B., Taylor, D., *et al.* (2012). Neonatal hypoglycaemia following maternal olanzapine therapy during pregnancy: a case report. Therapeutic Advances in Psychopharmacology **2**(6): 265–8.

Royal College of Physicians (2010). Passive smoking and children: A report of the Tobacco Advisory Group of the Royal College of Physicians. London, Royal College of Physicians.

Sacker, A., Done, D., Crow, T.J., *et al.* (1996). Obstetric complications in children born to parents with schizophrenia: a meta-analysis of case-control studies. Psychological Medicine **26**(2): 279–87.

Shah, N. and Howard, L.M. (2006). Screening for Smoking and Substance Misuse in Pregnant Women with Mental Illness. Psychiatric Bulletin **30**: 3.

Sherwood, R., Keating, J., Kavvadia, V., Greenough, A., and Peters, T.J. (1999). Substance misuse in early pregnancy and relationship to fetal outcome. European Journal of Pediatrics **158**(6): 488–92.

SIGN. (2012). Management of Perinatal Mood Disorders, SIGN, Scottish Intercollegiate Guideline Network, Edinburgh.

Skagerstrom, J., Chang, G., and Nilson, P. (2011). Predictors of drinking during pregnancy: A systematic review. Journal of Women's Health **20**(6): 901–13.

Stade, B.C., Bailey, C., Dzendoletas, D., *et al.* (2009). Pychological and/or educational interventions for reducing alcohol consumption in pregnant women and women planning pregnancy. Cochrane Database Systematic Review **15**(2): CD004228.

Stothard, K., Tennant, P., Bell, R., *et al.* (2009). Maternal overweight and obesity and the risk of congenital anomalies: a systematic review and meta-analysis. JAMA: Journal of the American Medical Association **301**(6): 636–50.

Taylor, D., Paton, C., and Kapur, S. (2012). The Maudsley Prescribing Guidelines in Psychiatry. Oxford, Wiley-Blackwell.

Taylor, T. and Hajek, P. (2001). Smoking Cessation Services for Pregnant Women. London, Health Development Agency.

Thornicroft, G., G.Strathdee, Phelan, M., *et al.* (1998). Rationale and design. PRiSM Psychosis Study I. The British Journal of Psychiatry **173**: 363–70.

Trevillion, K., Oram, S., Galley, H., *et al.* (2012). Domestic violence and mental disorders: systematic review and metal analysis. PlosOne **7**(12): e51740.doi: 10.1371/journal.pone.0051740.

Tsoi, D., Porwal, M., Webster, A.C., *et al.* (2010). Interventions for smoking cessation and reduction in individuals with schizophrenia. Cochrane Database of Systematic Reviews **16**(6: CD007253).

Vigod, S., Seeman, M., Ray, J.G., *et al.* (2012). Temporal trends in general age-specific fertility rates among women with schizophrenia (1996–2009): A population-based study in Ontario, Canada. Schizophrenia Research **139**(1–3): 169–75.

Webb, J.B., Siega-Riz, A.M., *et al.* (2008). Psychosocial determinants of adequacy of gestational weight gain. Obesity **17**(2): 300–9.

Webb, R., Abel, K., Pickles, A., *et al.* (2005). Mortality in offspring of parents with psychotic disorders: a critical review and meta-analysis. American Journal of Psychiatry **162**: 1045–56.

Webb, R., Abel, K., Pickles, A., *et al.* (2006). Mortality risk among offspring of psychiatric inpatients: A population-based follow-up to early adulthood. American Journal of Psychiatry **163**: 2170–7.

Webb, R., Pickles, A., King-Hele, S.A., *et al.* (2008). Parental mental illness and fatal birth defects in a national birth cohort. Psychological Medicine **38**: 1495–1503.

Webb, R.T., Wicks, S., Dalman, C., *et al.* (2010). Influence of environmental factors in higher risk of sudden infant death syndrome linked with parental mental illness. Archives of General Psychiatry **67**(1): 69–77.

Chapter 2

The psychoses of childbearing

Ian Brockington

Introduction

It is 50 years since the late Ralph Paffenbarger (1961) wrote a famous article on 'the picture puzzle of postpartum psychosis'. In order to solve this puzzle, it is necessary to clarify the term 'postpartum psychosis'.

One must first exclude a wide variety of disorders, occurring after childbirth, which are not 'psychoses'. This may seem obvious, but, at one time, some psychoanalysts included disorders of the mother-infant relationship under 'postpartum schizophrenia' (Zilboorg 1929).

Organic and non-organic psychoses

One must then draw a clear boundary between organic and non-organic psychoses. The birth process is so complex, and has so many complications, that there are (depending on definition) 15–18 distinct organic psychoses occurring in pregnancy, parturition or the puerperium (Brockington 2006). Nineteenth century alienists found it difficult to distinguish these from puerperal mania, and this was not finally achieved until the work of Chaslin (1895) & Bonhöffer (1910) at the turn of the twentieth century. Even the most common of these organic psychoses—eclamptic psychosis and infective delirium—are now rare in Europe, North America, and Japan; but these nations, where most of the research is done, contribute less than 10% of the world's births. In the rest of the world they may be important, and they may still interfere with epidemiological, genetic, and neuroscientific studies of non-organic psychoses.

As for the non-organic psychoses, a few are psychogenic, but most have manic depressive features. The term 'puerperal affective psychosis', however, does not suffice, because there is an extensive literature on 'atypical psychoses', under names like *hallucinatorische Irresein der Wochnerinnen* (Furstner 1875), amentia, cycloid psychosis, and acute polymorphic psychosis. That is why some psychiatrists still claim that 'puerperal psychosis' is a specific disorder, with its own clinical features—those 'specific features' are the polymorphic symptoms found in 'atypical psychoses', and occur in women at other times, and in men. Ralph Paffenbarger's 'picture puzzle', therefore, applies to the combined group of puerperal bipolar and acute polymorphic psychoses.

Menstrual psychosis

Marcé, rightly renowned for his *Traité de la Folie des Femmes Enceintes, des Nouvelles Accouchées et des Nourrices* (1858), made one contribution to the 'picture puzzle'—he drew attention to the importance of menstruation. At that time, little had been written about menstrual psychoses, but we now know they are similar to puerperal bipolar and polymorphic psychoses, having the same range of presentations and often occurring in the same women (Brockington 2008). It is likely that they share at least some elements of their aetiology. Channi Kumar achieved hormone challenge tests in the early puerperium in women with a history of puerperal psychosis (Wieck *et al.* 1991). Another approach is to study menstrual psychosis, which has the advantage that episodes are more frequent, and can be studied in women not recovering from the trauma of parturition. These psychoses are uncommon, but can be found if vigilant clinicians are aware of them.

Clinical methods

In biological studies, the devil is in the diagnosis. It is not enough to use structured psychiatric interviews and a set of diagnostic criteria. Because of the error in all psychiatric observation and measurement, multiple information sources and multiple raters must be used (Brockington and Meltzer 1982; Brockington *et al.* 1992). Because of the imperfection of our nosologies, the polydiagnostic approach and lifetime diagnoses are necessary, and because of the complexity of the psychiatry of motherhood, narrative descriptions are of great value. Until sophisticated neuropsychiatric studies are allied to equally disciplined clinical methods, the postpartum psychoses will remain 'a picture puzzle'.

References

Bonhöffer, K. (1910). Die symptomatische psychosen im Gefolge von akuten Infektionen und inneren Erkrankungen. Leipzig & Wien, Deutlicke.

Brockington, I.F. (2006). Eileithyia's mischief: the organic psychoses of pregnancy, parturition and the puerperium. Bredenbury, Eyry Press.

Brockington, I.F. (2008). Menstrual psychosis and the catamenial process. Bredenbury, Eyry Press.

Brockington, I.F. and Meltzer, H.Y. (1982). Documenting an episode of psychiatric illness: the need for multiple information sources, multiple raters and narrative. Schizophrenia Bulletin **8**: 485–492.

Brockington, I.F., Roper, A., Meltzer, H.Y., Altman, E., and Berry, R. (1992). Multiple raters. International Journal of Methods in Psychiatric Research 2: 187–190.

Chaslin, P. (1895). Confusion Mental Primitive, Stupidité, Démence Aiguë, Stupeur Primitive. Paris, Harmattan.

Furstner, C. (1875). Über Schwangerschafts- und Puerperalpsychosen. Archiv für Psychiatrie und Nervenkrankheiten. 5: 505–543.

Marcé L.V. (1857) Études sur les causes de la folie puerpérale. Annales Médico-psychologiques 3 s III p 562–584.

Paffenbarger, R.S. (1961). The picture puzzle of the postpartum psychoses. Journal of Chronic Diseases **13**: 161–173.

Wieck, A., Kumar, R., Hirst, A.D., *et al.* (1991). Increased sensitivity of dopamine receptors and recurrence of affective psychosis after childbirth. British Medical Journal **303**: 613–616.

Zilboorg, G. (1929). The dynamics of schizophrenic reactions related to pregnancy and childbirth. American Journal of Psychiatry **85**: 733–767.

Chapter 3

Personal reflections on the early development of the EPDS

John Cox

Introduction: first meeting with a Dr Kumar at The London Hospital

Shortly after returning to the London Hospital from Uganda in 1974, and still jet-lagged and culture-shocked, I had an unexpected call from a Dr Kumar at the Maudsley Hospital whose name was then unfamiliar to me. Stephen Wolkind (Child Psychiatrist at the London Hospital working with Professor Pond) had informed him that I had completed a study of postnatal depression in East Africa and had used Goldberg's Standardised Psychiatric Interview (SPI) translated into Luganda. Could we meet, and could I advise him on the use of the SPI? I was surprised, flattered and motivated by this request.

We met in Turner St, London E1. This was the beginning of a friendly and mutually respectful collaboration, which facilitated the later development of the Edinburgh Postnatal Depression Scale (EPDS) (Cox *et al.* 1987), helped launch the 1980 meeting in Manchester, when the Marcé Society was founded, and motivated Phase One of the International Transcultural Postnatal Depression Study. Channi Kumar was a fine team player, and as a leader had that knack of making you feel respected and at ease. His greeting 'Come in dear boy and have a seat' when he ushered you to a chair piled high with research papers, was characteristic of his style and productivity. We would then talk, not only about screening scales, but about College matters and the Perinatal Special Interest Group (which later became a Specialty Section), as well as our 'Blue Skies' research programmes.

Brice Pitt and the Uganda experience

My interest in perinatal psychiatry began when, as an impressionable medical student, I first met Brice Pitt at Claybury Hospital. He was carrying out a study of 'atypical' postnatal depression and was devising a self-report questionnaire to detect increases in depression scores after birth. This early experience, together with a postgraduate seminar some years later, must surely have been on my mind when I was asked by Allen German on my arrival in Uganda, what research I was planning to do. I replied that I wished to replicate Assael's finding (1972) that a quarter of pregnant women at Kasangati had mental health problems, and I was curious to know whether African women experienced depression as described by Pitt (1968)—and if not, what were the differences. This was the beginning of my formative transcultural research experience in Africa, which profoundly shaped my subsequent clinical and academic career.

Origins of the EPDS

The EPDS, interestingly, continues to be used in several major national screening programmes and research around the world (Gibson *et al.* 2009; Cox, Holden and Henshaw, 2014), and has been translated into over 50 languages. I want therefore in this chapter to describe the ideas, influences, and personalities that triggered its development and may not have been sufficiently emphasized in previous publications.In the early 1980s, the limitations of existing self-report questionnaires for use in community samples were beginning to be recognized. Philip Snaith (1981), for example, had acknowledged the need to modify existing scales for use in specialist settings; and Channi Kumar (1982), in Motherhood and Mental Illness Vol. 1, recognized that there was a need for

> . . . some form of simple self-administered scale . . . for use in antenatal and postnatal settings, to pick out potential cases of women with depression and anxiety. Existing questionnaires contain questions which are dissonant with the woman's pregnant or parturient state and, on the other hand, questions about her mental state, which take account of her condition, are lacking (p. 112).

In Edinburgh at that time, the serious limitations of existing self-report scales had become very apparent to us. Although we used the best available scale in our prospective study (Cox *et al.* 1982), the Anxiety and Depression Questionnaire (SAD) of Bedford and Foulds (1978), though having the advantage of brevity and few somatic items, failed to detect any increase in these symptoms in the first postpartum weeks, and the recommended cut-off score was completely inappropriate for use during pregnancy (Cox *et al.* 1983). Of the 13 pregnant women with a score of 6+, only 3 had any form of mental disorder, and some items lacked face validity for childbearing women. We concluded

> If these difficulties with the SAD are replicated by others using different self-report questionnaires, then the implications for the reliable detection of neuroses in childbearing women are considerable. It might for example be necessary to re-design or re-validate self-report scales specifically for use during pregnancy and again for use in the puerperium. (p. 6).

The intent of our grant application to the Scottish Home and Health Department in 1983 was therefore to develop and validate a screening scale specifically for use with childbearing women in the community, and also to carry out an intervention study by health visitors. We considered in our proposal the limitations of existing scales, as well as the published evidence that perinatal depression, and post-partum depression in particular, caused distress to the mother, was a threat to family cohesion and had an adverse effect on the growing infant. We described the relevance to our proposal of the studies of Pitt (1968), and Kumar and Robson (1978), as well as our prospective prevalence study in Edinburgh. Brice Pitt's 1968 finding that of 305 women attending routine obstetric clinics in East London, 33 (10.5%) developed a depressive illness 6 weeks after childbirth, and

4% remained depressed for at least 12 months, was seminal to our thinking. Likewise Kumar and Robson's (1978) Camberwell study was referred to, because they had interviewed 100 married women with the SPI and found 19 (11.6%) had psychiatric morbidity in the puerperium, which in 13 had an onset after childbirth. Similarly, in Scotland (Cox *et al.* 1982), of the 103 women included in a more representative antenatal sample, 13 were found to have a sustained postpartum depression, and a further 17 shorter depressive episodes. We also used the SPI, with which I was familiar, from the earlier Ugandan research. Each mother was interviewed by Yvonne Connor twice before delivery and at 1 week and 4 months after childbirth. The clinical characteristics of the 13 women with sustained postpartum depression were found to be very similar to those described by Pitt; and we particularly noted that in nine the onset had followed childbirth. Commonly, the mothers reported self-blame, inability to cope with family responsibilities, a sad mood, and were often tearful and anxious. Most said they were not their usual selves and were more likely than non-depressed mothers to report deterioration in their marriage with reduction in libido. Sustained clinical antenatal depression, as distinct from anxiety disorders, was much less common (4%). When 11 of the 13 depressed women were re-interviewed by a blind researcher three years later (Cox *et al.* 1984), all but four accurately recalled this earlier postnatal depression. Of the four women who did not, three had been pregnant again, and two of these three had experienced another postnatal depression and told us that the second puerperal depression was so bad that the first had been overlooked. Most of these young mothers had no formal therapy, and only two were recognised by their Health Visitor as needing extra help. It was these published findings, together with our clinical experience and the 'women's voices', that drove the subsequent development of the EPDS and led to the necessary financial support.

It is difficult to pin-point in retrospect the contribution of the Ugandan research (Cox, 1978, 1983) to the early development of the EPDS. However, my experience of working with Health Visitors at Kasangati, and particularly with their role in the prevention of depression and in infant nutrition, enabled optimal collaboration with health visitors in the UK and with other community health professionals. Also, the discipline of carrying out a controlled study of antenatal depression, and following up 183 women into the puerperium, sensitized me to the extent of both postnatal depression (10.5%) and antenatal depression and anxiety (20%) in a contrasting African context. The need to detect these vulnerable mothers was self-evident, as was the necessity of familiarity with local health beliefs and practices, including nuances of language and the understanding of spiritual and religious practices. I was thus sensitized to the limitations and ambiguities of transcultural research across language and cultural differences, and to the need to ensure that the questions being asked and the questionnaire items were each culturally appropriate. In this regard, when undertaking the pilot work on the EPDS, which was central to its success, we readily dismissed items from the Beck Depression Inventory, the Hospital Anxiety and Depression Scale (HAD), and the Irritability, Depression and Anxiety Scale (IDA) that lacked face validity for the puerperium (e.g. 'I can enjoy a good book or radio or television programme'; 'I have lost interest in my appearance', and 'I feel as if I am slowed down') as indicators of depression. Also, we omitted the item about libido and enjoyment of the baby, because in a self-report questionnaire honest answers implying that women had low libido or did not enjoy their babies were not likely.

This pilot process of reviewing with the mothers themselves, and with the community health professionals, the ordering of the items as well as their content was perhaps one of the key explanations for the satisfactory validation studies of the 13-, and then the 10,-item EPDS reported in the literature. The 13-item EPDS was derived from the 20 items pilot study, which had 7 items of our own construction, 3 from the IDA and 10 from the HAD. These items were never regarded as a symptom check list for depression, and their inclusion was due to their likelihood of increasing the hit positive rate for the overall total score. The subsequent removal of the three Irritability items from the 13 item EPDS was carried out, because in a factor analysis they were not correlated with the depression factor. This finding much interested Phillip Snaith (who reviewed our EPDS 1987 paper), as it supported his opinion that irritability was not always linked to clinical depression, but it surprised us—and Jeni Holden in particular.

The Edinburgh milieu

On return from Uganda I spent a year as a Lecturer in the London Hospital, where I started to write up my doctoral thesis under the mentorship of Desmond Pond (who had established one of the first mother and infant observation units) and John Orley, before moving with my family to Edinburgh in its academic professorial heyday. Bob Kendell had recently completed his, what he called, *preliminary* study of childbirth as an aetiological agent, using the Camberwell Birth Register (Kendell *et al.* 1976). Henry Walton (South African by birth) readily endorsed the transcultural elements of my African research, and Ian Oswald, then Head of Department, later signed off my grant application for £28K in 1983.

I knew I was looking at that time for a health visitor, who was also a psychologist, to work with me on this project. Fortunately Jennifer Holden, who had recently completed a psychology degree and was an experienced health visitor, was recommended by Kate Niven at a meeting of the Society of Reproductive and Infant Psychology. I was then working in general adult psychiatry with an interest in perinatal and liaison work, at the Royal Infirmary and the Western General Hospital, Edinburgh. Jeni Holden brought other advantages to our project team—she herself had experienced postnatal depression, and she had a keen eye for the detail of research methodology and good writing skills, which culminated in her own MPhil degree (1988), based on her intervention study (Holden *et al.*, 1989). She was therefore crucial to our skill mix and, with Ruth Sagovsky (then a senior registrar on a retainer scheme), Peter Holland (a GP) and myself, set out to develop a screening scale. This Edinburgh academic ambience in the tower block, which spanned the science and art of research and clinical work, suited us and so contributed to the success of our blue skies project. Robert Kendell continued with his work on the nature of puerperal psychosis and its links to bipolar disorder, and it was hoped that our two interests would come together to answer some of the then unanswered questions about the overall nature of the trigger for puerperal psychosis and for the non-psychotic mental disorders which remained the focus of my interests at that time.

In 1986 I moved to Keele University as the Foundation Professor of Psychiatry and established the Charles Street Parent and Baby Unit, whilst in 1991 Bob Kendell became Chief Medical Officer for Scotland. It was a surprise for both of us, I suspect, that several years later our paths again overlapped at the College, when Bob Kendell passed on the College Presidency to me in 1999. The College Perinatal Section had been inaugurated earlier in 1996 when I was College Dean.

Postnatal and antenatal depression: ambiguities of current usage

There is a current vogue to merge antenatal and postnatal depression into one concept of perinatal depression, but I am not sure if this is helpful—although it could be a pragmatic way around the linguistic muddle of a postnatal depression scale being used to identify antenatal depression, and in that context to use the EPDS as an acronym for perinatal rather than postnatal depression. Anticipatory anxiety with a realistic fear of death was a cogent explanation, particularly in unmarried women, for the higher rates of anxiety in the African pregnant women than in the controls. In Scotland we also found that the prevalence of antenatal depression was less than antenatal anxiety. The fear of birth and death, the world of fears and uncertainties associated with vulnerability was tangible, and not so far below the surface, in the women we interviewed in Edinburgh. In, up to, a quarter of the mothers identified as depressed postpartum, in both the Ugandan (Cox 1978, 1983) and Stoke-on-Trent. (Cox *et al.* 1993) controlled studies, the onset could be traced to the trimesters of pregnancy—although the depth of depression was often exacerbated after birth. It is for these reasons that we accepted, in certain circumstances, the ambiguity of referring to the EPDS as an Edinburgh *Perinatal* Depression scale.

More prospective controlled studies of both antenatal and postnatal mood disorder, using non-childbearing controls are still urgently needed, if we are to advance our field.

Concluding remarks

The 2012 Paris Marcé meeting was a major scholarly event and symptomatic of a rejuvenated international association. It did not only honour Louis Victor Marcé, but also his far sighted teacher Esquirol (1845), who observed a large number of women with mild to moderate puerperal mental illness who were cared for at home and so never recorded.

Channi Kumar well deserves the tributes to his legacy. He was a founder of the Marcé Society. Yet we should also recall the vision of others, including Ian Brockington, George Winokur, Ralph Paffenberger, Robert Kendell, James Hamilton, Gene Paykel, and Brice Pitt, who sowed the seeds for the Marcé Society as *the* main forum where new perinatal research is presented and clinical innovations evaluated.

As our work soon passes into history, I hope the readers of this chapter will be encouraged by our experience. The research culture is very different now, yet there must be space for the Blue Skies to beckon us, the unexpected to be discovered, and the satisfaction and solidarity that comes from adding to scientific knowledge that can contribute to improved well-being for the mother and father and their infant.

These values, I believe, can withstand the testing of time, whereas scales may come and go. Yet surprisingly, at the present time the EPDS has remained alive 30 years after its birth and would appear to have outlived some of its critics. It was deliberately short, user-friendly, and when used as intended, a valuable scale to assist the detection of perinatal depression. It is not a magic wand and only facilitates honest replies when administered in the context of a respectful relationship with the mother. It came from the pen of clinicians who had an integrative concept of psychiatry—and of the nature of persons and their relationships together.

When Members of Parliament could have an informed 3-hour debate in the House of Commons, where they displayed not only their knowledge but also their own experience of postnatal depression and severe psychosis (see Hansard 2012), then there has been much good public health work carried out since the EPDS was first conceived over 30 years ago.

References

Assael M.I., Namboze, J.M., German, G.A., Bennett, F.J. (1972). Psychiatric disturbances during pregnancy in a rural group of African Women. *Social Science and Medicine* **6**: 387–395.

Bedford, A. and Foulds. G. (1978). *Delusions—symptoms-states, State of Anxiety and Depression (Manual)*. Windsor, N.F.E.R. Publishing Company.

Cox, J.L. (1978). *Psychiatric Morbidity and Childbearing: a Study of 263 Semi-rural Ugandan Women.* Unpublished D M Thesis, Oxford University.

Cox, J.L. (1983). Postnatal depression: a comparison of Scottish and African women. *Social Psychiatry* **18**: 25–28.

Cox, J.L., Connor, Y.M., and Kendell, R.E. (1982). Prospective study of the psychiatric disorders of childbirth. *British Journal of Psychiatry* **140**: 111–117.

Cox, J.L., Holden, J. and Sagovsky, R. (1987). Detection of postnatal depression. Development of the 10-item Edinburgh Postnatal Depression Scale. *British Journal of Psychiatry* **150**: 782–786.

Cox, J.L., Holden, J. and Henshaw, C. (2014). *Perinatal Mental Health: the Edinburgh Postnatal Depression Scale Manual.* 2nd edn. London, Royal College of Psychiatrists.

Cox, J.L., Connor, Y.M., Henderson, I., McGuire, R.J., and Kendell, R.E. (1983) Prospective study of the psychiatric disorders of childbirth by self-report questionnaire. *Journal of Affective Disorders* **5**: 1–7.

Cox, J.L., Rooney, A., Thomas, P.F., *et al.* (1984). How accurately do mothers recall postnatal depression? Further data from a 3 year follow-up study. *Journal of Psychosomatic Obstetrics and Gynaecology* **3**: 185–189.

Cox, J., Murray, D., and Chapman, G. (1993). A controlled study of the onset, duration and prevalence of postnatal depression. *British Journal of Psychiatry* **1163**: 27–31.

Esquirol, E. (1845). *Mental Maladies: a treatise on Insanities.* Philadelphia, Blanchard.

Gibson, J., McKenzie-McHarg, K., Shakespeare, J., *et al.* (2009). A systematic review of studies validating the Edinburgh Postnatal Depression Scale in antepartum and postpartum women. *Acta Psychiatrica Scandinavica* **119**: 350–364.

Hansard (2012). House of Commons Hansard Debates for 14 Jun 2012 (pt 0004) http://www.publications.parliament.uk/pa/cm201213/cmhansrd/cm120614/debtext/120614–0004.htm.

Holden, J. (1988). *Counselling by Health Visitors in the Treatment of Postnatal Depression.* Unpublished M Phil Thesis, University of Edinburgh.

Holden, J., Sagovsky, R., and Cox, J.L. (1989). Counselling in a General Practice setting: a controlled study of Health Visitor intervention in the treatment of postnatal depression. *British Medical Journal* **298**: 223–226.

Kendell, R. E., Wainwright, S., Hailey, A. & Shannon, B. (1976). The influence of childbirth on psychiatric morbidity. *Psychological Medicine* **6**, 297–302.

Kumar, C. (1982). Neurotic disorders in childbearing women. In *Motherhood and Mental Illness.* Vol 1., Brockington, I. and Kumar, C.m. editors. London, Academic Press.

Kumar, C. and Robson, K. (1978). Neurotic disturbance during pregnancy and puerperium: preliminary report of a prospective survey of 119 primiparae. In: Sandler M (ed.) *Mental Illness in Pregnancy and Puerperium.* Oxford, Oxford University Press.

Pitt, B. (1968). 'Atypical' depression following childbirth. *British Journal of Psychiatry* **114**: 1325–1335.

Snaith, R.P. (1981). Rating Scales. *British Journal of Psychiatry* **138**: 512–514.

Chapter 4

Psychosocial and psychological interventions for the prevention of postpartum depression

An updated systematic review

Cindy-Lee Dennis and Therese Dowswell

Acknowledgments

The author gratefully acknowledges Dr Debra Creedy who assisted Dr Dennis with the first version of this review in 2004. The author also wishes to thank: (1) Julie Weston for her data extraction, independent evaluation of trial quality, contacting trial authors as necessary, and data entry; (2) Danni Li for translating Sun 2004; Tang 2009; and Xu 2003. Edward Plaisance Jr for translating Ajh 2006. Alison Balmfirth, Laura Wills, Ed Doragh, and Nivene Raafat for translating Bittner 2009. Aoife Fogarty for translating Kleeb 2005. Francesca Gatenby, Nick Jones, and Juliet Sheath for translating Urech 2009; and (3) the many study authors who were very helpful in responding to queries and providing additional data.

Introduction

Depression is a major cause of disability for all ages and both sexes worldwide. Postpartum depression is often defined as depression occurring within the first year following childbirth. In most studies this includes those women for whom the depression may be a continuation of that experienced during pregnancy, as well as those for whom it is a new onset. The *Diagnostic and Statistical Manual of Mental Disorders* (DSM-IV) does not recognize postpartum depression as diagnostically distinct from depression at other times, although does allow for the addition of a 'postpartum-onset specifier' in women with an onset within 4 weeks of birth. A recent systematic review of postpartum depression found the period prevalence of all depression to be 19.2% in the first 12 weeks postnatally, with a period prevalence for major depression of 7.1% (Gaynes *et al.* 2005). This review also identified depression to be common during pregnancy with a period prevalence of 18.4% across the 9 months of pregnancy, with 12.7% having an episode of major depression during this time. Not surprisingly, antenatal depression is a strong risk factor of postpartum depression.

The cause of postpartum depression suggests a multifactorial aetiology (Beck 2001; O'Hara and Swain 1996). Despite considerable research, no single causative factor has been isolated. However, meta-analytic findings consistently highlight the importance of psychosocial variables such as stressful life events, marital conflict, and the lack of social support. To address this issue, a variety of psychosocial and psychological interventions have been developed to treat postpartum depression (Dennis and Hodnett 2007). For example, randomized controlled trials evaluating cognitive behavioural counselling with antidepressants (Appleby *et al.* 1997), cognitive behavioural therapy and non-directive counselling (Cooper and Murray 1997; Cooper *et al.* 2003), health visitor-led non-directive counselling (Holden *et al.* 1989; Wickberg and Hwang 1996), peer support (Dennis 2003), and interpersonal psychotherapy (O'Hara *et al.* 2000) have all demonstrated the amenability of postpartum depression to treatment.

It is theoretically plausible that psychosocial and psychological interventions may also prevent postpartum depression, as many of the known risk factors are present during pregnancy and the immediate postpartum period. As such, these interventions may be provided to women antenatally or initiated early in the postpartum period. They may be individually based, focusing on specific maternal needs, or provided in a group setting that could incorporate peer support. Interventions may be intensive and include multiple contacts or be provided during a single session. They may be provided by a health professional, such as a midwife, nurse, psychologist, or lay individuals such as experienced mothers recruited from the community. Interventions may also target specific subgroups of women who are high risk, such as those with a history of abuse (Ross and Dennis 2009), young mothers (Brown *et al.* 2011), and migrant groups (Collins *et al.* 2011). The aim of the review presented in this chapter was to assess the effects of various psychosocial and psychological interventions compared with usual antepartum, intrapartum, or postpartum care to reduce the risk of postpartum depression. This systematic review is based on an updated full review to be published in 2013 in the Cochrane Library (Dennis and Dowswell 2013).

Methods

Searching

The Cochrane Pregnancy and Childbirth Group trials register was searched. This database contains trials identified from: monthly searches of the Cochrane Central Register of Controlled Trials, weekly searches of Medline, weekly searches of Embase, hand searches of 30 journals and the proceedings of major conferences, and weekly current awareness alerts for a further 44 journals. Secondary references and review articles were scanned and experts in the field were contacted. Trials published in all languages were considered.

Selection

Published and unpublished studies were eligible if they fulfilled the following criteria: were a randomized controlled trial; were methodologically strong based on a validity assessment; evaluated a psychosocial or psychological intervention in which the primary or secondary aim was a reduction in risk to develop postpartum depression; and included pregnant women and new mothers less than 6 weeks postpartum. Studies were excluded if they incorporated a quasi-randomized design; recruited participants where more than 20% of the sample were depressed at trial entry; or solely evaluated an educational intervention. For this review, a psychosocial or psychological intervention incorporated a variety of non-pharmaceutical strategies that were delivered antenatally and/or within the first month postpartum by a health professional or layperson via telephone, home or clinic visits, or individual or group sessions.

Validity assessment

Trial methodological quality was assessed according to the recommendations of the Cochrane Collaboration and examined: the generation of allocation sequence; allocation concealment; blinding of outcome assessors; completeness of follow up data; completeness of outcome reporting; and intention-to-treat analysis. Two reviewers independently assigned a quality rating to each trial; results were compared and differences discussed until agreement was obtained.

Data abstraction

Data were independently extracted by two reviewers and included: study design; participants (number and characteristics); intervention type, mode, onset, duration, and provider; outcomes measured; and results. Wherever necessary, unpublished or missing data were requested from the trial contact author and data were double entered into Review Manager version 5.1 (Cochrane Collaboration software).

Quantitative data synthesis

Meta-analyses were performed using relative risks as the measure of effect size for dichotomous outcomes; for continuous data, we used the mean difference if outcomes were measured in the same way between trials. We used the standardized mean difference to combine trials that examined the same outcome, but used different measures. For all outcomes, we carried out analyses, as far as possible, on an intention-to-treat basis (i.e. we attempted to include all participants randomized to each group in the analyses), and all participants were analysed in the group to which they were allocated, regardless of whether or not they received the allocated intervention. The denominator for each outcome in each trial was the number randomized minus any participants whose outcomes were known to be missing. We assessed statistical heterogeneity in each meta-analysis using the T^2, I^2, and χ^2 statistics. We regarded heterogeneity as substantial if T^2 was greater than zero and either I^2 was greater than 30% or there was a low P value (less than 0.10) in the χ^2 test for heterogeneity. We carried out statistical analysis using the Review Manager software. All trials were considered to include some form of 'talking therapy' and thus eligible to be combined in a meta-analysis. We used fixed-effect meta-analysis for combining data where it was reasonable to assume that the studies were estimating the same underlying treatment effect—i.e. where trials examined similar interventions, and the trials' populations and methods were judged sufficiently similar. If there was clinical heterogeneity sufficient to expect that the underlying treatment effects differed between trials, or if substantial statistical heterogeneity was detected, we used random-effects meta-analysis to produce an overall summary if an average treatment effect across trials was considered clinically meaningful. Eight a priori subgroup analyses were planned to estimate the effect of: psychosocial interventions, psychological interventions, intervention provider (e.g. professionally based and lay-based interventions), intervention mode (e.g. individual-based and group-based interventions), intervention duration (e.g. single-contact and multiple-contact interventions), intervention onset (e.g. antenatal only interventions, antenatal and postpartum interventions, and postpartum only interventions), and sample selection criteria (e.g. interventions targeting women with specific risk factors and the general population). We performed sensitivity analyses, for the primary outcome, in instances in which any of the following occurred: (1) a high risk of bias associated with the methodological quality of included trials; and (2) incomplete outcome data (more than 20% missing data) for any of the included trials.

Results

Twenty-eight trials, involving almost 17,000 women, contributed data to the review. There was an overall significant effect on the prevention of postpartum depressive symptomatology in the meta-analysis of all types of interventions (20 trials, 14,727 women; average relative risk (RR) 0.78, 95% confidence interval (CI) 0.66–0.93). Promising interventions include: (1) the provision of intensive, individualized postpartum home visits provided by public health nurses or midwives (RR 0.56, 95% CI 0.43–0.73), (2) lay (peer)-based telephone support (RR 0.54, 95% CI 0.38–0.77), and (3) interpersonal psychotherapy (standardized mean difference −0.27, 95% CI −0.52 to −0.01). Professional- and lay-based interventions were both effective in reducing the risk to develop depressive symptomatology. Individually based interventions reduced depressive symptomatology at final assessment (RR 0.75, 95% CI 0.61–0.92) as did multiple-contact interventions (RR 0.78, 95% CI 0.66–0.93). Interventions that were initiated in the postpartum period also significantly reduced the risk to develop depressive symptomatology (RR 0.73, 95% CI 0.59–0.90). Identifying mothers 'at-risk' assisted in the prevention of postpartum depression (RR 0.66, 95% CI 0.50–0.88).

Description of studies

Thirty trials, reported between 1995 and 2011, were identified and met the inclusion criteria (Table 4.1). Two trials (Austin *et al.* 2008; Heinicke *et al.* 1999) that were otherwise eligible for inclusion in the review did not report usable data for postpartum depression. In total, 28 trials, incorporating 16,912 women were included in the meta-analyses. The trials were primarily conducted in Australia and the UK; four trials were conducted in the USA (Feinberg and Kan 2008; Gjerdingen and Center 2002; Gorman 1997; Zlotnick *et al.* 2001), two trials were conducted in China (Gao *et al.* 2010; Tam *et al.* 2003), and one trial was conducted in each of the following countries: Canada (Dennis *et al.* 2009),

Germany (Weidner *et al.* 2010), and India (Tripathy 2010). Twelve of the trials targeted at-risk women based on various factors believed to put them at additional likelihood of developing postpartum depression (Armstrong *et al.* 1999; Brugha *et al.* 2000; Dennis *et al.* 2009; Gamble *et al.* 2005; Gorman 1997; Harris *et al.* 2006; Le *et al.* 2011; Stamp *et al.* 2011; Tam *et al.* 2003; Weidner *et al.* 2010; Zlotnick *et al.* 2001, 2006;), while the other 16 trials enrolled women from the general population.

Types of interventions

The studies were subgrouped into categories to examine specific types of psychosocial interventions, such as antenatal and postpartum classes/groups (Brugha *et al.* 2000; Feinberg and Kan 2008; Gjerdingen and Center 2002; Ickovics *et al.* 2011; Reid *et al.* 2002; Stamp *et al.* 1999; Tripathy *et al.* 2010), professional- (Armstrong *et al.* 1999; MacArthur *et al.* 2002) and lay-based (Cupples *et al.* 2011; Harris *et al.* 2006; Morrell *et al.* 2000) home visits, lay-based telephone support (Dennis *et al.* 2009), early postpartum follow-up (e.g. routine postpartum care initiated earlier than usual practice) (Gunn *et al.* 1998), continuity/models of care (Lumley *et al.* 2006; Sen 2006; Waldenstrom *et al.* 2000), and psychological interventions, such as debriefing (Tam *et al.* 2003; Gamble *et al.* 2005; Lavender and Walkinshaw 1998; Priest *et al.* 2003; Small *et al.* 2000), cognitive behavioural therapy (Le *et al.* 2011), and interpersonal psychotherapy (Gorman 1997; Weidner *et al.* 2010; Zlotnick *et al.* 2001, 2006). The interventions were provided by a variety of professionals, including nurses (Armstrong *et al.* 1999; Brugha *et al.* 2000; Lumley *et al.* 2006; Tam *et al.* 2003; Zlotnick *et al.* 2006), physicians (Gunn *et al.* 1998; Lumley *et al.* 2006), midwives (Gao *et al.* 2010; Gamble *et al.* 2005; Ickovics *et al.* 2011; Lavender and Walkinshaw 1998; Le *et al.* 2011; MacArthur *et al.* 2002; Priest *et al.* 2003; Reid *et al.* 2002; Sen 2006; Small *et al.* 2000; Waldenstrom *et al.* 2000), and mental health specialists (Gorman 1997; Weidner *et al.* 2010) including psychologists (Gjerdingen and Center 2002). In seven trials, the intervention was provided by lay individuals (Cupples *et al.* 2011; Feinberg and Kan 2008; Dennis *et al.* 2009; Harris *et al.* 2006; Morrell *et al.* 2000; Tripathy *et al.* 2010), including trained research staff (Le *et al.* 2011). In the majority of studies, the control group was reported to have received usual antenatal/postpartum care, which varied both between and within countries.

Definition of postpartum depression

In all trials but seven (Cupples *et al.* 2011; Feinberg and Kan 2008; Gjerdingen and Center 2002; Ickovics *et al.* 2011; Weidner *et al.* 2010; Zlotnick *et al.* 2001, 2006), postpartum depressive symptomatology was defined as a score above a specified cut-off point on a self-report measure; for many of the studies (*n* = 15) an Edinburgh Postpartum Depression Scale (EPDS) score >12 (also reported as a 12/13 cut-off score) indicated postpartum depression. Several studies also reported mean EPDS scores (Armstrong *et al.* 1999; Gorman 1997; Gao *et al.* Gunn *et al.* 1998; Ickovics *et al.* 2011; Le *et al.* 2011; Lumley *et al.* 2006; 2010; MacArthur *et al.* 2002; Morrell *et al.* 2000; Reid *et al.* 2002; Sen 2006; Small *et al.* 2000; Weidner *et al.* 2010). Three additional trials used the EPDS to measure

Table 4.1 Characteristics of included studies

Study	Methods	Participants	Interventions	Outcome	Notes
Armstrong et al. 1999	RCT—randomization was performed using a computer generated random numbers table and completed by clerical staff not involved in the eligibility assessment. Outcome assessor was blinded to group allocation. Nurses providing the intervention were also blinded to 6 weeks post partum (within usual care parametres). The 16-week attrition rate was 12%.	181 mothers (90 in the intervention group; 91 in the control group) who gave birth in one urban hospital in Queensland, Australia. Families were included where the child, for environmental (home/family) reasons, was at increased risk for poor health and development outcomes.	Intervention group: home visits by child health nurses with support from multidisciplinary team. The visits were weekly until 6 weeks post partum, every 2 weeks until 12 weeks and then monthly until 52 weeks. Control group: usual community care (which included choice of one home visit from the child health nurse) and a list of community resources.	EPDS >12 at 6, 16, and 52 weeks postpartum.	Only 63% of mothers completed the pre-trial screening questionnaire.
Austin et al. 2008	RCT—randomization was performed using a randomization table on a 2:1 basis to allow for more dropouts from the intervention group. No further details available from authors about process of randomization. Outcome assessors were blinded to group allocation. The 16-week attrition rate was 40%	277 pregnant women (191 in the intervention group; 86 in the control group) who attended antenatal clinics in an Australian hospital. Women were identified, by screening at the end of the first trimester, to be at an increased risk of postpartum depression.	Intervention group: information booklet and cognitive behavioural therapy group sessions. There were six weekly 2-hour sessions (and a later follow-up session) that were skills-based and led by a clinical psychologist. Control group: standard care which included an information booklet about postpartum anxiety and depression.	EPDS and MINI at 8 and 16 weeks postpartum.	No data from this trial were included in the meta-analyses

Table 4.1 (continued) Characteristics of included studies

Study	Methods	Participants	Interventions	Outcome	Notes
Brugha *et al.* 2000	RCT—randomization was performed using a computer-based stratification process with minimization on three prognostic factors (level of support, screening, and ethnic group). Outcome data were collected via interviews. The 12-week attrition rate was 9%.	209 pregnant women (103 in the intervention group; 106 in the control group) who attended antenatal clinics in a UK hospital between 12 and 20 weeks' gestation were identified, by screening, to be at an increased risk of postpartum depression.	Intervention group: 'Preparing for Parenthood'—six structured 2-hour weekly antenatal classes (preceded by an initial introductory meeting with the participant and her partner) and one 'reunion' class at 8 weeks post partum. Classes were provided by a trained nurse and occupational therapist and based on established psychological models for tackling depression together with emerging models for enhancing social support. Control group: routine antenatal care.	EPDS >10 at 12 weeks postpartum.	Only 45% of participants in the intervention group attended sufficient sessions to 'likely receive benefit'.
Cupples *et al.* 2011	RCT—randomization was performed using a computer-generated process of alternate blocks of 20 and 40 and completed by independent individuals at a remote location. Outcome assessor was blinded to group allocation. The 52-week attrition rate was 15%.	343 women (172 in the intervention group; 171 in the control group), pregnant with their first baby and less than 20 weeks' gestation, from Northern Ireland. They were 16–30 years old, had no co-morbidity and were from disadvantaged areas based on their postal code.	Intervention group: peer mentoring provided during home visits or phone calls. The peer mentors were non-health professionals. The mentoring sessions were offered twice monthly during pregnancy and monthly for the first postpartum year. Control group: routine ante natal and post partum care.	SF-36 mental health subscale at 52 weeks postpartum	

Table 4.1 (continued) Characteristics of included studies

Study	Methods	Participants	Interventions	Outcome	Notes
Dennis et al. 2009	RCT—randomization with stratification on self-reported history of depression was performed via the internet through a centrally controlled randomization service. Outcome assessors were blinded to group allocation. The 24-week attrition rate was 14%.	701 postpartum women (349 in the intervention group; 352 in the control group) from seven large health regions in Ontario, Canada. During the routine postpartum phone call (24–48 hours post-hospital discharge) public health nurses administered the EPDS and those scoring >9 and deemed to be high risk to develop postpartum depression were referred to the study.	Intervention group: standard community postpartum care plus telephone-based peer support from a mother with a history and recovery from postpartum depression. Telephone contact was initiated within 48–72 hours of randomization. Peer support mothers underwent a 4-hour training session and were asked to make a minimum of four contacts with each mother. Control group: standard community postpartum care including access to services from public health nurses and other providers (mother-initiated) and drop-in centres.	EPDS >12 and SCID at 12 and 24 weeks postpartum.	More women in control group were referred for treatment at 12 weeks so the 24-week results were not included in the meta-analyses.
Feinberg and Kan 2008	RCT—randomization was performed using a computer program and completed by a staff member, not involved in enrolment, based on the order of receipt of baseline data. Outcome data were collected via mailed questionnaires. The 24-week attrition rate was 10%.	169 couples expecting their first child (89 in the intervention group and 80 in the control group) who were recruited via antenatal education classes at two hospitals and doctors' offices in Pennsylvania, USA. They were heterosexual couples living together and were enrolled in second trimester of pregnancy.	Intervention group: eight group classes (four in the antenatal and four in the postpartum period), focusing on improving co-parenting by encouraging conflict management, sharing tasks and developing supportive roles in parents. The group sessions were in addition to the regular antenatal classes. Control group: regular antenatal classes and a mailed brochure about selecting child care.	CES-D at 24 weeks postpartum.	Only data collected from the mothers were used.

Table 4.1 (continued) Characteristics of included studies

Study	Methods	Participants	Interventions	Outcome	Notes
Gamble *et al.* 2005	RCT—randomization was performed using consecutively numbered, sealed, opaque envelopes. Outcome assessor was blinded to group allocation. The 12-week attrition rate was 0%.	103 mothers (50 in the intervention group; 53 in the control group) who were assessed for labour trauma risk in the immediate postpartum period in a Brisbane, Australia hospital.	Intervention group: one midwifery-led debriefing session before hospital discharge and another at 6 to 8 weeks postpartum. Control group: standard care with no midwifery-led debriefing session.	Outcomes EPDS >12 at 12 weeks postpartum.	
Gao *et al.* 2010	RCT—randomization was performed using a computer-generated table of random numbers. Unclear allocation concealment. Outcome assessor was blinded to group allocation. The 6-week attrition rate was 10%.	194 low-risk married women having their first babies (96 in the intervention group; 98 in the control group) who were <28 weeks of pregnancy and attending routine antenatal classes in a teaching hospital in China.	Intervention group: routine antenatal classes (as per control group); two 2-hour IPT-oriented group antenatal classes by trained midwives; and one telephone call at 2 weeks post partum from the same midwife. The extra classes were done immediately following the routine antenatal class and the group size was <10 participants. Control group: routine antenatal classes.	EPDS >12 at 6 weeks postpartum.	13.4% of overall sample had EPDS scores >13 at enrolment. 95.8% of women in the intervention group attended all the extra antenatal classes
Gjerdingen and Center 2002	RCT—randomization was performed using a computer-generated permuted block random number schedule and completed by a research assistant who randomly assigned couples to groups. Outcome data were collected via mailed questionnaires. The 24-week attrition rate was 13%.	151 couples having their first baby (77 in the intervention group and 74 in the control group) who were enrolled from prenatal classes in Minnesota, USA.	Intervention group: two 30-minutes breakout sessions run by a psychologist that occurred during the regular prenatal class program. One session dealt with supportive behaviours between the couple and the other discussed planned household work tasks. Control group: regular prenatal class programme which included a video about being a new parent and discussion of infant care during the breakout session times.	SF-36 mental health subscale at 26 weeks postpartum.	Only data from the mothers were used.

Table 4.1 (continued) Characteristics of included studies

Study	Methods	Participants	Interventions	Outcome	Notes
Gorman 1997	RCT—randomization was performed using a random numbers table and a blocking strategy based on the presence or absence of current or past history of depression. Outcome data were collected via interview and mailed questionnaires. The 24-week attrition rate was 18%.	45 pregnant women (24 in the intervention group; 21 in the control group) at-risk for postpartum depression who attending various obstetric clinics in Iowa City and St. Louis, USA.	Intervention group: five individual sessions based on interpersonal psychotherapy, beginning in late pregnancy and ending at approximately 4 weeks postpartum	EPDS >12 and SCID at 4 and 24 weeks postpartum.	
Gunn et al. 1998	RCT—randomization was performed via telephone through a centrally controlled randomization centre. Outcome data were collected via mailed questionnaires. The 12-week attrition rate was 30%.	683 healthy mothers (number of women randomised to each group not stated) who gave birth in 1 rural and 1 metropolitan hospital in Victoria, Australia. Women were excluded if they were patients of general practitioners who were the trial reference group, attended the teenage clinic, or delivered by an emergency Caesarean section.	All participants received a letter and appointment date to see a general practitioner for a check-up: the intervention group for 1 week after hospital discharge and the control group for 6 weeks postpartum.	EPDS >12 at 12 and 24 weeks.	

Table 4.1 (continued) Characteristics of included studies

Study	Methods	Participants	Interventions	Outcome	Notes
Harris et al. 2006	RCT—randomization was performed using consecutively numbered, sealed, opaque envelopes and completed by a research assistant not involved in enrolment. Outcome data were collected via interviews. The 12-week attrition rate was 44%.	117 pregnant women (61 in the intervention group; 56 in the control group) who were found to be at risk for depression during screening. Women with psychotic illness, serious suicidal risk or poor fluency in English were excluded. 71 of these women consented and completed baseline information at 30 weeks of pregnancy (32 in intervention group; 39 in control group). Three women in each group had major depression at baseline and were excluded at that time.	Intervention group: NEWPIN (New Parent Information Network). The NEWPIN program provides antenatal and postpartum social support with 1–1 befriending and psycho-educational group meetings by trained volunteer mothers. Control group: usual care.	SCAN at 12 weeks postpartum.	
Heinicke et al. 1999	RCT—randomisation was performed by a coin toss for every 2 families. No allocation sequence was used. Outcome assessors were blinded to group allocation. The 24-week attrition rate was 9%.	70 women receiving prenatal care in California, USA (35 in the intervention group and 35 in the control group) who were in their 3rd trimester of pregnancy. They were having their first baby, had no current mental illness and were identified as 'at-risk' by a social history interview. All participants were poor and lacked social support.	Intervention group: home visiting by mental health professionals, possible referral to community resources and the availability of a weekly mother-infant group. Visits were done for the first 2 years postpartum. They began at the end of pregnancy, were weekly during pregnancy and the first year, and every other week in the second year and 60 minutes in length. Telephone follow-up contacts were done in 3rd and 4th years. Control group: paediatric follow-up which entailed developmental evaluation, referrals as needed but no visits or access to the mother-infant group.	BDI at 4, 24, and 52 weeks postpartum.	No data from this trial were included in the meta-analyses.

Table 4.1 (continued) Characteristics of included studies

Study	Methods	Participants	Interventions	Outcome	Notes
Ickovics *et al.* 2011	RCT—randomization was performed using a computer-generated randomization sequence with stratification by site and expected month of delivery. Outcome assessors were blinded to group allocation. The 24-week attrition rate was 25%.	1047 medically low-risk pregnant women (653 in the intervention group; 394 in the control group) were recruited antenatally from 2 US hospital antenatal clinics in Atlanta, GA and New Haven, CT, USA. The women were 25 years old or less and <24 weeks' gestation at enrolment.	Intervention group: group prenatal care. Each prenatal visit was done in a group setting and led by a health professional (midwife or obstetrician). It was integrative prenatal care combining assessment, education, skill building and support. There were 10 2-hour sessions from 16–40 weeks of gestation (20 hours in total). Control group: usual prenatal care. Individual contact was made at the same time points as the group sessions. Each contact was 10–15 minutes (2 hours in total).	CES-D at 24 and 52 weeks postpartum.	For this review 2 groups that received group prenatal care were combined and considered to be the intervention group.
Lavender and Walkinshaw 1998	RCT—randomization was performed using computer-generated numbers and by opening consecutively numbered, sealed, opaque envelopes. Outcome data were collected via a mailed questionnaire. The 3-week attrition rate was 5%.	114 primiparous mothers (60 in the intervention group; 60 in the control group) in a UK teaching hospital. Inclusion criteria: singleton pregnancy, cephalic presentation, and spontaneous labour at term, normal vaginal delivery.	Intervention group: one debriefing session before hospital discharge, which lasted 30 to 120 minutes, provided by a midwife who received no formal training. Control group: standard care with no midwifery-led debriefing session.	HAD >10 at 3 weeks postpartum.	Atypical population - 59.6% were single mothers.

Table 4.1 (continued) Characteristics of included studies

Study	Methods	Participants	Interventions	Outcome	Notes
Le et al. 2011	RCT—randomization was performed using a coin toss and by opening consecutively numbered, sealed, opaque envelopes. Method for collecting outcome data is not stated. The 16-week attrition rate was 20%.	217 pregnant Latino women (112 in the intervention group; 105 in the control group) ≤24 weeks' gestation from a health-care centre and hospital clinic in Washington, DC. They were screened and considered to be at high risk of depression (CES-D ≥16 or self-report of personal or family history of depression) but did not currently have a major depressive illness.	Intervention group: cognitive behavioural group therapy sessions. Research staff provided 8 weekly sessions during pregnancy and three booster sessions at 6, 16, and 52 weeks post partum. Control group: usual prenatal care. This may have included services that participants chose for themselves.	BDI and Mood Screener measured post-intervention and at 6, 16, and 52 weeks postpartum	It is unknown how many women had a CES-D score >16 at recruitment.
Lumley et al. 2006	RCT with cluster design—randomization stratified on rural and metropolitan occurred within pairs and took place at a public event. No further details were provided. Outcome data were collected via mailed questionnaires. The 24-week attrition rate was 41%.	16 local government authorities (eight in the intervention group; eight in the control group) in Victoria, Australia who were matched on location (rural or metropolitan), size, rating of current and recent community activity, annual number of births, and non-contiguous boundaries. No individual consent was sought from participants. All women giving birth in the participating local government authorities over a 10-month period (19,193) were sent postal questionnaires (10,471 in the intervention group; 8,722 in the control group). A pre-paid reply envelope was included and reminder cards sent at 2 and 4 weeks.	Intervention group: The PRISM program which 'aimed to refocus the existing postpartum health care contact on maternal physical and mental health, to implement community strategies to increase the availability and accessibility of 'time-out', provide better information about common health problems and local services, with encouragement and incentives to use them'. It included an education programme for general practitioners and maternal child health nurses, and information kit given to new mothers at hospital discharge, a community information officer for 2 years, and local steering committees to help with local initiatives. Control group: usual care. No further details noted.	EPDS at 24 weeks postpartum.	

Table 4.1 (continued) Characteristics of included studies

Study	Methods	Participants	Interventions	Outcome	Notes
MacArthur et al. 2002	RCT with cluster design—randomization was performed using a customized, computer program in an independent clinical trials unit. 17 practices were randomised to the intervention group and 19 practices were randomized to the control group. Outcome data were collected via mailed questionnaires. The 16-week attrition rate was 27%.	The general practices had on average two or more general practitioners and ≥2 midwives. 17 practices were randomised to intervention group and 19 practices to the control group. 2,064 UK mothers (1,087 in the intervention group; 977 in the control group). Only mothers expected to move out of the general practice area were excluded.	Intervention group: flexible, individualized, extended home visits by a midwife to 28 days postpartum that included (1) screening with a symptoms checklist and the EPDS, (2) a referral to a general practitioner as necessary, and (3) a 10–12-week discharge visit. Control group: standard care that included 7 midwifery home visits to 10–14 days postpartum (may extend to 28 days) and care by health visitors thereafter. General practitioners completed routine home visits and a final check-up at 6 to 8 weeks postpartum.	EPDS >12 at 16 and 52 weeks postpartum.	
Morrell et al. 2000	RCT—randomization was performed using a random numbers table and by opening consecutively numbered, sealed, opaque envelopes. Outcome data were collected via mailed questionnaires. The 24-week attrition rate was 21%.	623 UK mothers (311 in the intervention group; 312 in the control group). Exclusion criteria: insufficient English to complete questionnaires and an infant in the special care unit for more than 48 hours.	Intervention group: postpartum care at home by community midwives plus up to 10 home visits in the first month postpartum lasting up to 3 hours provided by a community postpartum support worker. Control group: postpartum care at home by community midwives.	EPDS >12 at 6 and 24 weeks postpartum.	

Table 4.1 (continued) Characteristics of included studies

Study	Methods	Participants	Interventions	Outcome	Notes
Priest et al. 2003	RCT—randomization was performed within the strata of parity and mode of delivery. Each woman selected an envelope from a group of at least six sealed, opaque envelopes containing random allocation. Outcome data were collected via mailed questionnaires. The 52-week attrition rate was 19%.	1,745 Australian mothers (875 in the intervention group; 870 in the control group). Exclusion criteria: insufficient English to complete questionnaires, being under psychological care at the time of delivery, maternal age <18 years, and infant needing neonatal intensive care.	Intervention group: a single, standardized debriefing session provided in-hospital immediately after randomization or the next day; duration ranged from 15 minutes to 1 hour and all research midwives received training in critical incident stress debriefing. Control group: standard postpartum care.	EPDS >12 at 8, 24, and 52 weeks postpartum.	
Reid et al. 2002	RCT with a 2 × 2 factorial design— randomization was performed using a computer generated scheme with randomized permuted blocks, stratified by centre. Outcome data were collected via mailed questionnaires. The 12-week attrition rate was 27%.	1,004 UK mothers (503 in the intervention group; 501 in the control group). Inclusion criteria: all primiparous women attending antenatal clinics in two participating hospitals. Exclusion criteria: women whose infant subsequently died or was admitted to the Special Care Unit for more than 2 weeks.	Two postpartum interventions incorporating four groups: control, mailed self-help materials, invitation to support group, and self-help materials plus invitation to support group. Data analysed by pooling the four groups as self-help vs no self-help and support group vs no support group. The support groups were run on a weekly basis for 2-hours facilitated by trained midwives.	EPDS >11 at 12 and 24 weeks postpartum.	For this review, only the support group vs no support group comparisons were included. Only 18% of participants in the intervention group attended a support group session.

Table 4.1 (continued) Characteristics of included studies

Study	Methods	Participants	Interventions	Outcome	Notes
Sen 2006	RCT—randomization was performed using a web-based randomization service with randomized permuted blocks, stratified by parity. During the enrolment home visits, a laptop was connected to a mobile phone for access to the randomization service and the participant pressed the randomization button to obtain group allocation. Outcome data were collected via mailed questionnaires. The 24-week attrition rate was 18%.	162 pregnant women with an uncomplicated twin pregnancy were enrolled at <20 weeks' gestation (80 in the intervention group; 82 in the control group) from a hospital in the UK. Women having fetal or infant death were excluded (three in each group).	Intervention group: care, advice and support from a Twin Midwife Advisor which included: at least two home visits (1 antenatal and 1 in the early postpartum); specially designed antenatal preparation for parenting programme (four to five antenatal group classes and one postpartum class); care in-hospital and at outpatient hospital clinic. Control group: standard care and advice which included: shared antenatal care between general practitioner (GP) and consultant obstetrician at a twin clinic; allocation to a community midwife who may provide care in conjunction with GP; invitation to attend community-based antenatal education sessions (normally without a focus on twins); invitation to a breastfeeding workshop (rarely with focus on twins); self-referral to Childbirth Trust antenatal sessions (without focus on twins).	EPDS at 6, 12, 24, and 52 weeks postpartum.	

Table 4.1 (continued) Characteristics of included studies

Study	Methods	Participants	Interventions	Outcome	Notes
Small *et al.* 2000	RCT—randomization was performed via telephone using a computer-generated randomization schedule for each midwife. Outcome data were collected via a mailed questionnaire. The 24-week attrition rate was 12%.	1,041 mothers (520 in the intervention group; 521 in the control group) who had an operative delivery in a large maternity teaching hospital in Melbourne, Australia.	Intervention group: a midwifery-led debriefing session before discharge to provide women with an opportunity to discuss their labour, birth, and post-delivery events and experiences. Control group: standard care, which included a brief visit from a midwife on discharge to give a pamphlet on sources of assistance.	EPDS >12 at 24 weeks postpartum.	
Stamp *et al.* 1995	RCT—randomization was performed using consecutively numbered, sealed opaque envelopes stratified by parity. Outcome data were collected via a mailed questionnaire. The 24-week attrition rate was 13%.	144 pregnant women (73 in the intervention group; 71 in the control group) who screened at-risk for postpartum depression during antenatal clinic visits in Adelaide, Australia. Inclusion criteria: English-speaking, singleton fetus, and <24 weeks gestation.	Intervention group: routine antenatal care plus two antenatal and 1 postpartum midwifery-led group sessions. Control group: routine antenatal and postpartum care, which included a class at 6 weeks postpartum that incorporated a video on postpartum depression.	EPDS >12 at 6, 12, and 24 weeks postpartum.	A high number of women screened 'vulnerable' and only 31% of participants in the intervention group attended all 3 sessions.
Tam *et al.* 2003	RCT—randomization was performed using a random numbers table and consecutively numbered, sealed, opaque envelopes. The process of data collection in-hospital and at 6 weeks postpartum is not stated. The 6- and 24-week attrition rates are unclear.	560 in-hospital mothers (280 in each group) from Hong Kong, China, with at least one suboptimal outcome in the perinatal period ranging from antenatal complications requiring hospitalisation, elective Caesarean section, labour induction, postpartum haemorrhage, infant admission to special care unit, etc.	Intervention group: routine postpartum care plus 1 to 4 sessions of 'educational counselling' by a research nurse before hospital discharge that included information related to the adverse event and counselling to assist the mother to 'come to terms with her losses and find solutions to specific difficulties' (median total time of was 35 minutes). Twenty-four women also received one session by a physician.	HADS >4 at 6 and 24 weeks postpartum.	Health professionals were not blinded to group allocation.

Table 4.1 (continued) Characteristics of included studies

Study	Methods	Participants	Interventions	Outcome	Notes
Tripathy et al. 2010	RCT with cluster design—randomization with stratification by district and pre-existence of a women's group was performed and took place at a public event. Unit of randomization was geographic area. Outcome assessors were blinded to group allocation. The attrition rate is unclear.	Twelve clusters in each of three contiguous districts in eastern India (36 in total) (18 in the intervention group and 18 in the control group). The mean cluster size was 6,338 (range 3,605–7,467) and the proportion of Adivasis (indigenous groups) was 58–70%. The Adivasis are an underserviced population with lower rates of employment, lower rates of education for children, higher mortality rates and poorer access to health services than non-indigenous populations. Women were part of clusters based on where they lived. They attended a women's group (for those in the intervention group) during pregnancy if they wished to. Study consent was not required to attend the group. After delivery, women aged 15–49, living in the participating regions during study period were asked if they would consent to an interview. 19,030 women participated (9,770 in the intervention group and 9,260 in the control group.	Intervention group: existing women's groups expanded their function (172 groups) and 72 groups were created. Each group had a local leader and met monthly for a total of 20 meetings. The groups took part in a participatory learning and action cycle that identified problems, planned strategies, put strategies into practice, and assessed the effect. Clean obstetrics delivery practices and care-seeking behaviour were shared through stories and games at the groups. Control group: existing women's groups maintained their financial function but did not add anything else. Clusters without women's groups did not create any. In both groups health committees were formed so that community members could express their opinions about the design and management of local health services.	Kessler-10	Maternal depression was only measured in year 2 of the trial because of 'delays in identification of a contextually appropriate scale'.

Table 4.1 (continued) Characteristics of included studies

Study	Methods	Participants	Interventions	Outcome	Notes
Waldenstrom *et al.* 2000	RCT—randomization was performed via telephone using consecutively numbered, sealed, opaque envelopes. Outcome data were collected via mailed questionnaires. The 8-week attrition rate was 32%.	1,000 pregnant mothers (495 in the intervention group; 505 in the control group) attending an antenatal clinic in Melbourne, Australia. Inclusion criteria: >25 weeks gestation, English-speaking, and low medical risk.	Intervention group: team midwifery care provided antenatally and postnatally in hospital with a focus on continuity. Control group: standard antenatal and postpartum care by physicians and midwives with no focus on continuity.	EPDS > 12 at 8 weeks postpartum.	Demographic differences were found between questionnaire responders and non-responders.
Weidner *et al.* 2010	RCT—randomization was performed using a computer-based process and a list was generated by an independent institute at a university hospital. Outcome data were collected via mailed questionnaires. The 52-week attrition rate was 52%.	92 pregnant women admitted to a high-risk antenatal unit in Dresden, Germany (46 in the intervention group; 46 in the control group) with elevated scores on the HADS or the Giessen Subjective Complaints List. 17.4% had elevated depression scores, 40.2% had elevated anxiety scores and 77.2% had elevated complaints scores.	Intervention group: individualised psychosomatic intervention by trained psychologist or psychiatrist. 'The activation of resources and the dialogue about current conflicts are central aspects of the intervention.' One to five sessions were done while in-hospital and continuation on an outpatient basis could be done if needed. Control group: standard care.	HADS depression subscale at 52 weeks post-randomization.	15% of women in the intervention group were discharged before receiving the intervention.
Zlotnick *et al.* 2001	RCT—unclear randomization process. The method for collecting outcome data is unknown. The 12-week attrition rate was 6%.	37 pregnant women (17 in the intervention group; 18 in the control group) on public assistance who had at least one risk factor for postpartum depression and were attending a prenatal clinic at a general hospital in the northeast USA.	Intervention group: 'Survival Skills for New Moms', which involved four 60-minute group sessions over a 4-week period based on the principles of interpersonal psychotherapy. Control group: standard antenatal care.	SCID at 12 weeks postpartum.	50% of eligible women declined trial participation. 77% of participants were single women.

Table 4.1 (continued) Characteristics of included studies

Study	Methods	Participants	Interventions	Outcome	Notes
Zlotnick et al. 2006	RCT—unclear randomization process. The method for collecting outcome data is unknown. The 12-week attrition rate was 13%.	99 pregnant women (53 in the intervention group and 46 in the control group) who screened at-risk for postpartum depression during antenatal clinic visits in Rhode Island, USA. They were 23–32 weeks' gestation and on public assistance.	Intervention group: The ROSE Program (Reach Out, Stand strong, Essentials for new mothers) which involved 4 60-minute group session over 4 weeks and one 50-minute individual booster session post-delivery. The intervention was given by nurses who had received intensive training and supervision. Control group: standard antenatal care.	BDI at 12 weeks postpartum.	

BDI: Beck Depression Inventory; CES-D: Centre for Epidemiologic Studies Depression Scale; EPDS: Edinburgh Postpartum Depression Scale; HADS: Hospital Anxiety and Depression Scale; Kessler 10: MINI: Mini International Neuropsychiatric Interview; RCT: randomized controlled trial; SCAN: Schedules for Assessment in Neuropsychiatry; SCID: Structured Clinical Interview for DSM-IV; SF36: Short Form (36) Health Survey.

postpartum depression but incorporated a different cut-off score; one study used a 10/11 cut-off (Brugha *et al.* 2000) while another two studies selected a 11/12 cut-off (Morrell *et al.* 2000; Reid *et al.* 2002). It is important to note that the EPDS does not diagnose postpartum depression (as this can only be accomplished through a psychiatric clinical interview) but rather it is the most frequently used instrument to assess for postpartum depressive symptoms. Several other trials used a self-report measure other than the EPDS and included the Beck Depression Inventory (BDI) (Le *et al.* 2011; Zlotnick *et al.* 2001, 2006), Center for Epidemiologic Studies Depression Scale (CES-D) (Feinberg and Kan 2008; Ickovics *et al.* 2011), Hospital Anxiety Depression Scale (HADS) (Lavender and Walkinshaw 1998; Tam *et al.* 2003; Weidner *et al.* 2010), Kessler-10 (Tripathy *et al.* 2010), and the SF-36 Mental Health Subscale (Cupples *et al.* 2011; Gjerdingen and Center 2002), and five trials used a semi-structured diagnostic interview to provide a clinical diagnosis of depression(Gorman 1997; Brugha *et al.* 2000; Dennis *et al.* 2009; Harris *et al.* 2006; Zlotnick *et al.* 2001), with four of these trials using the Structured Clinical Interview for DSM-IV (SCID). The timing of the outcome assessments varied considerably between studies ranging from 3 (Lavender and Walkinshaw 1998) to more than 24 weeks (Armstrong *et al.* 1999; Cupples *et al.* 2011; Ickovics *et al.* 2011; MacArthur *et al.* 2002; Preist *et al.* 2003; Sen 2006). Due to the significant differences in the timing of outcome data, an additional outcome assessment point was included that used data 'at final study assessment'. Due to the complexity of the analyses, in this paper we only report depressive symptomology at final study assessment data. If this data were not available for a particular outcome then we reported standard mean differences (SMD). For a detailed report of the meta-analyses for each outcome, including depressive symptomatology across time, SMD, and clinical diagnosis of postpartum depression, please see the full systematic review (Dennis and Dowswell 2013).

Methodological quality

Randomization was performed most frequently by consecutively numbered, sealed, opaque envelopes (Groman, 1997; Tam *et al.* 2003; Gamble *et al.* 2005; Le *et al.* 2011; Stamp *et al.* 1995; Harris *et al.* 2006; Reid *et al.* 2002; Morrell *et al.* 2000; Waldenstrom *et al.* 1998; Lavender and Shaw, 1998; Priest *et al.* 2003). Various forms of computer-based randomisation was used by nine trials (Feinberg and Kan, 2008; Gjerdingen and Center, 2002; Gao *et al.* 2010; Weidner *et al.* 2010; Armstrong *et al.* 1999; Burgha *et al.* 2000; Ickovics *et al.* 2011; MacArthur *et al.* 2002; Cupples *et al.* 2011). Four trials incorporated a central, computerized randomization service accessed by telephone (Gunn *et al.* 1998; Small *et al.* 2000) or the internet (Dennis *et al.* 2009; Sen 2006) and two trials did the randomization of clusters at a public event (Lumley *et al.* 2006; Tripathy *et al.* 2010). Allocation concealment was unclear in four trials (Gao *et al.* 2010; Lumley *et al.* 2006; Zlotnick *et al.* 2001, 2006). In all but three trials (Brugha *et al.* 2000; Harris *et al.* 2006; Le *et al.* 2011), outcome data were collected by assessors blinded to group allocation or by mailed questionnaires; for three studies the method of collecting outcomes is unknown (Tam *et al.* 2003; Zlotnick *et al.* 2001, 2006). Six trials had a follow-up rate less than 80% (Gunn *et al.* 1998; Harris *et al.* 2006; MacArthur *et al.* 2002; Reid *et al.* 2002; Waldenstrom *et al.* 2000; Weidner *et al.* 2010); it is noteworthy that follow-up in all these trials except Harris *et al.* (2006) was done by mailed questionnaires. Trials were excluded for sensitivity analyses related to high susceptibility to bias due to methodological quality (Brugha *et al.* 2000; Harris *et al.* 2006; Le *et al.*2011; Tam *et al.* 2003; Weidner *et al.* 2010; Zlotnick *et al.* 2001, 2006) or follow-up losses greater than 20% (Harris *et al.* 2006; Gunn *et al.* 1998; MacArthur *et al.* 2002; Reid *et al.* 2002; Waldenstrom *et al.* 2000; Weidner *et al.* 2010).

Quantitative data synthesis

The main outcome measure for this review was postpartum depression at final study assessment. There was a beneficial effect on the prevention of postpartum depression in the meta-analysis of all types of interventions (20 trials, $n = 14,727$; relative risk (RR) 0.78, 95% confidence interval (CI) 0.66–0.93). There was significant heterogeneity among these trials ($I^2 = 64\%$, $T^2 = 0.07$). However, the removal of trials at risk of bias resulted in no substantial change to the conclusion. To assess the short- and longer-term effects of the preventive interventions, postpartum depression assessments were categorized as follows: 0 to 8 weeks postpartum—immediate effect; 9 to 16 weeks postpartum—short-term effect; 17 to 24 weeks postpartum—intermediate effect; and more than 24 weeks—long-term effect. Results suggested an immediate (13 trials, $n = 4907$; RR 0.73, 95% CI 0.56–0.95) and short-term (10 trials, $n = 3,982$; RR 0.73 95% CI 0.56–0.97) reduction in depressive symptomatology. While the preventative effect appeared to weaken at the intermediate postpartum time period between 17–24 weeks (9 trials, $n = 10,636$; RR 0.93; 95% CI 0.82–1.05), it was again significant when depressive symptomatology was assessed past 24 weeks postpartum (5 trials, $n = 2936$; RR 0.66, 95% CI 0.54–0.82).

Subgroup analyses

Effect of intervention type

In total, 17 trials evaluated a psychosocial intervention, of which 12 included a measure of depressive symptomatology. Overall, these interventions have a beneficial effect in decreasing the risk of developing postpartum depression at final study assessment (12 trials, $n = 11,322$; RR 0.83, 95% CI 0.70–0.99). No preventive effect was found with the following psychosocial interventions: antenatal and postpartum classes (4 trials, $n = 1488$; RR 1.01, 95% CI 0.77–1.32); postpartum lay-based home visits (1 trial, $n = 493$; RR 0.88, 95% CI 0.62–1.25); early postpartum follow-up (1 trial, $n = 446$; RR 0.90, 95% CI 0.55–1.49); or continuity/model of care (3 trials, $n = 7021$; RR 0.99, 95% CI 0.71–1.36). However, a clear beneficial effect was found when the intervention involved postpartum home visits provided by a health professional (2 trials, $n = 1262$; RR 0.56, 95% CI 0.43–0.73) and for postpartum lay-based telephone support (1 trial, $n = 612$, RR 0.54, 95% CI 0.38–0.77).

In total, 11 trials evaluated a psychological intervention. No preventive effect was found in relation to psychological debriefing (5 trials, $n = 3050$; RR 0.57, 95% CI 0.31–1.03) and cognitive behavioural therapy (1 trial, $n = 150$, RR 0.59, 95% CI 0.74–1.88), but a preventive effect was found in relation to interpersonal psychotherapy (5 trials, $n = 366$, SMD –0.27, 95% CI –0.52 to –0.01).

Effect of intervention provider

Nineteen trials evaluated an intervention provided by a health professional. The RR for depressive symptomatology at final assessment for professionally-based interventions was 0.78 (15 trials, n = 6790; 95% CI 0.60–1.00). Seven trials evaluated an intervention provided by a lay individual. The RR for depressive symptomatology at final assessment for lay-based interventions was 0.70 (4 trials, n = 1723; 95% CI 0.54–0.90).

Effect of intervention mode

Analysis of 14 trials evaluating individually-based interventions suggested reduction in depressive symptomatology at the last study assessment (n = 12,914; RR 0.75, 95% CI 0.61–0.92). When trials susceptible to bias were removed, the direction of the effect strengthened (11 trials, n = 10,653; RR 0.71, 95% CI 0.56–0.91). Of the six trials evaluating group-based interventions, there was no clear reduction in depressive symptomatology at final study assessment (n = 1,813; RR 0.92, 95% CI 0.71–1.19).

Effect of intervention duration

Only four trials evaluated single-contact interventions (e.g. psychological debriefing, early postpartum follow-up). The RR related to depressive symptomatology at final assessment was 0.70 (n = 2,877; 95% CI 0.38–1.28). In total, 24 trials evaluated a multiple-contact intervention. Of the trials 16 that included a measure of depressive symptomatology, a significant reduction was found at final study assessment (n = 11,850; RR 0.78, 95% CI 0.66–0.93).

Effect of intervention onset

Four trials evaluated an intervention that was conducted only in the antenatal period and the SMD at final study assessment was 0.03 (n = 1050; 96% CI 0.9–0.16). Eight trials evaluated intervention that were initiated antenatally and continued postnatally. The RR in relation to depressive symptomatology at final assessment was 0.96 (n = 1,941; 95% CI 0.75–1.22). A preventive effect was found for those trials evaluating an intervention initiated postnatally (12 trials, n = 12,786; RR 0.73, 95% CI 0.59–0.90).

Effect of sample selected

Trials selecting participants based on some 'at-risk' criteria had a reduction in postpartum depressive symptomatology at final study assessment (8 trials, n = 1853; RR 0.66, 95% CI 0.50–0.88). Twelve trials enrolled women from the general population. The RR related to depressive symptomatology at final study assessment was 0.83 (n = 12,874; 95% CI 0.68–1.02).

Discussion

This chapter summarizes the results of 28 trials involving almost 17,000 women. Currently, there is no clear evidence to recommend that the following interventions be implemented into practice in order to prevent postpartum depression: antenatal classes and postpartum classes, early postpartum follow-up, continuity of care models, and in-hospital psychological debriefing. While these interventions may be beneficial for other maternal outcomes at this time there is no evidence that they may prevent the development of postpartum depression.

The effectiveness of cognitive behavioural therapy (Le *et al.* 2011) and postpartum lay-based home visits (Morrell *et al.* 2000) remains uncertain. However, there is some evidence to suggest the importance of additional professional-based home visits provided postnatally. While one well-designed trial (Armstrong *et al.* 1999) suggested intensive nursing home visits with at-risk mothers was protective during the first 6 weeks postpartum, the beneficial effect was not maintained to 16 weeks. It is noteworthy that the 16-week assessment coincided with a decrease in intervention intensity from weekly to monthly nursing visits. Results from a cluster randomized controlled trial demonstrated that flexible, individualized midwifery-based postpartum care that incorporated postpartum depression screening tools also had a preventive effect (MacArthur *et al.* 2002). Individualized telephone-based lay support provided by peers postnatally (Dennis *et al.* 2009) is another promising intervention. Combined, these three trials decreased the risk to develop postpartum depression by almost 50% and provide accumulating evidence that additional individualized support early in the postpartum period may be an effective preventative intervention.

Another strategy that may assist in preventing postpartum depression is interpersonal psychotherapy. Interpersonal psychotherapy is a manual-based, time-limited psychotherapeutic approach with a basic premise that depression, regardless of aetiology, is initiated and maintained within an interpersonal context. The goal of interpersonal therapy is to achieve symptomatic relief for depression by addressing current interpersonal issues associated with its onset or perpetuation; it does not seek to attribute interpersonal problems to underlying personality characteristics or unconscious motivations. Interpersonal psychotherapy is primarily concerned with symptom functioning, presumed to have biological and psychological precipitants, and social functioning. There is a specific focus on social interactions. Given that a lack of support and marital conflict are two strong risk factors for postpartum depression (Beck 2001; O'Hara and Swain 1996), this intervention is theoretically congruent with preventing postpartum depression.

The trials can be further classified into different categories depending on the target population: *universal* interventions are designed to be offered to all women, *selective* interventions are designed to be offered to women at increased risk of developing depression, and *indicated* interventions are designed to be offered to women who have been identified as depressed or probably depressed (Mrazek and Haggerty 1994). While no trial that evaluated an indicated intervention was included in this review, to examine the effects of universal and selective interventions, subgroup analyses were conducted. The results suggested identifying mothers 'at-risk' may assist in the prevention of postpartum depression. However, currently there is no consistency in the identification of women 'at-risk' and a review of 16 antenatal screening tools suggests that there are no measures with acceptable predictive validity to accurately identify asymptomatic women who will later develop postpartum depression (Austin and Lumley 2003). This may partially explain why interventions initiated in the postpartum period may have a beneficial effect on reducing the risk to develop depressive symptomatology at final study assessment.

Other differences in intervention delivery were also examined. Women who receive a multiple-contact intervention were less likely to develop postpartum depression; it is noteworthy that the majority of trials provided a multiple-contact intervention. Individually based interventions were effective in significantly reducing the number of women with depressive symptomatology at final study assessment. Lastly, both professionally based and lay-based interventions were equally beneficial in reducing the risk to develop postpartum depression. The majority of the interventions included in this review were professionally based.

The methodological quality of the included trials was good to excellent. However, the reporting of the trials was often not comprehensive, lacking in terms of details in the training and qualifications of the intervention providers and in the description of adherence to the intervention protocol. There was also a failure to present details of the informational element of the interventions and on the background features of the care received by the control groups. While intent-to-treat data analyses were performed, trials involving group sessions had high (Brugha *et al.* 2000; Le *et al.* 2011; Reid *et al.* 2002) or unknown (Tripathy *et al.* 2010) levels of non-compliance with group attendance.

The diversity of preventative interventions and the widely differing study end-points should urge some caution in the interpretation of the pooled data. To partially address this issue, the meta-analyses included immediate-, short-, intermediate-, and longer-term effects where appropriate. Despite this caution and the sub-grouping of end-points, this review consistently demonstrated that women who received a preventive intervention were significantly less likely to experience postpartum depression than those who received standard care. Psychosocial and psychological interventions were both effective in reducing the risk to develop depressive symptomatology at final study assessment.

The long-term consequences of postpartum depression suggest preventive approaches are warranted. However, translating risk factor research into predictive screening protocols and preventative interventions is challenging, as complex interactions of biopsychosocial risk factors with individual variations need to be considered. The results from this review provide physicians and other health professionals with practice guidelines as well as recommendations for future preventive trials. To further address postpartum depression as a public health concern, the inclusion of ethnically and socioeconomically diverse women in these research efforts is critical to examining the differences in depression symptoms, response rate to interventions, and health service use. In addition, all future trials should include an economic analysis of the relative costs and benefits and more information about the development of preventive programmes.

Conclusions

Overall, psychosocial or psychological interventions significantly reduce the number of women who develop postpartum depression. Promising interventions include the provision of intensive, professionally-based postpartum home visits, telephone-based peer support, and interpersonal psychotherapy.

References

Appleby, L., Warner, R., Whitton, A., and Faragher, B. (1997). A controlled study of fluoextine and cognitive-behavioural counselling in the treatment of postnatal depression. British Medical Journal **314**: 932–6.

Armstrong, K.L., Fraser, J.A., Dadds, M.R., and Morris, J. (1999). A randomized, controlled trial of nurse home visiting to vulnerable families with newborns. Journal of Paediatrics & Child Health **35**(3): 237–44.

Austin, M. and Lumley, J. (2003). Antenatal screening for postnatal depression: a systematic review. Acta Psychiatrica Scandinavica **107**(1): 10–17.

Austin, M.P, Frilingos, M., Lumley, J., *et al.* (2008). Brief antenatal cognitive behavior therapy group intervention for the prevention of postnatal depression and anxiety: a randomised controlled trial. Journal of Affective Disorders **105**(1–3): 35–44.

Beck, C.T. (2001). Predictors of postpartum depression: an update. Nursing Research **50**(5): 275–85.

Brown, J.D., Harris, S.K., Woods, E.R., Buman, M.P., and Cox, J.E. (2011). Longitudinal study of depressive symptoms and social support in adolescent mothers. Maternal and Child Health Journal **16**: 894–901.

Brugha, T.S., Wheatley, S., Taub, N.A., *et al.* (2000). Pragmatic randomized trial of antenatal intervention to prevent post-natal depression by reducing psychosocial risk factors. Psychological Medicine **30**(6): 1273–81.

Collins, C.H., Zimmerman, C., and Howard, L.M. (2011). Refugee, asylum seeker, immigrant women and postnatal depression: rates and risk factors. Archives of Women's Mental Health **14**(1): 3–11.

Cooper, P. and Murray, L. (1997). The impact of psychological treatments of postpartum depression on maternal mood and infant development. In Postpartum depression and child development, Cooper, P. and Murray, L., editors. New York, Guilford, pp. 201–20.

Cooper, P.J., Murray, L., Wilson, A., and Romaniuk, H. (2003). Controlled trial of the short- and long-term effect of psychological treatment of post-partum depression. I. Impact on maternal mood. British Journal of Psychiatry **182**: 412–19.

Cupples, M.E., Stewart, M.C., Percy, A., *et al.* (2011). A RCT of peer-mentoring for first-time mothers in socially disadvantaged areas (the MOMENTS Study). Archives of Disease in Childhood **96**(3): 252–58.

Dennis, C.-L. (2003). The effect of peer support on postpartum depression: a pilot randomized controlled trial. Canadian Journal of Psychiatry **48**(2): 115–24.

Dennis, C. and Dowswell, T. (2013) Psychosocial and psychological interventions for preventing postpartum depression. Cochrane Database of Systematic Reviews (Issue 4. Art. No.: CD001134. DOI: 10.1002/14651858.CD001134.pub2).

Dennis, C.L. and Hodnett, E.(2007). Psychosocial and psychological interventions for treating postpartum depression. Cochrane Database of Systematic Reviews (4)(CD006116).

Dennis, C.-L., Hodnett, E.D., Kenton, L., *et al.* (2009). Effect of peer support on prevention of postnatal depression among high risk women: multisite randomised controlled trial. British Medical Journal **338**: a3064.

Feinberg, M.E. and Kan, M.L. (2008). Establishing family foundations: intervention effects on coparenting, parent/infant well-being, and parent-child relations. Journal of Family Psychology **22**(2): 253–63.

Gamble, J., Creedy, D., Moyle, W., *et al.* (2005). Effectiveness of a counseling intervention after traumatic childbirth: a randomized controlled trial. Birth **31**(1): 11–19.

Gao, L., Chan, S., Li, X., Chen, S., and Hao, Y. (2010). Evaluation of an interpersonal-psychotherapy-oriented childbirth education programme for Chinese first-time childbearing women: a randomised controlled trial. International Journal of Nursing Studies **47**: 1208–16.

Gaynes, B.N., Gavin, N., Meltzer-Brody, S., *et al.* (2005). Perinatal depression: prevalance, screening accuracy, and screening outcomes. Evidence Report Technology Assessment summary **119**: 1–8.

Gjerdingen, D.K. and Center, B. (2002). A randomized controlled trial testing the impact of a support/work-planning intervention on first-time parents' health, partner relationship, and work responsibilities. Behavioral Medicine **28**(3): 84–91.

Gorman, L.L. (1997). Prevention of postpartum difficulties in a high risk sample [dissertation]. Ames, University of Iowa.

Gunn, J., Lumley, J., Chondros, P., and Young, D. (1998). Does an early postnatal check-up improve maternal health: results from a randomised trial in Australian general practice. British Journal of Obstetrics & Gynaecology **105**(9): 991–7.

Harris, T., Brown, G.W., Hamilton, V., Hodson, S., and Craig, T.K.J. (2006). The Newpin antenatal and postnatal project: a randomised controlled trial of an intervention for perinatal depression. Poster prepared for the HSR Open Day, Institute of Psychiatry, King's College London. 6 July 2006.

Heinicke, C.M., Fineman, N.R., Ruth, G., et al. (1999). Relationship-based intervention with at-risk mothers: outcome in the first year of life. Infant Mental Health Journal **20**(4): 349–74.

Holden, J., Sagovsky, R., and Cox, J. (1989). Counselling in a general practice setting: controlled study of health visitor intervention in treatment of postnatal depression. British Medical Journal **298**: 223–26.

Ickovics, J.R., Reed, E., Magriples, U., et al. (2011). Effects of group prenatal care on psychosocial risk in pregnancy: results from a randomised controlled trial. Psychology & Health **26**(2): 235–50.

Lavender, T. and Walkinshaw, S.A. (1998). Can midwives reduce postpartum psychological morbidity? A randomized trial. Birth **25**(4): 215–19.

Le, H.N., Perry, D.F., and Stuart, E.A. (2011). Randomized controlled trial of a preventive intervention for perinatal depression in high-risk Latinas. Journal of Consulting & Clinical Psychology **79**(2): 135–41.

Lumley, J., Watson, L., Small, R., et al. (2006). Prism (program of resources, information and support for mothers): a community-randomised trial to reduce depression and improve women's physical health six months after birth. BMC Public Health **6**: 37.

MacArthur, C., Winter, H.R., Bick, D.E., et al. (2002). Effects of redesigned community postnatal care on womens' health 4 months after birth: a cluster randomised controlled trial. Lancet **359**(9304): 378–85.

Morrell, C.J., Spiby, H., Stewart, P., Walters, S., and Morgan, A. (2000). Costs and effectiveness of community postnatal support workers: randomised controlled trial. British Medical Journal **321**(7261): 593–8.

Mrazek, P.J. and Haggerty, R.J. (1994). Reducing risks for mental disorders—Frontiers for prevention intervention research. Washington, DC, National Academy Press.

O'Hara, M. and Swain, A. (1996). Rates and risk of postpartum depression - a meta-analysis. International Review of Psychiatry **8**: 37–54.

O'Hara, M.W., Stuart, S., Gorman, L.L., and Wenzel, A. (2000). Efficacy of interpersonal psychotherapy for postpartum depression. Archives of General Psychiatry **57**: 1039–45.

Priest, S.R., Henderson, J., Evans, S.F., andHagan, R. (2003). Stress debriefing after childbirth: a randomised controlled trial. Medical Journal of Australia **178**(11): 542–5.

Reid, M., Glazener, C., Murray, G.D., and Taylor, G.S. (2002). A two-centred pragmatic randomised controlled trial of two interventions for postnatal support. British Journal of Obstetrics & Gynaecology **109**(10): 1164–70.

Ross, L. and Dennis, C.-L. (2009). The prevalence of postpartum depression among women with substance use, an abuse history, or chronic illness: a systematic review. Journal of Women's Health **18**: 475–86.

Sen, D.M. (2006). A randomized controlled trial of midwife-led twin antenatal program—the Newcastle Twin Study [thesis]. Newcastle upon Tyne, University of Newcastle.

Small, R., Lumley, J., Donohue, L., Potter, A., and Waldenstrom, U. (2000). Randomised controlled trial of midwife led debriefing to reduce maternal depression after operative childbirth. British Medical Journal **321**(7268): 1043–7.

Stamp, G.E., Williams, A.S., and Crowther, C.A. (1995). Evaluation of antenatal and postnatal support to overcome postnatal depression: a randomized controlled trial. Birth 22(3): 138–43.

Tam, W.H., Lee, D.T., Chiu, H.F., *et al.* (2003). A randomised controlled trial of educational counselling on the management of women who have suffered suboptimal outcomes in pregnancy. BJOG: An International Journal of Obstetrics & Gynaecology 110(9): 853–9.

Tripathy, P., Nair, N., Barnett, S., *et al.* (2010). Effect of a participatory intervention with women's groups on birth outcomes and maternal depression in Jharkhard and Orissa, India: a cluster-randomised controlled trial. Lancet 375(9721): 1182–92.

Waldenstrom, U., Brown, S., McLachlan, H., Forster, D., and Brennecke, S. (2000). Does team midwife care increase satisfaction with antenatal, intrapartum, and postpartum care? A randomized controlled trial. Birth 27(3): 156–67.

Weidner, K., Bittner, A., Junge-Hoffmeister, J., *et al.* (2010). A psychosomatic intervention in pregnant in-patient women with prenatal somatic risks. Journal of Psychosomatic Obstetrics & Gynecology 31(3): 188–98.

Wickberg, B. and Hwang, C. (1996). Counselling of postnatal depression: a controlled study on a population based Swedish sample. Journal of Affective Disorders 39: 209–16.

Zlotnick, C., Johnson, S.L., Miller, I.W., Pearlstein, T., and Howard, M. (2001). Postpartum depression in women receiving public assistance: pilot study of an interpersonal-therapy-oriented group intervention. American Journal of Psychiatry 158(4): 638–40.

Zlotnick, C., Miller, I.W., Pearlstein, T., Howard, M., and Sweeney, P.A preventive intervention for pregant women on public assistance at risk for postpartum depression. American Journal of Psychiatry 163(8): 1443–5.

Chapter 5

Pregnancy prescribing of psychotropic drugs
Keeping pace in a contemporary landscape

Kathryn M. Abel

Introduction

Pregnant women and their fetuses are more likely than ever to be exposed to antipsychotic medications; perhaps to the newer agents in particular. Drugs like clozapine, olanzapine, risperidone, and quetiapine are increasingly used in women of reproductive age for a range of psychiatric and behavioural disorders other than schizophrenia (Buchanan *et al.* 2009). Reproductive safety data remain surprisingly incomplete and guideline recommendations lend limited support to clinical risk-benefit analyses (Howard 2005; McKenna *et al.* 2005; NICE 2007). This is a problem not least because the gold standard randomized controlled trial is considered unethical for assessing psychotropic medication use during pregnancy, while other available observational studies are generally underpowered, with biased samples and therefore remain unfit for purpose in a rapidly changing prescribing landscape (NICE 2007).

In a UK population approaching 66 million, –3,000–4,000 births per year may be exposed to antipsychotics or other psychotropic medications. This chapter provides a critical summary of current knowledge about potential risks of fetal antipsychotic and antiepileptic drug exposure and proposes how future observational studies might fill crucial gaps in the evidence.

A contemporary problem

Most incident cases of severe mental illness (schizophrenia, related disorders, and bipolar disorder) occur during the reproductive years and most are treated with continuous psychotropic pharmacotherapy (Buchanan *et al.* 2009). Better care, deinstitutionalization and the use of newer agents with fewer effects on fertility means that women with psychotic disorders maybe increasingly likely to become pregnant (Howard 2005; NICE 2007), while the use of newer 'atypical' antipsychotics for other mental disorders common among women of childbearing age is also expanding (McKenna *et al.* 2005). For these reasons, psychotropic medications is increasingly likely to be prescribed to mothers during pregnancy (Newport *et al.* 2007). It is surprising then that reproductive safety data for psychotropic agents remains so incomplete (Barnes 2008; Webb *et al.* 2004) and guideline recommendations lend limited support to women, their partners and their treating clinicians in difficult clinical risk-benefit analyses (NICE 2007). Recent reports conclude that prospective studies are needed which can access unbiased, reliable (large enough) samples of ill mothers exposed to psychotropic medication and take account of key maternal characteristics (e.g. psychiatric diagnosis, smoking, pre-pregnancy weight) in the estimation of risk (Barnes 2008; NICE 2007).

Two classes of drug primarily used to treat women with psychosis or severe behavioural disorder will be considered. These include first- (FGA) and second-generation antipsychotic (SGA) drugs and mood stabilizing or antiepileptic agents.

Antipsychotic studies

Studies of antipsychotic agents are limited in number and size and yield inconsistent findings for the following key outcomes.

Congenital malformations

Typical antipsychotics

In 1961, Sobel reported that women with psychotic illness were twice as likely as women in the general population to have a pregnancy resulting in congenital malformation or death, irrespective of chlorpromazine use in pregnancy. Currently, it is uncertain whether as a group antipsychotics lead to increases in congenital anomalies above the general population rate of ~2–4% (EUROCAT 2012; ONS 2008). Theoretically, offspring of psychiatric patients should be at increased risk of neural tube defects because of higher rates of obesity and reduced serum folate levels related to low dietary vitamin intake (Barnes 2008). A meta-analysis of older, mainly prospective cohort studies, reports small, but significant excess congenital malformations in infants exposed to phenothiazines ($n = 2,591$) compared with unexposed infants of well mothers ($n = 7\,1,746$) (odds ratio (OR) 1.21, confidence interval (CI) 1.01–1.45) (Altschuler *et al.* 1996). However, secular trends in some key outcomes suggest that estimates from more recent cohorts are likely to be more reliable. Table 5.1 summarizes only recent studies documenting the impact of antipsychotics on pregnancy and related outcomes in mothers with psychosis. Using a 10 year cohort of births (1995–2005) from Swedish national registers, Reis and Kallen (2008) report maternal antipsychotic use *overall* was associated with little or negligible excess risk of congenital malformation (OR 1.45, CI 0.99–1.41) compared to well population controls. Here, the excess was largely accounted for by cardiovascular anomaly (atrial or ventricular septal defects). Results were adjusted for concomitant antiepileptic use, but not for antidepressants, also associated with small increases in cardiovascular anomaly (Reis and Kallen 2010). Systematic review to July 2008 (Gentile 2010), however, concludes that risk of limb anomalies cannot be excluded with typical antipsychotics (i.e. haloperidol) exposure.

Table 5.1 Risks of adverse outcomes following antipsychotic (AP) exposure in pregnancy

Study	Outcome	Prenatal exposure	n	Findings
Bodén et al. (2012)	Gestational diabetes	All APs 1st trimester	507 exposed	2 × increased risk
	Prematurity			60% increased risk
	SGA			>twofold increased risk (but likely confounded)
Reis and Kallen (2008)	Severe CMs	All APs 1st trimester	576 exposed	50% increased risk
	Gestational diabetes			2 × increased risk
	LSCS			No increased risk
	Prematurity			70% increased risk
	SGA			50% increased risk
	LGA			No increased risk
Newham et al. (2005)	Prematurity	All APs 1st trimester		No increased risk
	SGA		70 exposed	No increased risk
	LGA			Increased risk for atypicals but very small numbers (n = 5)
Newport et al. (2007)	LBW	Atypical APs	41 exposed	No significant increase risk
	Hypoxia			
McKenna et al. (2005)	CMs	Atypical APs	151 exposed	No significant increase
	Spontaneous abortion			
	Prematurity			
	Pregnancy complications			
	LBW			
Lin et al. (2010)	Prematurity	All APs 1st trimester Compared to women with schiz on NO APs	242 exposed schizophrenia only	Twofold increase typical antipsychotics only
	LBW			No increased risk
	SGA/LGA			No increased risk
	Prematurity			No increased risk

Note: LBW low birthweight; SGA or LGA small or large for gestational age; CMs congenital malformations; APs antipsychotics.

Atypical antipsychotics

Although primarily used to treat schizophrenia and psychotic disorders, newer 'atypical' antipsychotics now treat a spectrum of disorders, including major depression, bipolar disorder, post-traumatic stress disorder (PTSD), and other anxiety disorders (McKenna *et al.* 2005). Far less data have accumulated for newer atypical agents: olanzapine, risperidone, quetiapine, aripiprazole, amisulpride and clozapine. Most data on reproductive safety for these agents is limited to manufacturers' case series and spontaneous reports, which are inherently biased by adverse outcomes reporting. Among reports of olanzapine-exposed pregnancies from the manufacturer, no increase in risk of major malformations is reported. In 523 clozapine-exposed pregnancies, 22 'unspecified malformations' were reported (4.2%) while in 151 quetiapine-exposed pregnancies, 8 infants had congenital anomalies (5.2%). Eight malformations were reported in infants born to 250 women taking risperidone (3.2%); however, pregnancy outcomes were unknown in many of these cases reported to the manufacturer (McKenna *et al.* 2005). Taken together, these reports do not suggest an increase in major malformation above that seen in the general population, nor do they indicate any specific pattern of abnormalities among atypical antipsychotic drug-exposed infants. This information does not suggest particular concerns for atypical antipsychotic use in early pregnancy, but conclusions can only be preliminary.

Individual antipsychotics

Most typical FGAs have been prescribed for emesis gravidarum rather than mental illness. This represents a potentially important (if not contemporary) control group which might allow distinction between effects of maternal illness from maternal medication. However, for emesis, FGAs tended to be used in much lower doses and intermittently limiting the benefit of using this as a comparison group. Restricting cases from relatively unbiased population samples, over 200 cases have been reported for olanzapine, haloperidol, or fluphenazine; 100–200 cases for risperidone or flupenthixol and less than 100 for all other antipsychotics, including chlorpromazine, clozapine, sulpiride, trifluoperazine and quetiapine (see Barnes 2008). Taken together, these limited data, and the considerable number of years that many compounds have been available, do not suggest antipsychotic drugs are major teratogens. However, the recent, and only systematic, review (Gentile 2010) concluded that risk of limb anomalies associated with early in utero exposure to haloperidol and penfluridol cannot be excluded (Barnes 2008; Gentile 2010; Garbis *et al.* 2005); no conclusions can be drawn about teratogenicity of fluphenazine, thioridazine and promethazine. To date, first-trimester exposures to aripiprazole is rarely reported including one child born with major congenital anomalies. No published information is currently available for sertindole, amisulpride, and zotepine.

Pregnancy and maternal outcomes

Typical antipsychotics

Reis and Kallen (2008) used births between 1995–2005 from the Swedish Medical Births register to report excess risk of prematurity (OR 1.73, CI 1.31–2.29), low birth weight (OR 1.67, CI 1.21–2.29), and trend increased risk of small for gestational age (OR 1.46, CI 0.99–2.15) for pregnancies exposed to any antipsychotic (*n* = 576) compared to well population controls. Bodén *et al.* (2012) use a different Swedish dataset, the Prescribed Drug Registry over a 4 year period (2005–2009) reporting that infants exposed to antipsychotics (*n* = 507) overall had higher risk of small for gestational age (OR 2.11, CI 1.29–3.47) and gestational diabetes (OR 2.78, CI 1.64–4.70). Further, infants exposed to any antipsychotics had a higher risk of being born small for gestational age for birth length (OR 2.29, CI 1.41–3.73) and for head circumference (OR 2.19, CI 1.33–3.62). All risks became non significant after adjusting for maternal factors e.g. smoking. Lin *et al.* (2010) report specifically Taiwanese schizophrenic mothers (*n* = 242) using any antipsychotics and who had given birth between 2001 and 2003. They only found excess risk of prematurity (OR 2.46, CI 1.50–4.11), and only in mothers receiving *typical* antipsychotics, but no excess risk of low birthweight, small or large for gestational age with early pregnancy antipsychotic exposure overall. No other outcomes were assessed. A far smaller UK study (Newham *et al.* 2008) reports that infants exposed to typical (*n* = 45) and atypical antipsychotics (*n* = 25) compared to unexposed controls had no significant risk of small for gestational age. Significantly more small for gestational age infants were exposed to typical drugs than the reference group; this difference disappeared after exclusion of mothers exposed to other weight-altering drugs. Finally, systematic review of studies to July 2008 (Gentile 2010) concluded that risk of perinatal complications (ranging from withdrawal symptoms to instability of body temperature) is associated with late in utero exposure to haloperidol and phenothiazines such as chlorpromazine.

Atypical antipsychotics

McKenna *et al* conclude that women exposed to atypical antipsychotics have significantly higher rates of low birthweight infants than controls (10% vs. 2%) whereas two subsequent studies reported excess of large for gestational age infants: Newham *et al.* (2008) report increase in infant birthweight and large for gestational age based on only five cases exposed to either clozapine or olanzapine. Bodén *et al.* (in press) report increased risk of gestational diabetes (OR 2.39, CI 1.12–5.13) and small for gestational age (OR for 2.42, CI 1.24–4.70) after early exposure to olanzapine and clozapine as a group. They examine risk of anabolic fetal growth with olanzapine and clozapine as a group, but do not find a significant effect. This latest study has the largest number of cases of women exposed to olanzapine or clozapine (*n* = 169) to date. No studies have been able to look separately at clozapine or other agents, such as olanzapine, quetiapine, and risperidone, which are fast becoming the most prescribed antispsychotics in the UK (HSCIC 2010; Downey *et al.* 2012). This is important because of placental passage (umbilical cord: maternal plasma concentration) of olanzapine was highest (mean 72.1%, SD = 42.0%) along with higher rates of either low birth weight and/or perinatal complications compared with other antipsychotics (Newport *et al.* 2007). See Table 5.1.

No studies examine quality of life, drug adherence, time to, risk of relapse in mothers with schizophrenia or related disorder who discontinue antipsychotic medication in pregnancy in powerful enough datasets.

Developmental outcomes

There is a remarkable absence of systematic studies of neonatal reaction following pregnancy exposure to antipsychotics. Several cases of neonatal extrapyramidal syndrome are reported in response to typical drugs (Gentile 2010), but there are no other consistent patterns of adverse effects in the literature. There are very limited data on potential longer-term neurobehavioural sequelae of fetal exposure to antipsychotics and it is not difficult to understand why. Such a follow-up study would be very hard to undertake, with a need to account for many postnatal risks associated with being the child of a mother with severe enough symptoms to warrant major psychotropic agents in pregnancy (McCabe *et al.* 2007). Most literature concerns high-risk children born to parents with psychotic illness (Niemi *et al.* 2003; Wan *et al.* 2008). Several older studies, where mothers may have been exposed to typical antipsychotics, report that deficits in infancy and early childhood have poor predictive value and are likely to have disappeared later in childhood (e.g. Sameroff *et al.* 1987). Two reviews of the older literature fail to find differences in behavioural functioning or IQ up to 5 years (Altshuler *et al.* 1996; Thiels 1987). Long-term cognitive, psychopathological, or developmental effects have not been examined. This is particularly important because much of the so-called 'high-risk' literature shows evidence that offspring of severely mentally ill parents are more likely to show poorer cognitive, social, and clinical outcomes (Niemi *et al.* 2003). Thus, Niemi *et al.* (2003) report on 145 children of mothers with psychosis and find them significantly more likely to have a severe academic problem (15%) than controls (8%). Impairments are more consistently reported in specific cognitive domains, such as verbal ability, executive functioning and processing speed (see Wan *et al.* 2008). However, none of this literature accounts for fetal psychotropic exposure and much cannot account for unmeasured family influences and counfounders.

Mood stabilizer studies

Nearly all studies concern mothers with epilepsy rather than mothers with psychotic or other severe behavioural disorder. In the UK, sodium valproate is licensed for treatment of acute mania; carbamazepine for prophylaxis of bipolar recurrence unresponsive to lithium; and lamotrigine for prevention of bipolar depression. These drugs are known collectively as mood stabilizers. They are now more commonly prescribed for bipolar disorder than antipsychotic drugs (Anderson *et al.* 2003; Baldessarini *et al.* 2007). Although severe affective disorders are more common than epilepsy in women of childbearing age, there is an almost complete absence of research on their reproductive safety in psychosis.

Congenital Malformations

Early studies in women with epilepsy (WWE) indicated that antiepileptic/mood stabilizer monotherapies are associated with risk of major congenital malformations; about 2–3 fold above population rates; this excess is not explained by seizure activity (Fried *et al.* 2004). Meador *et al.* (2009) conducted a systematic review of all cohort or pregnancy registry studies with more than 100 pregnancy outcomes of treated WWE and healthy control subjects. This included a recent Swedish study using the Swedish Medical Birth Registry (Wide *et al.* 2004). The incidence of births with congenital malformations in WWE after any antiepileptic exposure was significantly higher than in the controls (7.08% vs 2.28%) as was the incidence of perinatal deaths (1.30% vs 0.7 %). The incidence of congenital anomalies was highest for polytherapy (16.78%). In almost every category, more defects were detected in babies born to WWE than in babies born to those without epilepsy. However, the differences were only statistically significant for malformations of the ear/neck/face, cleft lip, and spina bifida. Antiepileptic drug monotherapy with the highest congenital malformation rate is valproate (10.73%), significantly different from the population (3.27%), and other monotherapies. Monotherapy with carbamazepine and lamotrigine did not significantly raise risk. However, there is no information available on the number of therapeutic abortions and all these figures derive from samples of WWE rather than from women with schizophrenia-like illness or bipolar disorder. In treated bipolar women, Bodén *et al.* (2012b) report 3.4% incidence of congenital malformations (mainly talipes/'clubfoot'), compared with 1.9% in untreated bipolar women and 2.0% in the well population control. However, even in this large population cohort, numbers were too small (n=12) to generate robust estimates Given the excess malformation rate in mentally ill women (Webb *et al.* 2008), prospective population studies are needed to disentangle medication effects from illness effects, particularly with the increasing use of mood stabilizers in women with psychosis. Added to this, most treated women receive a combination of mood stabiliser as well as an antipsychotic agent.

Maternal and pregnancy outcomes

Almost all the literature considering risk associated with intrauterine exposure to antiepileptics has focused on incidence of malformations. However, some adverse pregnancy outcomes are reported, including an excess risk of lower birth weight, birth length, and head circumference (HC), but there was no effect on gestational age, compared to newborns of women without epilepsy (Hvas *et al.* 2000) . These authors also found that none of these adverse effects was present in cases of untreated maternal epilepsy. Other studies have also reported a decrease in body dimensions, especially reduced HC, after antiepileptic exposure in utero, where polytherapy shows stronger growth reduction than monotherapy (Bertillini *et al.* 1987; Hiilesmaa *et al.* 1981; Wide *et al.* 2000). Studies all consist exclusively of mothers with epilepsy. Recently, Bodén *et al.* (2012b) report population data finding that infants of women with bipolar disorder had increased risks of prematurity, irrespective of whether the mother had received mood stabilisers. Furthermore, in treated bipolar women, risk of small for gestational age infants for weight, length, or head circumference was not significantly increased. Untreated women had an increased risk of having a symmetrically small for gestational age infant for both weight and length, but the estimate was attenuated and became imprecise after adjusting for confounding. There was an increased risk of microcephaly and neonatal hypoglycaemia, however, which was materially unchanged after adjustments. There was no significantly increased risk in treated women which may be related to the emerging reports that psychotropic drugs can increase fetal growth (Boden *et al.* 2012a).

Although fertility is reduced in bipolar disorder, bipolar women who become pregnant will do so while taking medication and most will not plan pregnancy. Therefore, women and fetuses may be exposed to medication in early pregnancy. Viguera *et al.* (2002) reported that abrupt withdrawal of medication in women with bipolar disorder was associated with unplanned pregnancies. In this small, but well designed study, they also looked at rates of relapse and time to relapse of illness. Among women who discontinued mood stabilizer treatment, risk of relapse was twice that of women who continued medication. Abrupt discontinuation was also associated with a much shorter time to relapse.

Developmental outcomes

Banach *et al.* (2010) conducted meta-analysis of 7 studies assessing intellectual development of children whose mothers were treated with antiepileptics in pregnancy. In total, 67 children were exposed to valproate and 151 to carbamazepine. There were 494 unexposed children born to healthy women or WWE. In the valproate group, verbal, performance and full scale IQ (FIQ) were significantly lower than controls; results were less clear for carbamazepine. Evidence for a differential effect of antiepileptics on intellectual development comes from the 'NEAD' (neurodevelopmental effects of antiepileptic drugs) study (Meador *et al.* 2009). This prospective study included exposure to monotherapy with carbamazepine: $n = 92$; lamotrigine: $n = 99$; phenytoin: $n = 52$; valproate: $n = 60$. Children exposed to valproate had significantly lower IQs (92) at age 3 than the children exposed to one of the other antiepileptic drugs (carbamazepine 98; lamotrigine 101; and phenytoin 99), whereas IQ scores did not differ significantly among children exposed to the other three antiepileptics (Meador *et al.* 2009). Other variables independently predicting child IQ were maternal IQ, maternal age, dose of antiepileptic, gestational age and maternal preconception use of folate. In a study subgroup cognitive fluency and originality was examined in relation to antiepileptic monotherapy at 4 years (McVearry *et al.* 2009). Children with fetal exposure to valproate had significantly lower performance scores in both measures compared to children exposed to carbamazepine and lamotrigine. These effects were independent of dose, maternal seizure type, maternal IQ, pregnancy risk factors, folate regimen, exposure to an antiepileptic by breastfeeding, the child's IQ, or gender. The strengths of the NEAD study are its prospective design and careful analysis of confounding factors. Although it is the largest prospective study of neurobehavioural toxicity to date, numbers of children exposed to each drug are small and all mothers are WWE. Studies in mental illness are needed to verify findings for valproate and delineate patterns of cognitive deficit. Evidence of the effects of carbamazepine or lamotrigine on intellectual development is also needed for mentally ill mothers.

Outstanding problems with the evidence base

The 'cohort effect'

Many studies quoted above are now relatively old. For a number of important reasons, the applicability of evidence gathered over a decade ago to a contemporary population is questionable.

Even the better population database studies relied on to some extent on midwife reporting. Thus, in the largest Swedish sample (Reis and Kallen 2008), rather low psychosis prevalences (<1 in 1,000) are reported in cohorts; this is likely due to lack of midwife awareness about psychosis. More modern Swedish data (1994–2013) reports somewhat higher prevalences (i.e. >1 in 1,000) (Personal communication).

Early studies are unable to examine risk from atypical drugs: either they were not on the market, the numbers of women prescribed were too small, the indications for drugs have changed through marketing by the pharmaceutical industry, or there have been changes in clinical practice as a result of marketing. Similarly, some outcomes of interest that occur in the general population may be affected by change in clinical practice over time, such as reducing rates of stillbirth or prematurity.

Perhaps of even greater relevance is that, in modern UK and US populations, women becoming pregnant on psychotropics today may be more likely to be obese (Barnes 2008; Bodén *et al.* 2012a), and to smoke, than in older samples and both maternal smoking and obesity independently increase risks of poor maternal and fetal outcomes.

Illness vs medication

In all studies (except Lin *et al.* 2010) analysing effects of maternal antipsychotic exposure, presence of either maternal or paternal mental disorder is not accounted for. This is important because studies which aim specifically to assess outcomes for children born to ill parents consistently demonstrate a significant relationship between maternal (and in some cases paternal) psychotic disorder and adverse pregnancy outcome (see Abel and Morgan 2011; McCabe *et al.* 2007). Thus, mothers with schizophrenia or bipolar are more likely than control mothers to have children with congenital malformations (Webb *et al.* 2008; Boden *et al.* 2012b). Stillbirth and neonatal death, low birthweight, and prematurity, are also all reported as more common in offspring of mothers with schizophrenia and bipolar disorder (Webb *et al.* 2008; McCabe *et al.* 2007). Heavy smoking is common among people with schizophrenia and bipolar disorder (Henriksson *et al.* 2005) and contributes to obstetric complications. Therefore, studies of maternal psychotropic exposure on pregnancy outcome based on patients with diverse types of mental disorders or other chronic disorders may confound findings. Many lifestyle factors associated with psychoses (e.g. smoking, substance misuse, poor nutrition, poor antenatal attendance) are also independent risk factors for many of the outcomes of interest e.g. congenital malformation, prematurity, small and large for gestational age. Lin *et al.* (2010) and Boden *et al.* (2012b) are the only studies to compare unexposed ill women, with unexposed well women. Unfortunately, Lin *et al.* (2010) used women with a diagnosis of schizophrenia who were not exposed to antipsychotics as the control group against which they calculated ORs for women exposed to typical and atypical agents, and well unexposed women in the general population. This meant that while it provided the excess risk of medication over and above illness alone, confounding by indication means that the ill unexposed women may have been a less unwell group with less inherent risk than the ill exposed group.

Adherence to medication

Adherence to medication is clearly important to assess when collecting these data, however, may be a particular problem in mental health settings where patients often lack insight into the need for treatment, especially when ill. Moreover, if a woman discovers she is pregnant, she may be especially likely to discontinue medication and not tell her clinician if she has a serious mental illness for fear of admission. However, little, if any of the previous literature on psychotropic exposure has assessed this. In the main, this is because datasets large enough to provide reliable information on exposure and outcomes do not contain the detailed information necessary to measure adherence. Ascertaining rates of refilling prescriptions is an accepted method of measuring adherence to medication (Osterberg and Blaschke 2005). Uniquely, the Swedish Prescribed Drug Register (Bodén *et al.* 2012a and b) contains information on all prescription fills in Sweden, including dispensed drugs using Anatomical Therapeutic Chemical codes (ATC), amount, formulation and date of prescribing and dispensing since July 1994. The Swedish Medical Birth Register contains data on almost all births in Sweden from 1973 and from the first, and all subsequent antenatal visits, information is obtained by midwives regarding current medication. Linking such data sources, it would be possible to validate self-reported medication use at antenatal visits with actual filling of prescription during pregnancy in order to examine adherence to medication.

Antipsychotic groupings

Prior literature confines analyses to exposure to all/any antipsychotics or, if numbers allow, to groupings of atypical and typical drugs. Because typical drugs differ in many properties, including efficacy, side effects and pharmacology, they do not form a homogeneous class; neither do 'atypicals' (Leucht *et al.* 2009). Heterogeneity in effect and side effects suggests that such 'improper grouping' may create confusion in an exposure. Although we shall adhere to the Commissioning Board's request to examine drug groupings as typical and atypical antipsychotics, we shall also examine individual drug differences or groups of drugs by side-effect profile. For example, if we look at susceptibility to metabolic side effects—e.g. maternal outcome weight gain, gestational hypertension, and gestational diabetes, low-potency typical drugs should be grouped with the -pines; thus, the 'typical' chlorpromazine might be considered in a grouping with atypical olanzapine and clozapine.

Potential confounders

A confounder is a risk variable associated (not necessarily equally) with both risk of exposure and of outcome. A good example in this context might be smoking acting as a potential confounder of the association between maternal mental illness and poor fetal growth. Mothers with mental illness are more likely to smoke and to have children with poor fetal growth; and smoking is more likely in mothers with mental illness and in offspring of women who smoke.

Similarly, compared with well unexposed women, a higher proportion of women who use psychotropics during pregnancy are immigrants, are older, not living with the father of the child, have more than one child and are smokers, with a high body mass index (Bodén et al. 2012a; Nilsson et al. 2002). Early studies tended to lack information on relevant maternal characteristics related to pregnancy outcome, such as smoking, alcohol, and other substance use, pre-pregnancy body mass index, and nutritional status. Only three population-based datasets (Medical Births & Prescribed Drug Registers in Sweden (Bodén et al. 2012a and b; Reis and Kallen 2008, 2010; Wide et al. 2004) and Taiwanese dataset (Lin et al. 2010)) have accounted for some of these potential confounders. Most studies, e.g. UK's NTIS dataset (Newham et al. 2008), do not have reliable recording of potential confounds. Moreover, because of limited sample sizes or statistical complexity, simultaneous administration of other agents is not generally considered. In addition, information on over-the-counter drug use has not been available.

Missing information

No studies have been able to look separately at clozapine or the antipsychotics now most commonly prescribed in the UK (olanzapine, quetiapine, risperidone) (HSCIC 2010; Downey et al. 2012). This is important because recent examination of placental passage of antipsychotics (umbilical cord: maternal plasma concentration) suggests olanzapine has highest passage (mean 72.1%, SD = 42.0%) and, also, higher rates of low birth weight and/ or perinatal complications than other antipsychotics (Newport et al. 2007). This means that, in an ideal world, we should be able to look at exposure to individual drugs. In some cases, it is also important to have enough power to take account of mono- versus polytherapy as this is much more likely to reflect the current clinical prescribing scenario (HSCIC 2010; Downey et al. 2012). Finally, no studies to date have examined quality of life in women taking psychotropic drugs during pregnancy. This is likely to be important for understanding and predicting drug adherence, or time to, or risk of, relapse in mothers with serious mental disorder who discontinue antipsychotic medication in pregnancy.

Conclusions

To fulfil the current research gap and support better, more consistent clinical decision making, future research is required using large enough databases with prospectively collected high quality clinical information in an unbiased and representative population. Such samples with small amounts of missing data on key variables, do exist in Scandinavian countries, Taiwan and Western Australia. However, these countries do not represent the majority of women likely to be exposed during pregnancy now or in the future. For the uniquely powered datasets required to assess rarer exposures and outcomes, global cooperation and administrative efforts are urgently needed. Such initiatives would combine disparate population datasets from developed and non developed countries on key common variable sets. This would allow proper assessment of factors such as ethnicity and migration alongside the ability to assess social and other non-biological factors in risk generation especially for the more common sets of pregnancy-related outcomes. In addition, creating a cohort that combined datasets may mean that future studies are able to take account of key confounders. Using sibling and intergenerational analyses, studies would also be able to account for other non-measured potential confounds. This is an ambitious task, but one increasingly relevant and increasingly urgent to growing numbers of exposed fetuses in the changing landscape of pregnancy care. In the meantime, women with serious mental illness appear at increased risk of a number of poor obstetric outcomes.

Clear local and national policies promoting pregnancy planning in women living with such illnesses and of reproductive age are required. Acknowledgement of the importance of this aspect of care in serious mental illness has been lacking; it is now time for multi-disciplinary teams to implement reproductive care planning for women with severe mental illness.

What should future studies do?

- ◆ Consider combining datasets on common exposure and outcome variables (diagnoses, maternal characteristics, common obstetric outcomes) to create cohorts large enough and representative enough of modern populations of exposed women.

- ◆ Develop cohorts powered to analyse exposures by trimester of pregnancy and for examination of individual drugs, as well as mono- versus polytherapy.

- ◆ Enable estimates to be adjusted for important potential confounders.

- ◆ Examine risk using both well and ill unexposed women as comparators

- ◆ Link widely available information obtained by midwives and self-reported medication use from antenatal visits with actual filling of prescription during pregnancy to examine adherence.

- ◆ Examine groups of drugs by side-effect profile rather than class of agent. For example, susceptibility to metabolic side effects, e.g. maternal weight gain, gestational hypertension and gestational diabetes, and low-potency FGA/typicals should be grouped with -pines; thus, e.g. the 'typical' chlorpromazine should be grouped with 'atypical' olanzapine and clozapine.

- ◆ Compare outcomes between siblings and generations can help account for other non-measured confounds or family-wide effects.

References

Abel, K.M. and Morgan, V.A. (2011). Mental illness, women, mothers, & their children. In Textbook in Psychiatric Epidemiology, Ming T. Tsuang, Mauricio Tohen, Peter B. Jones editors. Oxford, Wiley-Blackwell, UK pp. 483–514.

Altshuler, L.L., Cohen, L., Szuba, M.P., et al. (1996). Pharmacological management of psychiatric illness during pregnancy: dilemmas and guidelines. American Journal of Psychiatry **153**: 592–606.

Anderson, I.M., Haddad, P.M., and Chaudhry, I. (2004). Changes in pharmacological treatment for bipolar disorder over time in Manchester: a comparison with Lloyd et al. 2003. Journal of Psychopharmacology **18**: 441–4.

Baldessarini, R.J., Leahy, L., Arcona, S., *et al.* (2007). Patterns of psychotropic drug prescription for U.S. patients with diagnoses of bipolar disorders. Psychiatric Services **58**: 85–91.

Banach, R., Boskovic, R., Einarson, T., and Koren, G. (2010). Long-term developmental outcome of children of women with epilepsy, unexposed or exposed prenatally to antiepileptic drugs: a meta-analysis of cohort studies. Drug Safety **33**: 73–9.

Barnes, T.R. (2008). Evidence-based guidelines for the pharmacological treatment of schizophrenia: recommendations from the British Association for Psychopharmacology. Available from www.bap.org.uk/pdfs/Schizophrenia_Consensus_Guideline_ Document.pdf (accessed 30 August 2013).

Bertollini, R., Kallen, B., Mastroiacovo, P., and Robert, E. (1987). Anticonvulsant drugs in monotherapy effect on the fetus. European Journal of Epidemiology **3**: 164–71.

Bodén, R., Lundgren, M., Brandt, L., Reutfors, J., and Kieler, H. (2012a). Antipsychotics during pregnancy-relation to fetal and maternal metabolic effects. JAMA Psychiatry **69**(7): 715–21.

Bodén, R., Lundgren, M., Brandt, L., Reutfors, J., Andersen, M., Kieler, H. (2012b). Risks of adverse pregnancy and birth outcomes in women treated or not treated with mood stabilisers for bipolar disorder: population based cohort study. BMJ 2012 345–350.

Buchanan, R.W. *et al.* (2009). The 2009 schizophrenia PORT psychopharmacological treatment recommendations and summary statements. Schizophrenia Bulletin **36**(1): 71–93.

Downey, D., Hayhrust, K.P., Lewis, S.W., Brown, P. (2012). *SiGMA - Schizophrenia in Greater Manchester: Audit. Report 2011–2012.* Manchester: Greater Manchester Public Health Practice Unit.

EUROCAT (2012). EUROCAT classification of congenital malformations. Available from www.eurocat-network.eu/content/EUROCAT-Guide-1.3-Chapter-3.3-Jan2012.pdf (accessed 30 August 2013).

Fried, S., Kozer, E., Nulman, I., Einarson, T.R., and Koren, G. (2004). Malformation rates in children of women with untreated epilepsy: a meta-analysis. Drug Safety **27**: 197–202.

Garbis, H., *et al.* (2005). Safety of haloperidol and penfluridol in pregnancy: a multicenter, prospective, controlled study. Journal of Clinical Psychiatry **66**: 317–22.

Gentile, S. (2010). Antipsychotic therapy during early and late pregnancy. A systematic review. Schizophrenia Bulletin **36**: 518–44.

Henriksson, K.M., Larmark, G., and McNeil, T.F. (2005). Smoking in pregnancy and its correlates among women with a history of schizophrenia or affective psychosis. Schizophrenia Research **81**: 121–3.

Hiilesmaa, V.K., Teramo, K., Granstrom, M.L., and Bardy, A.H. (1981). Fetal head growth retardation associated with maternal antiepileptic drugs. Lancet **2**: 165–7.

Howard, L.M. (2005). Fertility & pregnancy in women with psychotic disorders. European Journal of Obstetetrics and Gynecology: Reproductive Biology; **119**: 3–10.

HSCIC (Health and Social Care NHS Information Centre), Prescription Cost Analysis—England (2010). Available from http://www.hscic.gov.uk/pubs/prescostanalysis2010 (accessed 24 September 2013).

Hvas, C.L., Henriksen, T.B., Ostergaard, J.R., and Dam, M. (2000). Epilepsy and pregnancy: effect of antiepileptic drugs and lifestyle on birthweight. British Journal of Obstetrics and Gynaecology **107**: 896–902.

Leucht, S., Corves, C., Arbter, D., *et al.* (2009). Second-generation versus first-generation antipsychotic drugs for schizophrenia: a meta-analysis. Lancet **373**: 31–41.

Lin, H.C., Chen, I.J., Chen, Y.H., Lee, H.C., and Wu, F.J. (2010). Maternal schizophrenia and pregnancy outcome: does the use of antipsychotics make a difference? Schizophrenia Research **116**: 55–60.

MacCabe, J.H. *et al.* (2007). Adverse pregnancy outcomes in mothers with affective psychosis. Bipolar Disorders **9**: 305–309.

McKenna, K. *et al.* (2005). Pregnancy outcome of women using atypical antipsychotic drugs: a prospective comparative study. Journal of Clinical Psychiatry **66**: 444–9.

McVearry, K.M., Gaillard, W.D., VanMeter, J., and Meador, K.J. (2009). A prospective study of cognitive fluency and originality in children exposed in utero to carbamazepine, lamotrigine, or valproate monotherapy. Epilepsy and Behaviour **16**: 609–616.

Meador, K.J., Baker, G.A., Browning, N., *et al*. (2009). Cognitive function at 3 years of age after fetal exposure to antiepileptic drugs. New England Journal of Medicine **360**: 1597–605.

National Institute for Health and Care Excellence NICE (2007). Antenatal and Postnatal Mental Health. Clinical Guideline 45. Available from www.nice.org.uk/CG045 (accessed 30 August 2013).

Newham, J.J. *et al*. (2008). Birth weight of infants after maternal exposure to typical and atypical antipsychotics: prospective comparison study. British Journal of Psychiatry **192**: 333–7.

Newport, D.J. *et al*. (2007). Atypical antipsychotic administration during late pregnancy: placental passage and obstetrical outcomes. American Journal of Psychiatry **164**: 1214–20.

Niemi, L.T., Suvisaari, J.M., Tuulio-Henriksson, A., and Lönnqvist, J.K., *et al*. (2003). Childhood developmental abnormalities in schizophrenia: Evidence from high-risk studies. Schizophrenia Research **60**: 239–58.

Nilsson, E., *et al*. (2002). Women with schizophrenia: pregnancy outcome and infant death among their offspring. Schizophrenia Research **58**: 221–9.

Office for National Statistics (2008). ONS Congenital Anomaly Statistics, England and Wales (Series MB3), No. 23, 2008 Available from http://www.ons.gov.uk/ons/rel/vsob1/congenital-anomaly-statistics–england-and-wales–series-mb3-/no–23–2008/index.html (accessed 30 August 2013).

Osterberg, L. and Blaschke, T. (2005). Adherence to medication. New England Journal of Medicine **353**: 487–97.

Reis, M. and Kallen, B. (2008). Maternal use of antipsychotics in early pregnancy and delivery outcome. Journal of Clinical Psychopharmacology **28**: 279–88.

Reis, M. and Kallen, B. (2010). Delivery outcome after maternal use of antidepressant drugs in pregnancy: an update using Swedish data. Psychological Medicine **40**: 1723–33.

Sameroff, A., Seifer, R., Zax, M., and Barocas, R. (1987). Early indicators of developmental risk: Rochester longitudinal study. Schizophrenia Bulletin **13**: 383–94.

Sobel, D.E. (1961). Infant mortality and malformations in children of schizophrenic women. Psychiatric Quarterly **35**: 60–4

Thiels, C. (1987). Pharmacotherapy of psychiatric disorder in pregnancy & during breastfeeding: a review. Pharmacopsychology **20**: 133–46.

Tomson, T., Battino, D., Bonizzoni, E., Craig, J., and EURAP (2011). Dose-dependent risk of malformations with antiepileptic drugs: an analysis of data from the EURAP epilepsy and pregnancy registry. Lancet **1474–4422**: 70107–7.

Viguera, A.C., Cohen, L.S., Bouffard, S., Whitfield, T.H., and Baldessarini, R. (2002). Reproductive decisions by women with bipolar disorder after prepregnancy psychiatric consultation. American Journal of Psychiatry **159**: 2102–4.

Wan, M.W., Abel, K.M., and Green, J. (2008). Transmission of risk to children from mothers with schizophrenia: A developmental psychopathology model. Clinical Psychology Reviews **28**: 613–37.

Webb, R.T. Howard, L., and Abel, K.M. (2004). Antipsychotic drugs for non-affective psychosis during pregnancy & postpartum. CD004411.

Webb, R.T. *et al*. (2008). Parental mental illness and fatal birth defects in a national cohort. Psychological Medicine **38**: 1495–503.

Wide, K., Winbladh, B., Tomson, T., and Kallen, B. (2000). Body dimensions of infants exposed to antiepileptic drugs in utero: observations spanning 25 years. Epilepsia **41**: 854–61.

Wide, K., Winbladh, B., and Källen, B. (2004). Major malformations in infants exposed to antiepileptic drugs in utero, with emphasis on carbamazepine and valproic acid: a nation-wide, population-based register study. Acta Paediatrica **93**: 174–6.

Section 2

Perinatal psychiatry across the world

Chapter 6

Perinatal depression across the world
Prevalence, risk factors, and detection in primary care

Michael W. O'Hara and Lisa S. Segre

Dedication

This chapter, like the entire volume, is dedicated to the memory of Channi Kumar. I first met Channi in August 1984 in Oakland, California, at the biennial meeting of the Marcé Society, hosted by James Hamilton. I had already been impressed by Channi's research but knew him only through his published work. In person, the man did not disappoint. He was elegant and kind, a man who treated everyone with respect. Over the years, my affection and admiration for Channi grew through many stimulating discussions and delightful social occasions. Even our last series of meetings focused on a new, exciting initiative of Channi's: the 'Transcultural Study', which he envisioned as a way to harmonize the detection, assessment, and treatment of perinatal mood disorders, across western Europe and even the United States, Asia, and Africa. Through experiences like these, Channi made my life richer, personally and professionally; and I greatly miss him as a mentor and a friend, and feel privileged, along with my colleague Lisa Segre, to contribute a small piece to honor this great psychiatrist and humanitarian.
Michael W. O'Hara

Introduction

Perinatal depression is a significant mental health problem that afflicts women around the world at a time when they are highly vulnerable—pregnant or managing a new infant. In one form or another, perinatal depression has been recognized for thousands of years; however, only in the past 50 years has there been a sustained focus on the non-psychotic mental illnesses experienced by some during pregnancy and the postpartum period. The literature of the 1960s contains only a few papers with the words postpartum depression, postnatal depression, or perinatal depression. Not until the 1970s did these terms come into common use. Indeed, a search for at least one of these terms on the PsycNET database (from entries catalogued between 1884 and 9 September 2012) revealed the vast majority (2,743 or 75%) of 3,651 papers, books, and book chapters on perinatal depression were published after 2000. These findings show how work in the field of perinatal mental illness has expanded exponentially.

'What is so special about postpartum depression?' This was a question one of us (M.W.O.) posed in one of our many discussions about perinatal depression. We wondered what distinguished perinatal depression from depression in general, a problem common among women from menarche until menopause; indeed, the risk factors, symptoms, and treatment for postpartum depression seemed not much different than for other depressions. Although in recent years, these facts have changed, to some degree, we still ask ourselves what is special about post partum depression.

Why do we care?

Quite simply, we care about perinatal depression because women and their children suffer. This suffering has an impact on the fetus during pregnancy and on the infant after delivery. This suffering impairs a woman's functioning in a variety of important life domains, particularly in family life and parenting, so it is imperative to determine the best opportunities for prevention, early intervention, and tertiary care. This is often not as straightforward as it seems it should be. Clearly, the perinatal period offers excellent opportunities for medical intervention, because women frequently visit the health system during pregnancy and with their child; still, women find choosing treatment complicated by concerns about their children. Women worry that psychotropic medication could harm their fetus or breastfeeding infant, or that too much time and expense would be diverted to psychological interventions (if these treatment options are even offered).

However, with the expansion of research, new insights from neuroscience are providing clues as to a biological basis (in addition to the well-known psychological factors) for some perinatal depressions. For all of these reasons, clinicians and researchers alike find the area of perinatal mental illness to be compelling.

Perinatal depression and its bounds

The perinatal period includes pregnancy and the postpartum period. The bounds of pregnancy are obvious, but not so regarding what is considered the 'postpartum or postnatal period.' For example, the DSM-5 (American Psychiatric Association 2013) assigns 'with peripartum onset' to episodes of depression if onset of mood symptoms occurs during pregnancy or in the 4 weeks following delivery. The ICD-10 (<http://apps.who.int/classifications/icd10/browse/2010/en#/F53.9>) uses a 6-week timeframe for 'mental and behavioural disorders associated with the puerperium, not elsewhere classified.' Despite any official diagnostic nomenclatures, studies have included women up to one year after delivery. In sum, what constitutes the extent of the postpartum period is unsettled and will probably vary depending upon the nature of the research or clinical questions: Biologically oriented studies will likely use a short timeframe; whereas, social and clinical studies will probably use a longer one.

The definition of perinatal depression also varies. For example, some clinicians and investigators use the DSM or ICD definitions, which impose relatively stringent standards as to what is considered a mental disorder. Others use self-report symptom scales, such as the Edinburgh Postnatal Depression Scale (Cox *et al.* 1987), to index severity of depressive symptoms. Such questionnaires for new mothers, and their sliding-scale answer formats, demonstrate that the severity of postpartum depression can vary from mild to severe. Threshold scores then establish that a woman might require intervention. In some settings, women who exceed a specified threshold are interviewed to diagnose depression; while in others a self-report measure that shows the threshold is exceeded suffices to prompt referral for treatment.

Another facet of the definition and diagnosis arises given what is known about the comorbidity of depression and anxiety. It is likely that postpartum depressed women will also have an anxiety disorder or be experiencing significant symptoms of anxiety. In fact, in a recent review Fisher *et al.* (2012) entitled their article 'Prevalence and determinants of common perinatal mental disorders . . .' thereby blurring the distinction between depression and anxiety. Until now anxiety disorders have been relatively neglected, both as stand-alone disorders or comorbid with depression; thus the definition of postpartum depression is evolving.

It is well established that depression is common among women. A recent epidemiologic study of adult women reported the prevalence rate of major depression during a one-year period is 10.1% (Eaton *et al.* 2012), revealing that many women enter pregnancy while experiencing a major depression. In addition, many are in any variety of subthreshold depressions, often with a comorbid anxiety disorder. Others develop a new-onset depression during pregnancy that may end during pregnancy or carry over to the postpartum period. Of course, new episodes may develop in the postpartum period. The reality is that what is classified as perinatal depression includes recurrent depressions unrelated to childbearing, depressions that have some aetiological link to the biology of pregnancy or parturition, and depressions with features of both. Accordingly, it is not clear whether making a distinction between 'true' postpartum depression and 'coincidental' postpartum depression has any practical significance with respect to detection, prevention, and treatment.

The prevalence of perinatal depression

Pregnancy

The prevalence of perinatal depression has been the focus of a number of literature reviews (O'Hara and Swain 1996; Bennett *et al.* 2004; Gavin *et al.* 2005; Fisher *et al.* 2012). Using interview and self-report data Bennett *et al.* (2004) reported that the rates of perinatal depression were 7.4% in the 1st trimester, 12.8% in the 2nd trimester, and 12% in the 3rd trimester; for lower socioeconomic status women the rate was even higher, at about 36% across pregnancy (all three trimesters). Reporting only on studies using clinical assessment during pregnancy (i.e. using diagnostic criteria), Gavin *et al.* (2005) reported a point prevalence range of 8.5% to 11% for major and minor depression, respectively (range 3.1% to 4.9% major depression only). In a recent review of studies of women in low- and lower-middle-income countries, Fisher *et al.* (2012) reported a weighted-mean prevalence (based on self-report or clinical interview) of 15.9% (95% confidence interval (CI):15.0–16.8%); when the estimate was limited to data drawn from studies that used diagnostic assessments, the prevalence was 21.7% (95% CI: 19.8–23.7). These findings converge to suggest that depression during pregnancy is common both in the developed and the developing world.

The postpartum period

Studies on the prevalence of postpartum depression were first reviewed in an article published in 1996 (O'Hara & Swain 1996); this review included articles based both on self-report and clinical interview, and reported an overall prevalence of 13%. Gavin *et al.* (2005) reported a point prevalence range of 6.5% to 12.9% (1.0 to 5.9% major depression only) over the first year postpartum; period prevalence, for the first 3 months postpartum, was reported to be 19.2% (7.1% major depression only). The authors also argued that, in the studies they reviewed, the great majority of postpartum depressions were new onset after delivery. In lower and lower-middle income countries the prevalence of postpartum depression, based on pooled estimates across all studies, was 19.8% (95% CI: 19.2–20.6) (Fisher *et al.* 2012). If estimates were limited to studies that used diagnostic assessments, then the prevalence was 16.1% (95% CI: 14.6–17.6).

The take-away message is that perinatal depression is common, particularly during pregnancy and through the first 3 months after delivery. Nevertheless, very few studies of prevalence have included large representative samples. In developed countries, studies often used convenience samples, based on the local setting of the investigator; these might range from a college town in the State of Iowa to a low-income community in south London. Studies in developing countries obtained samples from a range of settings, including rural communities with little modern health care, as well as provincial centers where clinical and research resources are available (Fisher *et al.* 2012). Still, in both developed and developing countries, large scale, epidemiologic studies designed to specifically address postpartum depression have never been done. When they are, they must include representative samples.

Risk factors for postpartum depression

Many hundreds (perhaps thousands) of studies have examined risk factors for postpartum depression. Four major meta-analyses summarized this literature, three for research conducted primarily in developed countries (Beck 2001; O'Hara and Swain 1996; Robertson *et al.* 2004) and one for research conducted in developing countries (Fisher *et al.* 2012). The meta-analyses of studies in developed countries converge on three conclusions: Risk factors with medium to large effect sizes include history of depression, depression or anxiety during pregnancy, negative life events, and lack of social support. Risk factors that have medium effect sizes include marital adjustment and neuroticism. Risk factors that have small effects include socioeconomic status and obstetric complications. For women in developing countries the most important risk factors would appear to be past history of mental illness or mental illness during pregnancy, being unmarried, polygamous marriage, adverse reproductive outcomes, grief over death of an infant, poor family and social relationships, poor-quality relationship with the partner, and low socioeconomic status (Fisher *et al.* 2012). Many of the risk factors for depression in developed and developing country are similar, such as those relating to history of psychopathology, poor social support, partner violence and lack of access to economic resources. Others are more idiosyncratic to specific cultural settings (e.g. polygamous marriage, gender preference). In drawing conclusions from these reviews, it is important to consider that specific features of a study can greatly influence the variables that emerge as risk factors. For example, if a study sample is homogeneous (e.g. with respect to status, age, ethnicity, or parity), then it cannot capture the full spectrum of risk factors, no matter how great the associated risk.

The following composite of a woman describes the prototypical pregnant woman from a developed country at risk for postpartum depression. She most likely occupies a lower social stratum; however, women representing middle and upper social strata will also be abundantly represented. She is very likely to have experienced life stressors during pregnancy and may have had a more difficult than normal pregnancy or delivery. She will be experiencing marital difficulties and experience her partner as providing little in the way of social support. Compounding the life stress she is experiencing and her poor marital relationship will be her perception that others in her social network are not particularly supportive of her. Finally, her history will show evidence of psychopathology, in most cases major depression or dysthymia; and she will show evidence of being at least mildly depressed and anxious, and excessively worried.

Risk factors for postpartum depression provide a window into targets for preventive and secondary interventions. Certainly, the major identifiable risk factor for postpartum depression is depression during pregnancy or emerging depression symptoms during the early postpartum period. It is to this discussion of detection, treatment, and follow-up in primary that we now turn.

Detection of depression in primary care: public policy

The United States Preventive Services Task Force (USPSTF) demonstrated that screening for depression in the general population improves patient outcome only if screening results are *coordinated with follow-up and treatment*, prompting them to issue the following recommendation: screen 'adults for depression when staff-assisted depression-care supports are in place to assure accurate diagnosis, effective treatment, and follow-up (USPSTF 2009, p. 784).' While postpartum women were included in this general recommendation, other recommendations specific to depression screening in perinatal women have not yet been issued in the US. In what might be characterized as a 'soft' recommendation, the Committee on Obstetric Practice of the American Congress of Obstetricians and Gynecologists (ACOG) suggested such practice should be strongly *considered*; but concluded that currently the empirical evidence is insufficient to support a firm recommendation for universal antepartum or postpartum screening (Committee on Obstetric Practice 2010). Concurrent with this conclusion, the president of the ACOG designated perinatal depression as a presidential initiative. This high-profile designation highlighted the importance of three areas of future research: (1) determining the true prevalence and incidence of postpartum depression, by setting uniform definitions of the disorder in research; (2) developing precise screening tools, and (3) developing evidence-based guidelines for screening (Joseph 2009). Despite the somewhat conservative stance of ACOG, several high-profile health organizations have issued position statements supporting the screening of perinatal women, including the National Association of Pediatric Nurse Practitioners (2003), the American College of Nurse Midwives (2002), and the Association of Women's Health, Obstetric and Neonatal Nurses (2008).

In the UK, however, the National Institute for Health and Care Excellence (NICE 2007) issued recommendations for depression identification specifically for perinatal women. These guidelines advise practitioners (obstetricians, midwives, health visitors, and general practitioners) to ask women about their mental health at their first prenatal contact, as well as postnatally (usually 4 to 6 weeks and 3 to 4 months). Further, they recommend that healthcare professionals use two screening questions: (1) During the past month have you been bothered by feeling down, depressed, or hopeless? (2) During the past month have you been bothered by having little interest or pleasure in doing things? If the woman answers yes to either of these questions, the recommendation suggests follow-up with a third question: (3) Is this something for which you feel you need or want help? For women who respond in the affirmative to these questions, referrals are made for further evaluation for treatment.

Detecting depression in primary care: practical considerations

Although use of a tool can increase the chances of detecting depression, when the feasibility of screening in primary care is evaluated, the results regarding success are mixed. In the obstetric setting, screening rates with prenatal or postpartum patients ranged from 67% in an OB-GYN practice in an academic medical setting, to 100% in a large obstetric-care practice (Gordon *et al.* 2006; Rowan *et al.* 2012). In contrast, screening rates were found to vary widely in pediatric settings, when screening was done during well child visits (Olson *et al.* 2006; Sheeder *et al.* 2009). Finally, although depression screening on the maternity unit has been described in conference presentations (Brassil *et al.* 2011), we could locate no published evaluations of screening rates obtained in this key perinatal setting.

Key implementation steps

Little evidence is available on whether perinatal depression screening improves outcome. Nevertheless, screening is generally supported in many countries (but not all) as good clinical practice. In general, however, even evaluations that show it is generally feasible offer little detailed guidance on how to implement depression screening (Kemper *et al.* 2007).

Although, in theory, implementation seems to be a relatively straightforward task (e.g. select a depression screening tool and have staff administer it), in practice, the complexity of implementation has been duly noted: 'Its introduction into primary care is anything but simple. In its wake it carries widespread system change as well as a new philosophy' (Elliott 1994, p. 229). Even recommended procedures for implementing screening will be markedly influenced by local context and health system structures, so, depending on local health and social services, care pathways will differ around the world. Nevertheless, a few key programmatic elements always need to be in place to successfully implement depression screening, in any context. The purpose of this more pragmatically oriented section, therefore, is to summarize these elements.

Provider education

Ideal settings for implementing depression screening and referral are the primary care clinics serving perinatal women; however, these venues are not staffed with depression specialists. Nevertheless, nurses (Segre *et al.* 2010) and physicians (LaRocco-Cockburn *et al.* 2003; Olson *et al.* 2002) recognize screening for depression in new mothers as a legitimate part of their practice but often report that they do not feel educationally prepared to screen (Olson *et al.* 2002). Depression education can arm providers with the knowledge and confidence they need to implement a screening programme. This idea is highlighted by the finding that nurses were more likely to comply with a screening programme if they had been trained about perinatal depression and screening procedures (Massoudi *et al.* 2007).

In response to this educational need, several approaches to teaching health and social service staff about perinatal depression have been developed, including face-to-face group training (Segre *et al.* 2012a), web-based resources (Baker *et al.* 2009), one-to-one professional consultation (Segre *et al.* 2012b), and a train-the-trainer model (Segre *et al.* 2011). When deciding which educational format would be best for the venue under study, consideration should be given to which format is sustainable for educating new personnel.

Depression screening protocol

To implement perinatal depression screening the screening procedures must include key protocol elements:

Screening tool. Compared to informal clinical assessment, which often fails to detect depression in perinatal women, a depression screening tool increases the number of women who are identified as possibly depressed (Georgiopoulos *et al.* 2001). Additionally, a screening tool gives providers an easy way to invite women to discuss their emotional well-being. Two screening tools, commonly used in primary care settings are the Patient Health Questionnaire or PHQ-9 (Kroenke *et al.* 2001) and the two-question screen (Whooley *et al.* 1997). Two other tools were developed for and validated with perinatal women specifically: the Edinburgh Postnatal Depression Scale (EPDS; Cox *et al.* 1987) and the Postpartum Depression Screening Scale (PDSS; Beck and Gable 2000).

Cutoff score. Cutoff scores standardize the point where clinical action is taken. For example, in the case of the two-question screen, the cutoff that indicates a need for referral is set when two criteria are met: the positive endorsement of either loss of interest or sad mood *and* the patient indicating a desire to receive help. For any self-report screening tool, the cutoff scores should be based on tool-specific psychometric data showing the sensitivity and specificity of the tool *as well as the implementation context*. For example, the British validation studies of the EPDS designated the optimal cutoff score as 13 or above (Cox *et al.* 1987); however, numerous other cutoff scores, ranging from greater than 8 to greater than 14, have been used with this same tool (Matthey *et al.* 2006). Notably, however, not all of these cutoff scores were validated for use in clinical practice or research (Matthey *et al.* 2006).

Pragmatic considerations also may influence the choice of cutoff score. For example, in settings where women can be repeatedly screened (e.g. prenatal visits), a lower cutoff score might be adopted *with the proviso* that a lower score will prompt a repeat screening, with referral made only after a repeatedly elevated score. In contrast, in settings where women can only be screened once, a cutoff that is too low might overuse limited referral resources. Finally, in hospital settings where depression screening is conducted in multiple clinics, a hospital-wide cutoff score has many practical advantages and should be considered. In brief summary, the cutoff score should be tailored to each setting and depends on the joint consideration of psychometric data for the tool, the screening schedule, practices in other clinics, and the availability of services.

Screening schedule. A third key aspect of developing a depression screening protocol is specifying when and how frequently screening is implemented. While screening within the first 3 months of delivery seems warranted, epidemiological evidence does not indicate a particular time of increased risk, so does not guide us in choosing the best time(s) to screen (Gavin *et al.* 2005). Depressive symptoms in both pregnant and postpartum women, however, are known to be relatively common, which suggests screening could be conducted throughout this period. Therefore, the specification of when and how frequently to screen should be tailored to the specific service context. For example in an obstetric clinic, opportunities to screen are broadly defined by the pre- and postpartum obstetric visit schedule; thus, a major task in developing a screening schedule for this context would be to determine the frequency of the screenings. In contrast, the very short window of opportunity in the maternity unit setting predetermines both the timing and number of screens.

Referral sources

One of the most challenging parts of developing a perinatal depression screening protocol can be identifying referral sources. Yet, a referral system needs to be in place before screening commences; indeed, there is no point in identifying depressive symptoms if the woman cannot access effective interventions. Depending upon the severity of the depression, a woman may need antidepressant medication and care from a physician (perhaps her family doctor) or a psychiatrist. Alternatively, psychological care may be provided by a range of mental health professionals, including psychologists and social workers. It is very helpful if these professionals, physicians and non-physicians alike, have experience in treating perinatal depression and anxiety. (It is still true that many professionals minimize perinatal depression and provide inadequate care to depressed perinatal women.) These issues may also be complicated in cases in which women are unwilling or unable to access professional mental health care; here, alternative approaches must be considered.

For some women, providing an educational brochure may suffice (Heh and Fu 2003). In 2006, the US Health Resources and Services Administration (HRSA) made such an informational brochure widely available. This booklet, written for women, family, and friends, provides a complete and accurate description of perinatal depression in an easy-to-understand and visually appealing format. The information covered includes, the definition of perinatal depression, a description of the full range of perinatal mood disorders (blues, depression, and psychosis), the negative effects of depression, and an adapted checklist version of the EPDS. A range of treatment options are described, including recommending increased attention to self-care, support groups, and professional mental health treatment. This brochure is available in English and Spanish and can be obtained free of charge from HRSA (<http://mchb.hrsa.gov/pregnancyandbeyond/depression/index.html>).

Postpartum Support International (<http://www.postpartum.net/>), a non-profit organization addressing the needs of perinatal women with depression or anxiety symptoms, provides numerous, accessible, helpful options, including but not limited to a 'warm line' to which distressed new mothers can call for help, educational brochures, and DVDs, and the 'chat with an expert' on-line forum. A referral list might also include support groups or home-visiting services provided by organizations or programmes specifically serving perinatal women. Whatever the form of intervention, it is incumbent upon the primary care provider to follow up with women to ensure they are engaged in treatment and ask whether the treatment is ameliorating the depressive symptoms.

Hidden tasks

Finally, developing a screening protocol requires specifying a few additional procedures that do not fit neatly into the above categories. First, consideration should be given to identifying which staff will screen and whether that staff will also provide the referral. In many settings, the person who screens will likely also provide referrals. In some instances it might be more appropriate for a different staff member, who is more familiar with treatment resources, to offer referrals and link women to services directly .

Second, particular attention must be paid to any screening scale items assessing suicidal feelings. A number of decisions need to be made. For example, what score on the suicide item will be considered elevated? Recent evidence suggests that the 'yes, quite often' response on the suicide ideation item (#10) of the EPDS is associated with other indicators of suicidal risk (Howard *et al.* 2011). Once a woman is identified as at risk for suicide, what procedures should screeners follow to keep a woman safe? Some settings have suicide protocols already in place, while others will need to develop this before implementation.

Third, where will documenting information be stored? In adult clinic settings, the medical record is the likely place; however, here the question might be raised whether the entire

Table 6.1 Depression screening protocol development worksheet

---

Introducing and supervising screening programme

1. Who will propose the implementation of depression screening and what is his/her position?

2. Who will supervise the implementation of depression screening and what is his/her position?

Administration procedures

1. Which programme staff will provide maternal depression screening?

2. What depression screening tool will be used?

3. What cutoff score will be used?

Procedure after a high EPDS

1. Will one elevated score be sufficient to receive a referral or will one elevated score require a repeat assessment (after what time period?) Describe the procedure for determining when a referral will be made in detail.

2. When will clients be screened for the first time?

3. Will clients be screened more than once, if so, at what time points? What happens if a woman misses a screening appointment? Should the screening staff wait for the next screening period?

Referral procedures

1. Who will make the referral? The staff member providing the screening or another programme staff member?

2. Where will clients be referred?

3. You will need a list of treatment resources in your community.

4. What procedures will be used to follow-up with referred clients? (What happens if the woman is identified at her last regular visit?)

Referral: elevated suicide item

1. What score on an item assessing suicidal thoughts will be considered elevated?

2. Who should the screener contact if the woman is considered suicidal? What additional backup personnel are available if the contact person is not available? Is there an emergency number in the community that could be used?

Recording/charting

1. Where will the completed screening scale forms be kept?

2. Where will staff members record the information that a client has been screened and the outcome of that screening?

3. Where will staff members record the information regarding referrals?

4. Where will the follow-up information be documented?

5. Would a 'mental health tracking form' for each client be helpful? What information would be recorded on this form?

---

completed form will be kept or just the screening score. Storing a mother's screening information in a paediatric setting might prove challenging.

Fourth, consideration must be given to training new personnel about perinatal depression screening. Specifically, who will provide this education? Will it be provided to each new staff member individually as they are hired, or to all new staff, in a group format, annually or semi-annually? Finally, any plan must establish who will supervise depression screening on an ongoing basis; this person must collect screening data and provide feedback to staff on screening performance.

Protocol-development worksheet

Depression screening protocols are not 'one-size-fits-all' programmes, but must be tailored to suit each organizational context. Developing tailored protocols benefits from the input of on-site health care professionals, who are intimately familiar with local routine; yet, such professionals are not usually experts in perinatal depression. To meet this shortfall, we have developed a program for training on-site providers in our Maternal Depression Screening: Train-the-Trainer Program (Segre *et al.*, 2011). Based on our experience disseminating depression screening, below we provide a worksheet that was useful in guiding primary health care and social service professionals in developing their own, tailored screening protocols (Table 6.1).

Summary and conclusions

Perinatal depression is prevalent in high, middle, and low-income countries around the world, creating a significant health burden for women and their families. Risk factors for perinatal depression are largely similar across cultures, with local variations. The major factors include psychiatric illness and psychological distress, negative life events (including violence), poor social relationships and relationship discord, and social deprivation.

Detecting perinatal depression in primary care can be a daunting task because it requires several steps, including educating providers, identifying a screening tool, determining scores on the tool that lead to further action, developing a screening schedule, identifying referral sources, and arranging for follow-up after treatment. All of these elements must be in place to optimize health and mental health care for the pregnant and postpartum woman.

The World Health Organization has identified improving maternal health as one of its Millennium Development Goals (no. 5) (<http://www.who.int/topics/millennium_development_goals/maternal_health/en/index.html>). It cites the strong link between maternal mental health and physical health. The WHO also argues that it is fundamentally important that mental health problems of pregnant women and mothers be integrated into the existing maternal health programs and activities, an opinion that can be summarized very simply: 'There is no health without mental health.' This should be recognized as the charge to all of us who provide care to perinatal women. This is the charge that animated the clinical and research career of Channi Kumar.

References

American College of Nurse-Midwives (2002). Depression in women: Position statement Available from http://www.midwife.org/siteFiles/position/Depression_in_Women_05.pdf (accessed 10 September 2013).

American Psychiatric Association (2013). *Diagnostic and Statistical Manual of Mental Disorders*, 5th ed. Arlington, VA, American Psychiatric Association.

Association of Women's Health Obstetric and Neonatal Nurses. (2008). The role of the nurse in postpartum mood and anxiety disorders. Available from http://www.awhonn.org/awhonn/content.do?name=05_HealthPolicyLegislation/5H_PositionStatements.htm (accessed 10 September 2013).

Baker, C.D., Kamke, H., O'Hara, M.W., and Stuart, S. (2009). Web-based training for implementing evidenced-based management of postpartum depression. Journal of the American Board Family Medicine **22**: 588–9.

Beck, C.T. (2001). Predictors of postpartum depression: An update. Nursing Research **50**: 275–85.

Beck, C.T. and Gable, R.K. (2000). Postpartum Depression Screening Scale: Development and psychometric testing. Nursing Research **49**: 272–82.

Bennett, H.A., Einarson, A., Taddio, A., Koren, G., and Einarson, T.R. (2004). Prevalence of depression during pregnancy: Systematic review. Obstetrics and Gynecology **103**: 698–709.

Brassil, M.L., Magri, E., Calvo, A., *et al.* (2011). Perinatal mood disorders: Implementation of a hospital-based screening program. Journal of Obstetric and Gynecological Nursing **40**: s44–s45.

Committee on Obstetric Practice (2010). Screening for depression during and after pregnancy. Obstetrics and Gynecology **115**: 394–5.

Cox, J.L., Holden, J.M., and Sagovsky, R. (1987). Detection of postnatal depression: Development of the 10-item Edinburgh Postnatal Depression Scale. British Journal of Psychiatry **150**: 782–6.

Eaton, N.R, Keyes, K.M., Krueger, R.F., *et al* (2012). An invariant dimensional liability model of gender differences in mental disorder prevalence: Evidence from a national sample. Journal of Abnormal Psychology **121**: 282–8.

Elliott, S.A. (1994). Uses and misuses of the Edinburgh Postnatal Depression Scale in primary care: a comparison of models developed in health visiting. In Perinatal Psychiatry: Use and Misuse of the Edinburgh Postnatal Depression Scale. Cox, J. and Holden, J., editors. London, Gaskell, pp. 221–32.

Fisher, J., de Mello, M. C., Patel, V., *et al.* (2012). Prevalence and determinants of common perinatal mental disorders in women in low- and lower-middle-income countries: a systematic review. Bulletin of the World Health Organization **90**:139–49.

Gavin, N.I., Gaynes, B.N., Lohr, K.N., *et al.* (2005). Perinatal depression: A systematic review of prevalence and incidence. Obstetrics and Gynecology **106**: 1071–83.

Georgiopoulos, A.M., Bryan, T.L., Wollan, P., and Yawn, B.P. (2001). Routine screening for postpartum depression. The Journal of Family Practice **50**: 117–22.

Gordon, T.E.J., Cardone, I.A., Kim, J.J., Gordon, S.M., and Silver, R.K. (2006). Universal perinatal depression screening in an academic medical center. Obstetrics and Gynecology **107**: 342–7.

Heh, S.-H. and Fu, Y.-Y. (2003). Effectiveness of informational support in reducing the severity of postnatal depression in Taiwan. Journal of Advanced Nursing **42**: 30–6.

Howard, L.M., Flach, C., Mehay, A., Sharp, D., and Tylee, A. (2011). The prevalence of suicidal ideation identified by the Edinburgh Postnatal Depression Scale in postpartum women in primary care: Findings from the RESPOND trial. BMC Pregnancy and Childbirth **11**: 57 doi:10.1186/1471-2393-11-57

Joseph, G.F. (2009). Transitions. Obstetrics and Gynecology **114**: 4–6.

Kemper, K.J., Kelleher, K., and Olson, A.L. (2007). Implementing maternal depression screening. Pediatrics **120**: 448–9.

Kroenke, K., Spitzer, R.L., and Williams, J.B.W. (2001). The PHQ-9: Validity of a brief depression severity measure. Journal General of Internal Medicine **16**: 606–13.

LaRocco-Cockburn, A., Melville, J.L., Bell, M., and Katon, W. (2003). Depression screening attitudes and practices among obstetrician-gynecologists. Obstetrics and Gynecology **101**: 892–8.

Massoudi, P., Wickberg, B., and Hwang, C.P. (2007). Screening for postnatal depression in Swedish child health care. Acta Paediatrica **96**: 897–901.

Matthey, S., Henshaw, C., Elliott, S., and Barnett, B. (2006). Variability in use of cut-off scores and formats on the Edinburgh Postnatal Depression Scale—implications for clinical and research practice Archives of Women's Mental Health **9**: 306–15.

National Association of Pediatric Nurse Practitioners (2003). The PNP's role in supporting infant and family well-being during the first year of life: Position statement. Journal of Pediatric Health Care **17**: 19A–20A.

National Institute for Health and Care Excellence (2007). Antenatal and postnatal mental health: Clinical management and service guidance: National Collaborating Centre for Mental Health. London, NICE.

O'Hara, M.W. and Swain, A.M. (1996). Rates and risk of postpartum depression-A meta-analysis. International Review of Psychiatry **8**: 37–54.

Olson, A.L., Dietrich, A.J., Prazar, G., and Hurley, J. (2006). Brief maternal depression screening at well-child visits. Pediatrics **118**: 207–216.

Olson, A.L., Kemper, K.J., Kelleher, K.J., *et al.* (2002). Primary care pediatricians' roles and perceived responsibilities in the identification and management of maternal depression. Pediatrics **110**: 1169–76.

Robertson, E., Grace, S., Wallington, T., and Stewart, D.E. (2004). Antenatal risk factors for postpartum depression: a synthesis of recent literature. General Hospital Psychiatry **26**: 289–295.

Rowan, P., Greisinger, A., Brehm, B., Smith, F., and McReynolds, E. (2012). Outcomes from implementing systematic antepartum depression screening in obstetrics. Archives of Women's Mental Health **15**: 115–20.

Segre, L.S., O'Hara, M.W., Arndt, S., and Beck, C.T. (2010). Nursing care for postpartum depression: Part 1 Do nurses think they should offer both screening and counseling? MCN The American Journal of Maternal Child Nursing **35**: 220–225.

Segre, L.S., Brock, R.L., O'Hara, M.W., Gorman, L.L., and Engeldinger, J. (2011). Disseminating perinatal depression screening as a public health initiative: A train-the-trainer approach. Maternal and Child Health Journal **15**: 814–821. doi: PMID: 20640494.

Segre, L.S., O'Hara, M.W., Brock, R.L., & Taylor, D. (2012b). Depression Screening of Perinatal Women by the Des Moines Healthy Start Project: Program Description and Evaluation. Psychiatric Services **63**: 250–255

Segre, L.S., O'Hara, M.W., & Fischer, S.D. (2012a). Perinatal depression screening in Healthy Start: An evaluation of the acceptability of technical assistance consultation. *Community Mental Health Journal.* Available from http://www.springerlink.com/content/r125m3gm88206um3/fulltext.pdf (accessed 10 September 2013).

Sheeder, J., Kabir, K., and Stafford, B. (2009). Screening for postpartum depression at well-child visits: Is once enough during the first 6 months of life? Pediatrics **123**:e 982–e988. Available from http://pediatrics.aappublications.org/content/123/6/e982.full.pdf+html (accessed 10 September 2013).

US Preventive ServicesTaskForce (2009). Screening for depression in adults: US Preventive Services Task Force recommendation statement. Annals of Internal Medicine **151**: 784–92.

Whooley, M.A., Avins, A.L., Miranda, J., and Browner, W.S. (1997). Case-finding instruments for depression: Two questions are as good as many. Journal of General Internal Medicine **12**: 439–45.

Chapter 7

Perceptions of postnatal depression across countries and cultures

From a TransCultural Study of PostNatal Depression (TCS-PND), initiated by Channi Kumar

Nine M.-C. Glangeaud-Freudenthal

Introduction

Professor Channi Kumar was the initiator and leader of a 'Transcultural Study of Postnatal Depression within European Health Systems: Harmonisation of research methods and promotion of mother-child health'. A project management team (PMT)[1] was coordinated by Channi Kumar from 1998 until his death in September 2000, and then by Maureen Mark until 2004, and run in collaboration with 19 centres located in 14 countries (Table 7.1).

Results from the TCS-PND study on 'Development and testing of harmonised research methods' were published in 2004 (Marks et al. 2004; Asten et al 2004; Oates et al. 2004; Gorman et al. 2004; Bernazzani et al. 2004; Bifulco et al. 2004; Gunning et al. 2004; Chisholm et al. 2004)[2].

Qualitative methods of the Transcultural Study of Postnatal Depression

The aim of the qualitative part of the TCS-PND project, developed in this chapter, was to explore perceptions of postnatal depression (PND) by: (a) lay and professional key informants, specifically regarding description of symptoms, awareness of this pathology, and of possible care; (b) women, their partners, and their own mothers about their perception of happiness and mental health difficulties and care during pregnancy and postpartum.

Most of this methodological section was written in 2001, by Asten and colleagues. Extracts from their text, never published before, are quoted in the following sections.

> The qualitative study was an investigation into women's concepts of happiness and unhappiness during pregnancy and after birth, understanding and beliefs about postnatal illness, related health services and pathways to obtaining care in different countries and cultures'.

Table 7.1 List of co-ordinators within the "Transcultural Study of Postnatal Depression" (TCS-PND) research group initiated by Channi Kumar (1998–2000)

Country	Centre	Co-ordinator
England:		
	Keele	John Cox
	Nottingham	Margaret Oates
	London	Paul Asten
	Manchester	Louis Appleby
Ireland	Dublin	Siobhan Barry
United States	Iowa	Michael O'Hara and Laura Gorman
France		
	Bordeaux	Anne-Laure Sutter
	Paris	Nine Glangeaud-Freudenthal
Italy	Florence	Paola Benvenuti and Vania Valoriani
Austria	Vienna	Claudia Klier
Switzerland	Zurich	Martin Kammerer
Sweden	Goteborg	Birgitta Wickberg
Japan		
	Kyushu	Keiko Yoshida
	Mie	Tadaharu Okano
Uganda	Kampala	Stella Neema
Portugal	Porto	Barbara Figueiredo
Brazil	Sao Paolo*	Antonio Vieira
United Arabic Emirates	Dubai	Rafia Ghubash
China	Hong Kong	Dominic Lee

*Centre member of the management team that did not contribute to qualitative data collection.

Developing the study

After discussing and after consultation with qualitative research experts[3], it became clear that the question we wanted to answer was: How do concepts of happiness and unhappiness during pregnancy and after birth differ between countries and cultures. An understanding of what normally makes people happy or unhappy during this period would help us to understand the context of people's understanding and beliefs about postnatal illness. Furthermore, we wanted to know about related health services and pathways to obtaining care in different countries and cultures. We were interested in the meaning that people give to the concept of postnatal depression phenomena and how these different factors (normal feelings of happiness and unhappiness, cultural influences, knowledge and availability of services) interact to produce that specific meaning.

With such an objective in mind, the most appropriate study methodology was therefore a 'grounded theory' approach (Corbin and Strauss1990), a general methodology for developing theory that is grounded in data systematically gathered and analysed (Glaser and Strauss 1967).

Such an approach has many advantages, because the data collection and analysis techniques employed provide well-grounded, rich descriptions of processes in identifiable local contexts from the perspective of the people under study. It can help researchers to go beyond initial conceptions and generate and revise conceptual frameworks and, very importantly, it can improve competence of research centres (Miles and Huberman 1984).

A common method is to use different sources of information to corroborate each other, a form of methodological 'triangulation' (Mason 1996). With this in mind, three separate sources of information were identified: Focus groups of recent mothers, relatives of recent mothers, and healthcare professionals with influence in planning or providing healthcare.

By the time the study had been funded by the European Union, the project management team had begun to develop research probes for the study, and at the first TCS-PND workshop, in Keele in 1998, England, they presented these to the group. They had also conducted some pilot interviews and focus groups in Keele, Nottingham, and Kampala to test the research probes.

We will not develop here in detail of the pilot process of using a long questionnaire for healthcare professionals which was then modified to a less directive questioning «to allow the informant to offer their knowledge on the subject, rather than answer specific questions presented by the interviewer. Similarly, the creation of the draft discussion guide for focus groups, piloted in Uganda, requiring a certain level of knowledge and understanding, was contradictory to the grounded theory approach of information arising only from the data. Thus, a set of broader open-ended probes were developed for focus groups', 'that would not assume any prior knowledge of childbirth or understanding of postnatal illness, but would allow for cultural differences to be clearly seen.

The final prompts used are as below for focus groups and relative key informants (those for professionals key informants are not reported in this chapter):

1 Happiness–unhappiness

- What brings happiness to women during pregnancy?
- What brings unhappiness to women during pregnancy?
- What brings happiness to women after childbirth?
- What brings unhappiness to women after childbirth?

2 What do people (you) know/understand about being emotionally unwell following birth (PND) [Probe for causes] [Probe for local terms]

3 When a woman is emotionally unwell during the postpartum period, what can be done to help her? [Probe for health/help seeking behaviour]

4 What suggestions do you have for improving health care for these mental health concerns?

The researchers

After method training,

'where possible, the same researchers interviewed all subjects and were present at all focus groups. The average size of research team was 3 (median), the notable exceptions of this being Florence with 7 and Iowa with 10 researchers. The research teams were on the whole an experienced group of researchers, the vast majority with previous research experience of at least one year (70%), although not necessarily in qualitative research, with less than a third (28%) having previously conducted qualitative research.'

Sample selection

After three more workshops in Paris, France in November 1998, in Tyrol, Austria 1999, and in London in July 1999 a clear protocol had been developed

> regarding sampling subjects and interviewing and group moderation techniques, and analysis methods.

The three sources of information (for triangulation) used in this study, were (i) new mothers of babies, (ii) fathers and grandmothers, and (iii) *the third data source were general practitioners (or equivalent) and planners/administrators in positions of influence'*. We will not give results from this third source of data here.

In each centre new mothers were invited to focus group discussions, and prompted to discuss the topics outlined above.

> Mothers were not recruited specifically because they had personal experience of PND. Rather it was thought that accessing the experiences of a wider range of mothers would result in a rich supply of data that would be representative of the normal experiences of mothers in each culture and society, from which an understanding of unhappiness and depression could be contextualized.

To substantiate the information from the focus groups, the second data source was key informant interviews with a sample of recent fathers and grandmothers, who were relatives of new mothers, to also *'allow for an analysis of the differences in perceptions of the perinatal experience between genders, between mothers and fathers, and between generations, between mothers and grandmothers'.*

The pre-defined criteria for subject selection were that:

(i) Focus groups should consist of between four and six women between 5 and 7 months postpartum. Groups should be recruited until there is 'theoretical saturation' of emerging themes (Corbin and Strauss 1990).

(ii) Three fathers and three grandmothers of babies between 5 and 7 months old should be interviewed in each centre as lay (relative) key informants.

Whilst there were predefined criteria for subject selection, there were inevitably differences between centres in sample selection and interview and analysis techniques that may have been due to researchers, institution or to cultural differences.

> The greatest variation in selection and recruitment methods was for the focus groups of new mothers. The most common method of recruitment for focus groups was through a health centre, as in Kampala, Kyushu, and Porto, and specifically through midwives or health visitors, as in two UK centres, Keele and Nottingham. Four centres recruited through parental support groups, Dublin, Gothenburg, Florence, and Vienna, whilst the two centres in France, Paris and Bordeaux, recruited through nurseries or crèches. Four centres, Dubai, Iowa, London, and Zurich, recruited women from the community by sending letters to women on a recent birth register or by posters inviting people to attend groups.
>
> Recruitment of relatives for key informant interviews was done in one of three ways, often by recruiting relatives of the women both the partners of women and grandmothers from focus groups (Gothenburg, Nottingham, Paris, and Vienna). Other centres recruited both fathers and grandmothers through a health centre (Kampala, Keele, London, Porto, and Zurich). In Kyushu and

Dublin they recruited fathers through the focus group women but grandmothers through health centres. In Dubai, the fathers were friends or acquaintances of the research team, and the grandmothers a random sample taken from those who accompanied patients (not patients themselves) at a private clinic. At the other three centres, Bordeaux, Florence, and Iowa, both the fathers and grandmothers were recruited through friends or acquaintances of the research team. There will inevitably be differences in data collected . . . and this should be borne in mind in analysis.

There were some interesting issues that arose in some centres, however, with regards to sample recruitment of mothers for focus group discussions and lay (relatives) key informants. In Keele they originally tried evening groups without children but there were not enough volunteers, so they changed to daytime groups and had to arrange child-minders but still had trouble recruiting'. In London they had difficulty recruiting all subjects, and found it difficult to get minimum of four mothers to a group. Also, as they were in an inner city multiethnic centre, they could not control for ethnicity of members or social class factors, and they felt that some groups were biased by self-selected members—e.g. middle-class mothers. In Nottingham the Mirpur women invited to focus groups were often unable to gain permission or approval of their husbands and families to attend. Possibly owing to stigma attached in the South Asian population with regards to mental health issues, many mothers either refused outright or did not turn up for the group. Those women who attended groups were very distrustful of the presence of the lay translator/note keeper (confidentiality issues) and this was therefore dropped from later groups. Bordeaux and Paris had similar problems recruiting in crèches for focus groups and it took a lot of time first to get permission.

A common concern amongst researchers was how they could obtain focus group samples representative of their area and country, which would provide data reflective of their country or culture.

Some centres tried to get samples that they thought would be representative, they tried to include people from different social background. Thus, they approached all consecutive women with including criteria or random samples in community centres.

Conducting interviews and focus groups

Interviews were always conducted in the native language and consent was obtained from all informants being interviewed and all focus groups participants. The interviewer's role was to be neutral and facilitating, so long or multiple-phrase questions were avoided. Various techniques were employed by centres to ensure their study was data driven, using techniques such as summarizing the main points that each group had brought up during the course of the group for comments, or feeding back answers from previous groups or interviews at the end of sessions for comments and then probing in subsequent groups/interviews to ensure that such themes were saturated.

'Nearly half of the study centres conducted their focus groups with mothers in health centres or community centres, as in Porto, Dublin, Keele, Nottingham, Kyushu, Vienna, and Kampala. A hospital was the setting for groups in Zurich and London, and a university research centre in Florence and Iowa. Both French centres, Paris and Bordeaux, held their groups in nurseries, as this was where they had recruited subjects. In Gothenburg and Dubai they held groups in the home of one of the parents, although some groups in Gothenburg were at the Child Health Services, and some Dubai groups were held at the house of the researcher.

The most common setting for interviews with fathers and grandmothers was in their own home, except for Kampala and Porto, where interviews took place at the same health centres as they used for focus groups. Some centres used a variety of other settings for their interviews.

The same demographic information was collected on all relatives and focus group participants. This was done either as a short form or set of questions and included age, current/usual job, highest level of education, ethnicity, marital status, other children, and current medical treatment (if any).

This information was included in the discussion of the results.

All interviews and focus groups were tape-recorded and transcribed, and written notes were made of non-verbal responses to supplement verbatim transcripts. When tape-recording was not possible the interview was recorded by a note-taker and a near-verbatim account written within 24 hours of the interview.

Analysis

It was important to understand the methods of analysis of qualitative data, in order to analyse each set of data as it was obtained. To this end, following the third workshop in Tyrol, Austria, the project management team circulated guidelines on analysis techniques produced from the literature and discussion with experienced qualitative researchers.

The basis of analysing grounded theory data, is in the coding technique of extracting key sentences, concepts or formulations, which allow the researcher to articulate the data analytically. The six relative informant interviews, six professional interviews and the four to six focus groups were all analysed separately. Analysis was on-going and was carried out as transcripts became available, so each analysis could help inform the next interview.

Analysis should have been done by someone present at the focus groups or interviews, in consultation with other team members who were present. In most research centres analysis was done by the majority of team members (median = 90% of research team), although in a few centres (n = 3) analysis was done by a single researcher.

Many centres reported having used techniques to check theme extraction and thus improve the validity and reliability of their data. The most common method was double-checking theme extraction with colleagues or by other means such as software and arriving at a consensus decision about extracted themes.

A key factor in analysis of qualitative data is that it should take into account typical patterns and not just variations (Corbin and Strauss 1990), and it is these common patterns that would be most insightful in understanding what part of the perinatal experience is a truly human experience and what is a cultural manifestation of the experience.

This led to the question of negative cases or outliers, when one person said something very different to everyone else. Centres dealt with this in a variety of ways, most usually by trying to identify such statements during group sessions, and checking these statements with the rest of the group for comment and noting affirmation or disagreement. Where there was no agreement, this was noted and considered in analysis as to whether the statement appeared to be a very personal and special idea of only one person related to a precise event that was not relevant to the discussion but may bring a new statement to be tested in a next session.

Coding and analysis continued until themes were reduced to 6–10 cluster groups representing all statements in the data. From this, a final table was produced with a list of the themes for each topic. For focus groups, data from all groups was combined to produce a set of themes representing views from women from all groups.

After discussions at an international workshop in Florence, Italy in May 2000 *'the final tables of themes were internally revalidated in each centre'* and translated into English when necessary. Copies of all data were gathered by the study coordinator.

Reflection on the research process

> It had been suggested by the project management team that those involved in the research should have been persons who knew sufficient about clinical conditions and services to be able to clarify answers in interviews, but should not have been a psychiatrist known locally for his or her special interest as this might have biased the responses. However, even with such guidelines, there would still inevitably be an influence on data collection and analysis of an individual's status.

The centres were asked, *'What was your awareness of yourself as a health professional on the research process? Did you think you influenced responses to any of the questions because of your status as a psychiatrist/psychologist etc.?'*

Some qualitative results

In March 2001, seven centres of the TCS-PND group presented their results in a symposium during the first World Congress on Women's Mental Health in Berlin, Germany, on 'Perceptions of postnatal depression across countries and cultures: From a TransCultural Study of PostNatal Depression (TCS-PND)'. The symposium was dedicated to the memory of Professor Channi Kumar and abstracts published in Archives of Women's Mental Health (Asten *et al.* 2001).

A workshop in Dublin, Ireland (2–4 April 2001), added to contributions from those seven centres; 11 other centres[4] also presented their contribution to a book on the qualitative data by the TCS-PND group, which alas, was never published—*Perceptions of postnatal depression across countries and cultures: From a TransCultural Study of PostNatal Depression (TCS-PND) by seven centres of the TCS-PND group.*

The qualitative data for the seven centres were supplemented with sociodemographic data to address the issues of: (i) whether perceptions of PND are related to some specific cultural perception of mental health and/or of status of parenthood and (ii) how high or low levels of general care and specificity of health policy relate to differences in perception of needs for care. In addition, it was shown that PND is a well-recognized condition by recent mothers in all countries in this study, even though it is not described with the same words and the word postpartum depression does not exist in some countries.

The next sections are very short summaries of results from focus groups of postpartum women and on fathers' interviews in the six countries and one result concerning general practitioners, patients and planners. They illustrate some similarities and differences in perceptions and the main concerns in those countries.

Pregnancy, delivery, and post-partum experiences: similarities and differences in Portuguese mothers

Eight focus groups were formed, each one with four to six participants. The sample of 35 women had quite heterogeneous social and demographic characteristics. The majority of the mothers had their first (45.7%) or the second child (45.7%), about 6 months prior to the study. The mothers were invited to participate by the nurses responsible for the vaccination in the medical centres where the focus groups were held in the presence of two researchers. Focus groups were audio-taped, then transcribed and mothers' statements were categorized using the IN-VIVO program (Figueiredo and Alegre 2001).

This Portuguese sample—together with the advantages of using a qualitative methodology when conducting a study with this kind of purpose—shows the great importance of on one side of the quality of the relationship and support from the extended family and husband to the happiness of Portuguese women during pregnancy and postpartum, and on the other side the negative effect of the intrusiveness of the family after delivery. Moreover, as far as PND is concerned, and having regard to the causes, almost all the mothers stated that overwork and lack of support from their husband and their mother might lead to depression after delivery.

What do Swedish mothers and fathers think about happiness, unhappiness and mental health in the transition to parenthood period?

Data from six focus groups with 28 mothers were collected from the regular parental groups offered to all parents at 1 to 5 months postpartum by the child health services in Sweden. Relative key informant fathers and grandmothers were also interviewed (Wickberg and Nordström 2001).

An effect of Swedish cultural perceptions[5] could be that the fathers talked about their own feelings instead of those of their partners. (1) Happiness during pregnancy for fathers meant: a good relationship; talking a lot with the partner; feeling ready to have a baby; having enough time. (2) Unhappiness during pregnancy meant worries and sad mood. (3) Happiness in postpartum meant: long parental leave; having grandparents near; good hospital care; sharing baby care; partner support.

The mothers also stressed that (1) for happiness during pregnancy the partner relationship is as important as feelings of proudness and self-esteem. Many focus groups consider childbearing as a miracle and giving meaning to life. (2) Unhappiness meant: worries about baby's health; not being able to cope as a mother; and worries about partner relationship. (3) Happiness postpartum meant: sharing experiences with partner; successful breastfeeding; not being self-centred; following the development of the baby. (4) Unhappiness postpartum meant: vulnerability; worries about not coping as a mother; stress; not having enough time; tiredness and birth complications.

Mother's perception of postpartum depression in France—Is it different from father's perception?

Data presented are from interviews of three postpartum men and focus groups of 17 postpartum women recruited in crèches (casual day baby-care centres) and in maternal and infant protection centres (PMI), in Paris and in the suburbs, in order to have different socioeconomic backgrounds. The main results are (Glangeaud-Freudenthal *et al.* 2001):

1 Happiness (or no unhappiness) during pregnancy. For women, it was: having no health problems; feeling the baby's movements; having a joint project of a child with partner; having family around; not being alone; not having marital conflicts; and being understood at work (women also described anxiety about delivery and baby's health). Men

spoke of being able to feel the baby through their partner's belly, being a supportive partner, having financial and material comfort, and about the importance of having a child for continuity of generations.

2 After childbirth. For women, it was: becoming a family; having a good relationship with their own mother and partner still interested in you. Women also talked about difficulty to care at the same time for baby, partner, work, and family. Both men and women spoke of: pride of having a healthy growing baby; successful nursing; having family support and joys; not being alone; and confidence in childcare. For men only this meant: being together at birth; having direct contact with the baby; woman's returning to work; and re-establishing a normal rhythm of life.

3 Understanding postnatal depression. For women this meant: having a difficult baby; different from what you had expected; lack of sleep with a crying baby; and being over-loaded with other children, can all cause depression. For migrant women: a far-away family was also perceived as a possible cause for depression. Although, telling that they do not to know very much about PND, men were able to describe quite well the symptoms and causes of PND.

4 How to help a depressed mother. For women this meant having support and under-standing from their mother and from other women after birth. Both men and women stressed the importance of practical help of someone at home and said medical consultation was needed only in very severe cases of depression. Men insist, first of all, on their help and understanding for the women, and next on other women's support for her. They were keener to express ideas on how to help to 'avoid depression' than on what to do if their partner is depressed.

The 'Italian father'—comparison between mothers' expectations and men's experiences

Data were collected from five focus groups and from semi-structured interviews with fathers. One of the main themes for women, related to happiness and unhappiness during pregnancy and after childbirth, is the expectation of the presence, empathy, and effective support from one's own partner. This expectation is strongly prevalent in respect to other possible forms of support (i.e. from one's own parents, friends, etc.). It seems that the women in our sample consider their partner as the only figure able to support them, implicitly loading him down with responsibilities (Benvenuti et al. 2001).

The fathers, while realizing this, express some personal difficulties. The availability for a practical support clearly emerges together with sharing responsibilities related to take decisions and daily needs. Fathers' difficulties concern the assumption of the paternal role, the changes in the couple's relationship, and feelings of exclusion.

The apparent contradiction between mothers' and fathers' perceptions corresponds to different idealized points of view of the importance of their own roles. On one side the mothers pretend to be the exclusive focus of attention, on the other, the fathers experience feelings of jealousy, affective deprivation, and low acknowledgement of their attempts.

Postnatal depression in Japanese women: modern and traditional aspects[6]

Data from focus groups of mothers (four groups with 17 women in total, from 5 to 8 months postnatal, all married) and three key informants in each category (fathers, grandmothers) were collected through one local health centre located in the catchment area of our university hospital (Yoshida *et al.* 2001).

To highlight different perceptions of PND, which are related to specifically Japanese cultural perceptions, the following were noted. (1) Happiness during pregnancy means: having a baby boy (focus group); socially accepted (father, grandmother); attending a traditional ceremony for pregnancy (father); being proud of having a pregnant daughter (grandmother). (2) Unhappiness during pregnancy means: husband's affair during wife's absence. (3) Happiness after birth means: being accepted by mother-in-law (focus group); going to shrine with a baby (father). (4) Understanding of PND.

Many focus group mothers discussed PND as to be something like being depressed; however they confused it with maternity blues. Fathers and grandmothers did not know much about this so they did not give any particular answers, and nothing culturally relevant.

An obvious gap between somatic and psychosocial treatment in pregnancy, delivery, and postpartum, in Austria[7]

Qualitative research was employed to study the views of healthcare planners, mothers, grandmothers, and fathers on PND with regard to symptoms, causes and desired treatment (Schmidt-Siegal *et al.* 2001).

Professional key informants do know about the psychosocial and biological causes of PND, about clinical symptoms and the repercussions for child development and the family. There is agreement that a high quality of medical services should be maintained, that the high prevalence of PND is not recognized, and that there is a lack of public awareness, information, psychotherapeutic services, and specific facilities such as mother–baby units.

Results of the focus groups show that women are fairly well aware of the symptoms and causes of PND, what treatment options should be available and what should be done to improve services. It can only be speculated about why Austrians are so well informed or if this represents a sample selection bias.

Health services provision for patients with perinatal–psychiatric problems in Switzerland[8]

Kammerer *et al.* (2001) addressed two research questions:

+ What is the structure of perinatal–psychiatric service provision in Switzerland from the top–down perspective of the ministries of health?[9]

+ What are the met and unmet needs in the eyes of service planners, patients, clinicians, specialists for child protection, health visitors, mothers, fathers and grandparents?

Qualitative data were obtained by focus discussion groups of women with perinatal psychiatric problems and key informant interviews. The qualitative data suggest that pregnant patients may experience dangerous situations on psychiatric wards and that mothers with babies may have to face long waiting times until the hospital can provide joint mother and baby admission under safe circumstances. On the ward they may find it difficult to look after the baby, especially breastfeeding, while patients without babies may behave in an inappropriate way (from patients' interviews). Health visitors report difficulties in identifying outpatient services that have a constant interest in the perinatal-psychiatric health service. The interest of the institutions and the quality of the perinatal-psychiatric service may depend too much on the individual doctor's interests; this means that the quality of service may fluctuate (from health visitors, social workers, doctors). Systematic quantitative research in order to establish the pathways of care and the outcome of perinatal-psychiatric patients in Switzerland is necessary.

Conclusion

To conclude with a personal thought—all these results are just a small part of the many results that should be discussed in the cultural context of each country. There are many more results from those 17 centres that were generated by this study that should be edited and published. However, Channi Kumar's enthusiasm, energy, bright ideas, and leadership is missed for many of us to achieve this (Glangeaud-Freudenthal 2002, 2003).

Notes

1 Project Management Team (PMT) in 2001:
   Central Administration: Maureen Marks (London), Paul Asten (London, until 2001) and Sue Conroy (London, from 2001)
   Qualitative study: John Cox (Stock on Trent), Emma Hirst (Manchester) and Stella Neema (Kampala),
   Clinical study: Laura Gorman (Iowa), Michael O'Hara (Iowa), Nicole Guedeney (Paris),
   Health Services Research Study: Margaret Oates (Nottingham), Nine Glangeaud-Freudenthal (Paris), Daniel Chisholm (Geneva)
   Psychosocial (C.A.M.E.) Study: Odette Bernazzani (Canada)
   Mother-Infant interaction Study: Melanie Gunning (Reading).

2 Marks *et al.* (2004).

3 For instance, Maurice Eisenbuch and two anthropologists from Uganda: John Orley and Stella Neema (note by John Cox).

4 Centres that collected data for the transcultural study:
   For parents focus groups and descriptors (added to the 7 centres that presented in Berlin)
   • Nottingham UK Margaret Oates, Neelam Sisodia, and J. Stewart
   • Keele,UK Sue Hacking and Carol Henshaw
   • London, UK Trudy Seneviratne, Paul Asten and Sue Conroy
   • Manchester, UK Emma. Hirst and Louis Appleby
   • Bordeaux, France Anne-Laure Sutter-Dallay, and Elisabeth Glatigny
   • Kampala, Uganda Stella Neema and Grace Nakasi
   • Dublin, Ireland Sioghan Barry and Mary Smith
   • Iowa, USA Michael W O'Hara, Laura L. Gorman, Carol Mertens and Shelley Whitcher

For national descriptors of perinatal illness and care:

- Mie, Japan Tadaharu Okano
- Dubai, United Arab Emirates Rafia Ghubash and Valsa Eapen
- Hong Kong, China Dominic T.S. Lee

5   Equality in working life (80 % of mothers of pre-school children are employed) and in family policy is highly valued in Sweden. The ideal of family life is one of parents sharing infant care and responsibility. In reality, only 10% of the parental leave is used by fathers. In the perinatal period, however, the main support person for the woman is her partner with 90 % of fathers taking 10 days parental leave after the birth. the generational support system has become less important.

6   Japanese childbearing women are well educated and want to establish their career rather than trying to get married quickly. On the other hand, many modern Japanese women keep traditional concepts of marriage. About half of women get married through the traditional arranged marriage system and tend to quit work at marriage or after pregnancy. They often choose a traditional support system for perinatal women (called *Satogaeri bunben*), staying a few months prenatally at her own family house to get sufficient support, especially from their own mothers.

7   In 1974 a standardized prevention programme was introduced that consists of medical check-ups for pregnant women and children until the age of 4. All check-ups are free of charge, a financial incentive for mothers was given until 1995 (95% of pregnant women attended). This programme is the main reason for the good physical health of mothers and babies and the low perinatal mortality rate (4.4/1,000 in 1999). Although in Austria there are a mean of 10.1 contacts with health professionals during pregnancy, no regular psychosocial assessments are performed for mothers during pregnancy and after child birth. The healthcare system was studied using the statistical yearbooks and information provided by the ministry of health.

8   In Switzerland there is a non-gatekeeper system. Outpatients are looked after by both adult and child psychiatrists and psychologists in private practice and by adult and child psychiatric hospital outpatient services. Pregnant women who need inpatient services obtain treatment on general wards for women (or for both sexes). Mothers with babies are provided joint mother and baby admission for psychiatric treatment on general wards for women (or for both sexes) in at least one hospital of nearly every canton.

References

Asten, P., Marks, M.N., Oates, M.R., and the TCS-PND Group (2004). Aims, measures, study sites and subject samples of the Transcultural Study of Postnatal Depression (TCS-PND). In Transcultural Study of Postnatal Depression (TCS-PND): Development and testing of harmonised research methods. British Journal of Psychiatry **184**(suppl 46): 3–9.

Asten, P., Oates, M., Figureido, B., *et al.*, and the TCS-PND Study Group (2001). A comparison of understanding of postnatal depression in different countries and cultures: Focus group study. Archives of Women's Mental Health, 3 (suppl 2): 52–4.

Benvenuti, P., Poggiolini, D., Ardito, M., *et al.* (2001). The father's role between mother's expectations and the man's experience: From a Transcultural Study of Postnatal Depression (TCS-PND). Archives of Women's Mental Health 3(suppl 2): 53 (Abstract).

Bernazzani, O., Conroy, S., Marks, M.N., *et al.*, and the TCS-PND Group (2004). Contextual assessment of the maternity experience: development of an instrument for cross-cultural research. In Transcultural Study of Postnatal Depression (TCS-PND): Development and testing of harmonised research methods. British Journal of Psychiatry **184**(suppl 46): 24–30.

Bifulco, A., Figueiredo, B., Guedeney, N., *et al.*, and the TCS-PND Group (2004). Maternal attachment style and depression associated with childbirth: preliminary results from a European and US cross-cultural study. In Transcultural Study of Postnatal Depression (TCS-PND): Development and testing of harmonised research methods. British Journal of Psychiatry 184(suppl 46): 31–37.

Chisholm, D., Conroy, S., Glangeaud-Freudenthal, N.M.C., *et al.*, and the TCS-PND Group (2004). Health services research into postnatal depression: results from a preliminary cross-cultural study. In Transcultural Study of Postnatal Depression (TCS-PND): Development and testing of harmonised research methods. British Journal of Psychiatry 184(suppl 46): 45–52.

Corbin, J. and Strauss, A. (1990). Grounded theory method: procedures, canons and evaluative criteria. Qualitative Sociology, 13: 3–21.

Chisholm, D., Conroy, S., Glangeaud-Freudenthal, N.M.C., *et al.*, and the TCS-PND Group (2004). Health services research into postnatal depression: Results from a preliminary cross-cultural study. British Journal of Psychiatry suppl 46: 45–52.

Figueiredo, B. and Alegre, C. (2001). Pregnancy, delivery and post-partum experiences: similarities and differences in Portuguese mothers: From a Transcultural Study of Postnatal Depression (TCS-PND) Archives of Women's Mental Health 3(suppl 2): 53 (Abstract).

Glangeaud-Freudenthal, N.M.-C. (2002). Channi Kumar's contribution to perinatal psychiatry. A personal tribute from France. Psychological Medicine 32: 559–561.

Glangeaud-Freudenthal, N.M.-C. (2003). Channi Kumar and the History of the Marcé Society. Archives of Women's Mental Health 6(suppl 2): 79–82.

Glangeaud-Freudenthal, N., Garcia, S., Cukier-Hemeury, F., Dutilh, P., and Guedeney, N. (2001). Mother's perception of postpartum depression in France—is it different from father's perception? From a Transcultural Study of Postnatal Depression (TCS-PND). Archives of Women's Mental Health 3(suppl 2): 54 (Abstract).

Glaser, B. and Strauss, A. (1967). The discovery of grounded theory: Strategies for qualitative research. Chicago, Aldine.

Gorman, L.L., O'Hara, M.W., Figueiredo, B., *et al.*, and the TCS-PND Group (2004). Adaptation of the SCID for assessing depression in pregnant and postnatal women across countries and cultures. In Transcultural Study of Postnatal Depression (TCS-PND): Development and testing of harmonised research methods. British Journal of Psychiatry 184(suppl 46): 17–23.

Gunning, M., Conroy, S., Valoriani, V., *et al.*, and the TCS-PND Group (2004). Measurement of mother—infant interactions and the home environment in a European setting: Preliminary results from a cross-cultural study. In Transcultural Study of Postnatal Depression (TCS-PND): Development and testing of harmonised research methods. British Journal of Psychiatry 184 (suppl 46): 38–44.

Kammerer, M., Kammerer, E., Bollag, C., *et al.* (2001). Health services provision for patients with perinatal-psychiatric problems in Switzerland: From a Transcultural Study of Postnatal Depression (TCS-PND). Archives of Women's Mental Health 3(suppl 2): 53–4 (Abstract).

Marks, M.N. (2004). Introduction: Channi Kumar (1938–2000). In Transcultural Study of Postnatal Depression (TCS-PND): Development and testing of harmonised research methods. British Journal of Psychiatry 184(suppl 46): 1–2.

Marks, M., O'Hara, M., Glangeaud-Freudenthal, N. M.C., Guedeney, N., Klier, C., Figueiredo, B., and Benvenuti, P. (editors) (2004). Transcultural study of postnatal depression (TCS-PND): Development and testing of harmonised research methods. British Journal of Psychiatry, vol 184, (suppl 46).

Mason, J. (1996). Qualitative researching. London, Sage.

Miles, M.B. and Huberman, A.M. (1984). Qualitative data analysis: A sourcebook of new methods. Beverly Hills, CA, Sage.

Oates, M.R.Cox, J.L., Neema, S., *et al.* and the TCS-PND Group (2004). Postnatal depression across countries and cultures: A qualitative study. In Transcultural Study of Postnatal Depression

(TCS-PND): Development and testing of harmonised research methods. British Journal of Psychiatry **184**(suppl 46): 10–16.

Schmid-Siegel, B., Klier, C.M., Kumpf-Tonrsch, A., and Lenz, G. (2001). A obvious gap between somatic and psychosocial treatement in pregnancy, delivery and post-partum, in Austria: From a Transcultural Study of Postnatal Depression (TCS-PND). Archives of Women's Mental Health **3**(suppl 2): 53 (Abstract).

Wickberg, B. and Nordström, B. (2001). What do Swedish mothers and fathers think about happiness, unhappiness and mental health in the transition to parenthood period? From a Transcultural Study of Postnatal Depression (TCS-PND) Archives of Women's Mental Health **3**(suppl 2): 52–53 (Abstract).

Yoshida, K. (2001). Postnatal depression in Japanese women: modern and traditional aspects: From a Transcultural Study of Postnatal Depression (TCS-PND). Archives of Women's Mental Health **3**(suppl 2): 52 (Abstract).

Chapter 8

Development of the perinatal mental health service in Kyushu Japan

Research and clinical perspective

Keiko Yoshida, Hiroshi Yamashita,
and Shigenobu Kanba

Introduction

Postnatal depression (PND) in Japan, despite a traditional support system for perinatal women and cultural differences, is no less common than in western countries. Our previous two studies, which began in the 1990s, found that PND was experienced by about 15% of Japanese women. First, 98 Japanese women living in England (Yoshida *et al.* 1997) and then 88 Japanese women living in Japan (Yamashita *et al.* 2000) were recruited into two prospective studies of PND from late pregnancy to 3 postnatal months. Using the same research protocol and diagnostic method, (Schedule for Affective Disorders and Schizophrenia, Research Diagnostic Criteria), the incidence of PND was 12% and 17% respectively.

We have a traditional support system for perinatal women called *Satogaeri Bunben*. *Satogaeri* means returning to their home towns where their families of origin live and *Bunben* means delivery. Pregnant women return to their home towns several weeks prior to their delivery and remain there, with their babies, after delivery for a couple of months. It seems to be a very supportive system. However, *Satogaeri Bunben* itself did not lower the incidence of PND in either of the groups mentioned above. A disadvantage of *Satogaeri Bunben* is that a woman cannot be monitored by the same midwife or obstetrician and her husband has to work and live separately until their reunion in their marital home (Yoshida *et al.* 2001).

Most mothers with PND are unlikely to access psychiatric care, even though their depressive symptoms are serious (McIntosh 1993). Therefore neonatal home visits by health visitors were seen as a potentially useful opportunity for detecting mothers with PND. Luckily, a home visit system by community health visitors has been well organized throughout Japan since the late 1940's. In the past, the focus was on reducing infant death and promoting infant growth and development. In our city, the neonatal home visit service is provided for mother–baby dyads where (a) a baby's birth weight is less than 2500 g, (b) first-born babies with a birth weight of less than 2800 g, (c) babies with perinatal or pediatric physical health problems. In addition, mothers who request a home visit, mostly due to having difficulties in baby care or parenting problems, can also utilize this service. As mentioned earlier, health visitors tend to focus on the babies' physical health rather than on any potential psychological problems that the mothers may have. A lack of concern for the mothers' mental health seemed to be common and mental problems were easily overlooked even by those professionals unless a mother asked for their help.

One of my colleagues carried out a pilot study whose aims were to elucidate whether or not mothers who receive neonatal home visits tend to suffer from depressive disorders during the first postpartum year and to examine what kinds of factors were related to the postnatal depression observed in these mothers (Ueda *et al.* 2006). The subjects consisted of 70 Japanese mothers who received neonatal home visits and completed the one-year study. At 12 months postpartum, a diagnostic interview using the Structured Clinical Interview for DSM-IV (SCID, American Psychiatric Association 1994) was performed by a psychiatrist to confirm the maternal diagnosis. Nineteen mothers (27%) were categorized as having had a new onset of depression. In comparison to the non-depressed mothers, infant-related health problems that required either outpatient treatment or hospitalization were significantly related to postnatal depression. As a result, neonatal home visits by health visitors were seen as a potentially crucial opportunity to give emotional support, particularly for mothers with the extra burden of having to care for prematurely born babies or sick infants. Having found an important role of health visitors to detect postnatal women with depression and to support them, we developed an education and training system for health visitors covering the whole of Japan, using three simple, self-report questionnaires. These are: (1) a self-developed check list to pick up women who have risk factors for onset of PND, such as lack of emotional support, adverse life events, infant problems, and a past psychiatric history; (2) Edinburgh Postnatal Depression Scale for Japanese use with a cut-off point of 9 or more (Cox *et al.* 1987; Okano *et al.* 1996); and (3) a Japanese version of the Mother-to-Infant Bonding Scale (Yoshida *et al.* 2012). This nation-wide training showed substantial progress between the years 2004 and 2006 when funding was granted by the Ministry of Health and Labour (Grant holder: Yoshida), and the educational effect has been confirmed by one of our co-researchers (Kamibeppu *et al.* 2007, 2009).

Development of our mother–baby mental health clinic: care from pregnancy

Postnatal mental care has been developed little by little, based on research and practical trial. However, developing a service starting in pregnancy with collaborating obstetric specialists was a challenge for our university staff. In the field of mother–child mental health research and practice, knowledge of genetic influences, of developmental disorders such as attention deficit/hyperactivity disorder, has increased the opportunities for understanding the influence of the maternal stress during pregnancy (Glover 2011). It is recognized that a comprehensive estimation of the cumulative effect of various risk factors is essential for clinical research and the development of preventive interventions for mother–child mental health problems. The Mother–Infant Mental Health Clinic in Kyushu University Hospital has been providing pregnant women with specialist psychiatric care since 2002. We have investigated the clinical features of women who received assessment and care and the obstetric and developmental outcomes of their infants.

Staff and clinical services

The clinic consists of the staff working in the university hospital; obstetricians and midwives from the obstetric department and psychiatrists (Yoshida and Yamashita) and clinical psychologists from the Department of Child Psychiatry. Our services include; psychotherapy, providing information on the fetal risk factors of psychotropic drugs if pregnant women are on medication, optimal psychotropic drug administration for the mother and fetus, assessment and support for (mothering parenting), and evaluation of the infant's growth and development.

Recruitment

All pregnant women booked to deliver in our university hospital, who had no plan for artificial abortion and who had reached 30 weeks' to gestation were eligible for the study. The recruitment criteria were: (1) women with a current mental disorder, most of whom were receiving psychiatric treatment including psychopharmacotherapy; (2) women with a past psychiatric history; and (3) women who were in trouble or had psychosocial difficulties in domains such as lack of emotional support or apparent problems in parenting their baby. Women meeting any of these criteria are identified by the midwives or obstetricians and recommended to visit our clinic. All women gave written informed consent to accept referral to our service and to be monitored. The recruitment was carried out from 2002 to 2009.

Instruments and procedures

The prospective data collection and clinical care were carried out as follows. The Structured Clinical Interview for DSM-IV (SCID) was performed during the third trimester of pregnancy. Obstetric and paediatric data were obtained at delivery and at 1 postnatal month. The Edinburgh Postnatal Depression Scale (EPDS, Cox *et al.* 1987) was completed during late pregnancy, and at 5 days, 1 month, 4 months, and 7 months postnatally. At 1 month and 4 months postnatally, the Japanese version of the Mother-to-Infant Bonding Scale (MIBS, Yoshida *et al.* 2012) was administered. At 7 months, children's developmental outcomes were examined by the Denver Development Scale for their cognitive developmental level, including infants whose mothers took psychotropic drugs during their pregnancy.

Results of clinical survey

Psychiatric characteristics

One hundred and nine women and their infants were consecutively recruited and received our service. Women were categorized as having a mood disorder ($n = 29$) an anxiety disorder (*n* = 27), schizophrenia (*n* = 10), other psychiatric diagnoses (*n* = 21) (which were dissociative disorders, eating disorders, adjustment disorders, and personality disorders), or no major psychiatric disorder reaching diagnostic criteria according to DSM-IV but fulfilling 'other conditions that may be a focus of clinical attention' (APA 2000), such as relational problems, or abuse or neglect of a child (*n* = 22).

Maternal depression and bonding score

The proportion of women in each diagnostic group who scored at or over our chosen cut-off point on the EPDS during pregnancy and at one and four months post delivery, is shown in Table 8.1, together with the scores on the Mother-to-Infant Bonding Scale. There were statistically significant differences between all diagnostic groups for each of the scores (Kruskal–Wallis test, ** $p < 0.05$).

Infant's birth data in different categories of psychiatric diagnosis and developmental outcome

As shown in Tables 8.2 and 8.3, there was no obvious impact of mood or anxiety disorders on infant obstetric or developmental outcome. One child with developmental disorder was observed in both the mood disorder and schizophrenia groups.

Discussion and conclusions

The impact of mood or anxiety disorders on infant development was not obvious in our sample of mothers. Concern should be paid to the infants of mothers with schizophrenia due to their lower birth weight and possible risk of suffering from poor parenting from their mothers (Wan *et al.* 2008; Yoshida *et al*, 1999). Kumar *et al.* (1994) investigated 100 consecutive admissions to a mother and baby unit and reported that the proportion separated from their infant on discharge was 50% among the group with schizophrenia, and the proportion was much higher compared to the group with affective psychosis or non-psychotic disorders (8% and 4%, respectively). Kumar's in-patient subjects were more severely ill compared to our outpatient subject. Most of our subject mothers were married and all of them, including the mothers with schizophrenia, had a stable relationship with their partner.

Table 8.1 Maternal depression and bonding score

Diagnosis	EPDS score mean (SD)			Mother to Infant Bonding Mean (SD)	
	Late pregnancy	Postnatal 1 month	Postnatal 4 month	Postnatal 1 month	Postnatal 4 month
Mood disorder	18.3 (6.4)	12.4(7.8)	9.9 (6.5)	6.8 (6.9)	5.0 (7.0)
Anxiety disorder	14.6 (4.8)	10.0 (6.1)	9.3 (3.3)	4.0 (4.6)	2.2 (2.2)
Schizophrenia	9.0 (7.9)	7.7 (5.0)	5.3 (3.0)	4.4 (5.3)	2.3 (2.5)
Other diagnosis	15.5 (7.8)	10.5 (7.0)	9.3 (6.0)	2.9 (4.2)	3.3(5.8)
Other conditions	11.2 (5.8)	8.0 (4.0)	9.2 (5.9)	4.6 (5.4)	5.7 (6.7)

Table 8.2 Infant birth data according to maternal psychiatric diagnosis

Diagnosis	Gestation (weeks)	Body weight (g)		Apgar score	
		At birth	1 month	1 minute	5 minutes
Mood disorder	39.0	3077.6	3948.3	8.3	8.8
Anxiety disorder	38.6	3039.8	3998.2	8.5	9.0
Schizophrenia	38.4	2789.5	3784.6	7.8	8.8
Other diagnosis	38.2	2804.2	3548.2	7.8	8.6
Other conditions	39.1	2906.0	39.401	8.0	8.6

Table 8.3 Infant development according to maternal psychiatric diagnosis

Diagnosis	Denver Developmental Screening Test		
	Normal	Delayed	Not examined
Mood disorder	13	1	15
Anxiety disorder	15	0	12
Schizophrenia	6	1	3
Other diagnosis	5	0	16
Other conditions	14	1	7

Additionally, some of our patients were taking medication during pregnancy and also breast-fed their babies postnatally. Although no adverse outcome was observed among the infants, the range of treatment observed in this study means it is difficult to draw conclusions about the impact of specific medications on infant outcome.

Nevertheless, perinatal women and their infants should be monitored for a longer period of time than was possible in this study, because both mothers and infants are vulnerable in the context of the biological and psychological aspects of perinatal metal health problems.

References

American Psychiatric Association (1994). Diagnostic criteria from. DSM-IV-TR. Washington, DC, American Psychiatric Press.

Cox, J.L., Holden, J.M., and Sagovsky, R. (1987). Detection of postnatal depression. Development of the 10-item Edinburgh Postnatal Depression Scale. British Journal of Psychiatry **150**: 782–6.

Glover, V. (2011). Annual Research Review: Prenatal stress and the origins of psychopathology: an evolutionary perspective. Journal of Child Psychology and Psychiatry **52**(4): 356–67.

Kamibeppu, K., Nishigaki, K., Yamashita, H., Suzumiya, H., and Yoshida, K. (2007). Factors associated with skills of health visitors in maternal-infant mental health in Japan. BioScience Trends **1**(3): 149–55.

Kamibeppu, K., Furuta, M., Yamashita, H., *et al.* (2009). Training health professionals to detect and support mothers at risk of postpartum depression or infant abuse in the community: A cross-sectional and a before and after study. BioScience Trends **3**(1): 17–24.

Kumar, R., Marks, M., Platz, C., and Yoshida, K. (1994). Clinical survey of a psychiatric and baby unit characteristics of 100 consecutive admissions. Journal of Affective Disorders **33**: 11–22.

Mclntosh, J. (1993). Postpartum depression: women's help-seeking behaviour and perceptions of cause. Journal of Advanced Nursing **18**: 178–84.

Okano, T., Murata, M., Masuji, F., *et al.* (1996). Validation and reliability of Japanese version of EPDS (Edinburgh Postnatal Depression Scale). (in Japanese with English summary) Archives of Psychiatric Diagnosis and Clinical Evaluation. **7**: 525–33.

Ueda, M., Yamashita, H., and Yoshida, K. (2006). Impact of infant-related problems on postpartum depression: Pilot study to evaluate a health visiting system. Psychiatry and Clinical Neurosciences **60**(2): 182–9.

Wan, M.W., Moulton, S., and Abel, K.M. (2008). A review of mother-child relational interventions and their usefulness for mothers with schizophrenia. Archives of Women's Mental Health **11**(3): 171–9.

Yamashita, H., Yoshida, K., Nakano, H., and Tashiro, N. (2000). Postnatal depression in Japanese women. Detecting the early onset of postnatal depression by closely monitoring the postpartum mood. Journal of Affective Disorders **58**: 145–54.

Yoshida, K., Marks, M.N., Kibe, N., *et al.* (1997). Postnatal depression in Japanese women who have given birth in England. Journal of Affective Disorders **43**: 69–77.

Yoshida, K., Marks, M.N., Craggs, M., Smith, B., and Kumar, R. (1999). The sensorimotor and cognitivedevelopment of infants of mothers with schizophrenia. British Journal of Psychiatry **175**: 380–7.

Yoshida, K., Yamashita, H., Ueda, M., and Tashiro, N. (2001). Postnatal depression in Japanese mothers and the reconsideration of 'Satogaeri bunben'. *Pediatrics International* **43**: 189–93.

Yoshida, K., Yamashita, H., Conroy, S., Marks, M., Kumar, C. (2012). A Japanese version of Mother-to-Infant Bonding Scale: factor structure, longitudinal changes and links with maternal mood during the early postnatal period in Japanese mothers. Archives of Women's Mental Health **15**: 343–52.

Chapter 9

Maternal depression and child health

The case for integrating maternal mental health in Maternal and Child Health (MCH) Programmes

Atif Rahman

Introduction

While the physical health of women and children is emphasized in international policy guidelines, the mental dimensions of their health are often ignored, especially in developing countries. However, recent and strong evidence suggests that the mental and physical health of mothers and children is inextricably linked, and the one cannot be possible without the other (Prince *et al.* 2007). This chapter reviews the evidence and suggests directions for policy and research in this area.

Maternal depression in developing countries

Depression is the fourth leading cause of disease burden and the largest cause of non-fatal burden, accounting for almost 12% of all total years lived with disability worldwide. Depression around childbirth is common, affecting approximately 10–15% of all mothers in Western societies (O'Hara and Swain 1996). Epidemiological studies from the developing world have reported increasingly high rates of postnatal depression in diverse cultures across the developing world. An early pioneering study by Cox (1979) in a semirural Ugandan tribe found rates of 10% based on the ICD-8 criteria. Two decades later, a community study by Cooper *et al.* (1999) in a periurban settlement in South Africa, found rates of 34.7%, an increase of over threefold. Hospital-based studies have found rates of 23% in Goa, India (Patel *et al.* 2002), 22% in eastern Turkey (Inandi 2002) and 15.8% in Dubai, United Arab Emirates (Goubash and Abou-Saleh 1997). A rural-community study in Rawalpindi, Pakistan, reported over 25% women suffering from depression in the antenatal period and 28% in the postnatal period (Rahman *et al.* 2007). Over half these women were found to be still depressed a year later (Rahman and Creed 2007). A recent meta-analysis shows that the rates in low- and middle-income countries (LAMIC) are higher than high income countries, ranging from 18–25% (Fisher *et al.* 2012). Risk factors identified include previous psychiatric problems, life events in the previous year, poor marital relationship, lack of social support, and economic deprivation. Female infant gender was found to be an important determinant of postnatal depression in India, but not in South Africa. Importantly, postnatal depression was found to be associated with high degrees of chronicity, disability and disturbances of mother–infant relationship.

Can maternal depression increase infant risk of growth impairment and illness in developing countries?

Depression is a debilitating disorder, with symptoms such as depressed mood, tiredness, insomnia, lack of energy, low self-esteem and a lack of interest in the environment. It is also a disabling disorder. Patel and colleagues (Patel *et al.* 2002) found that postnatal depressed mothers scored significantly higher on the Brief Disability Questionnaire (an eight-item questionnaire that rates current problems in carrying out daily activities), spending about twice the number of days in the previous 30 days unable to complete their daily activities. Maternal competence in child care is likely to play a greater role in the child's physical well being and survival chances in developing countries, as the environment is frequently more hostile than in the developed world. Overcrowding, poor sanitation and food insecurity are common, with suboptimal maternal care potentially resulting in a greater risk to the physical health of a child. There is likely to be a particularly high risk during the first year of life, not only because this is a time of increased susceptibility of mothers to a depressive episode (a state which often becomes chronic) but also because it is during this period that the infant requires most care. Unlike a 2-year-old, and certainly a 5-year-old child, who might be able to seek food for themselves, the young infant is completely dependent on their carer to meet their every need. It is therefore at this age that deficiencies in care are most likely to manifest in a child's physical well being.

Two other bodies of evidence add plausibility to this question. The first is the large litera-ture documenting the effects of maternal depression on the psychological development of children. Four decades ago, Michael Rutter in a seminal monograph highlighted risks to the development of children of parents with a psychiatric disorder (Rutter 1966). Since then, studies have shown that maternal depression adversely effects the child's psychological de-velopment, intellectual competence, psychosocial functioning, and rate of psychiatric mor-bidity (Goodman and Gotlib 1999). The Avon Longitudinal Study of Parents and Children in the southwest UK also provides evidence that antenatal stress and postnatal depression in mothers leads to behavioural and emotional problems in their children (O'Connor *et al.* 2002). However, almost all of these studies have been carried out in developed countries, and the outcomes studied in children have usually been psychological rather than physical.

The second line of investigation has examined the quality of emotional care and psycho-social environment of the infant, showing an association with infant growth and well-being. Early observational studies by Widdowson (1951) in German orphanages indicated that the emotional quality of childcare influenced their growth. Kerr *et al.* (1978) in Kingston, Jamaica, found evidence of poor psychosocial functioning in mothers of malnourished children. These mothers had more chronically disrupted lives, unsupportive partners and fewer social contacts. Many of these mothers were described as 'apathetic' and 'dependant' by the authors. O'Callaghan and Hull (1978) compared 40 Caucasian children, ages between 3 months and 3 years, whose weights were below the 3rd centile, with 34 children from a similar background whose weights were between the 25th and 75th centile. In 23 out of the 40 malnourished children, organic illness was considered to be insufficient to explain the child being underweight. Three factors occurred more frequently in the malnourished group. The mother perceived herself as having disturbed mood and used the word 'depression' to describe these feelings. She also tended to come from a lower social class than the mother in the comparison group, and her infant had lower birthweight. While it is to be expected that infants with low birthweight would have greater chances of being underweight later in life, it is notable that women who are prenatally depressed give birth to babies with lower birthweight than normal mothers (Copper *et al.* 1996). Montgomery *et al.* (1997) studied a 1958 British cohort from the National Child Development Study and concluded that slow growth in childhood is associated with family conflict and this is independent of socioeconomic circumstances. It is therefore widely accepted that an adverse family and social environment can retard physical growth and development.

However, maternal depression as a risk factor for the child's physical health has so far received little attention, especially in developing countries where the parameters of infant health are dismally poor.

Recent evidence from south Asian and global studies

Two south Asian countries, namely Pakistan and India, have very high rates of maternal depression, and almost half the population under 5 years of age suffers from malnutrition, in spite of food sufficiency achieved by these countries. The region thus provides ideal settings to examine this question, and a number of studies have been carried out in the last 5 years (Patel *et al.* 2004). In Goa, India, Patel and colleagues (2003) carried out a hospital-based cohort study of mothers who had been diagnosed postnatal depression at 6–8 weeks after birth. Their infants were weighed and measured at 6 months age. Infants of mothers with depression had a relative risk of about 2 (95% confidence interval (CI) 1.1–4.7) for being underweight and about 3 (95% CI 1.3–6.8) for being short for age. These associations remained statistically significant after adjustment for other variables influencing growth, such as birth-weight and exclusive breast-feeding.

In Rawalpindi, Pakistan, we carried out a case–control study of healthy and age-matched infants brought to an immunization clinic for their 8-month measles vaccine. (Rahman *et al.* 2004a). Mothers of 82 malnourished and 90 well-nourished infants were administered the self-reporting questionnaire (SRQ-20), a psychiatric screening instrument. Mental distress determined by World Health Organization (WHO) SRQ-20 was associated with increased risk of undernutrition in infants (odds ratio 3.9, 95% CI 1.95–7.86). The association remained significant after adjustment for birth weight, economic status, maternal age and literacy, sex of infant and family structure.

In a community based case–control study of risk factors for malnutrition in children aged 6–12 months in Tamil Nadu, India (Anoop *et al.* 2004), the odds ratio for postpartum depression was 7.4 ($p = 0.01$). This association remained significant after adjustment for maternal intelligence, birth weight, breast feeding, immunization and economic status.

Further strong evidence of the link between maternal depression and infant outcomes is provided by our 1-year prospective cohort study of 320 mothers and their infants in Rawalpindi, Pakistan (Rahman *et al.* 2004b) It showed that infants of antenatally depressed mothers had poorer growth than controls. The relative risk for being underweight (weight-for-age *z*-score < –2SD) was 4.0 (95%CI 2.1–7.7) at 6 months and 2.6 (95% CI 1.7–4.1) at 12 months, while the risks for stunting (length-for-age *z*-score < –2SD) was 4.4 (95%CI 1.7–11.4) at 6 months and 2.5 (95% CI 1.6–4.0) at 12 months. Chronic depression (depression persisting for over a year) carried a greater risk for poor outcome than episodic depression. The associations remain significant after adjustment for confounders by multivariate analyses. The data suggests that the population-attributable risk of stunting at the age of 1 year (i.e. the proportion by which the incidence of infant stunting would be reduced if maternal depression were eliminated from the population), is 30%. Infants of depressed mothers also have lower birth weight, higher rates of diarrhoea, and are less likely to be immunized. Thus, maternal depression makes an important and possibly major contribution to poor infant growth outcomes and morbidity in less resourced countries.

This evidence has been strengthened by recent reviews which include studies from all over the world, showing that maternal depression has strong and independent associations with preterm birth and low birthweight (Grote *et al.* 2010), undernutrition in the first year of life (Surkan *et al.* 2011; Stewart 2009), higher rates of diarrheal diseases, and early cessation of breastfeeding (Wachs *et al.* 2009).

Possible mechanisms linking maternal depression to infant morbidity

There are a number of possible mechanisms that could link maternal depression to physical morbidity in their young children (Rahman *et al.* 2002). The first is through the risks that antenatal depression could pose to the unborn infant. In developed countries it has been shown that depressed women are more likely than non-depressed women to obtain inadequate antenatal care (Pagel *et al.* 1990). This is likely to be a consequence of social withdrawal and poor problem solving skills associated with depression. Studies in developed countries have also found increased rates of premature births and lower birth weight among the infants of depressed versus non-depressed mothers (Hedegaard *et al.* 1993; Hoffman and Hatch 2000). In developing countries where antenatal care is more difficult to acquire, depression in mothers could influence the level of care received, increasing the incidence of low birth weight, and subsequent infant morbidity and mortality. Depression is also associated with risk taking lifestyles such as smoking and unhealthy eating (Milberger *et al.* 1996), which could further increase the risks to the fetus.

The second set of mechanisms involves the direct impact that depressive symptoms have on parenting. Depressed mothers in developed countries have been observed to provide less quantity and poorer quality of stimulation for their infants (Cooper *et al.* 1999) and to be slower in responding and less responsive to them (Livingood *et al.* 1983). Depressed mothers are also more likely to have negative views of themselves as parents, seeing themselves as having less personal control over their child's development, and less able to positively influence their children (Goodman and Gotlib 1999). It might therefore be expected that in developing countries these symptoms could influence maternal care behaviours, which in turn increase the child's susceptibility to illness. For example, in Thailand, mothers who washed their hands before breastfeeding, gave their child food immediately after cooking, and warmed infant foods before meals, had infants with significantly less diarrhoea compared to those who did not. This is also true for other care activities of mothers such as breastfeeding practice, preparation of appropriate weaning foods, uptake of immunizations, and care-seeking behaviours when children are ill. It could be expected that depression in mothers could adversely influence these activities.

A third potential mechanism linking maternal depression to physical morbidity in children is through its links with negative life events and chronic psychosocial difficulties. There is evidence that depressed mothers can act in ways that increase the risks that their children will experience adversity. For example, longitudinal research from the USA suggests that the children of depressed mothers are exposed to a much greater number of stressors, such as family discord, than the children of nondepressed mothers (Goodman and Gotlib 1999). As mentioned above, psychosocial adversity and family conflict in childhood has been associated with poor growth, particularly stunting, in children.

There are likely to be complex interactions between factors in the child's social and economic environment, home environment, mother and the child. While the interaction between these factors may be more important than any one individual risk factor, poor maternal mental health may be a common denominator and thus an important indicator, as well as a mechanism, of risk to the child. Furthermore, depression is a treatable disorder and therefore its possible association with poor child health assumes even greater public health implication, as potential intervention strategies could have a bearing on health outcomes of both mother and child.

Further exploratory research

Further epidemiological and anthropological studies can help identify important moderators, many of which may be culture-specific. Women's status in society, their own and society's perceptions of their role in childcare, and the inter-relationship of their mental and physical health would be important areas for further exploration. The gradual erosion of the traditional extended family and the impact of this on childcare practices, family support, and maternal psychological state in societies undergoing rapid transition may be important to understand.

Such studies also need to explore the mediating effects of mother–infant interactions in malnourished infants of depressed mothers. High maternal responsiveness to child's needs for food and comfort may have a direct bearing its growth, while increased stimulation may improve the child's exploratory behaviour, levels of physical activity and improved general health. It also needs to be considered that mother–infant interactions are two-way. Thus the child's innate temperament may influence maternal mood and behaviour in ways that affect the nutritional outcome in the infant.

The important mediating effects of feeding behaviour in maternal depression have not been fully explored (Tomlinson and Landman 2007). Along with duration of breastfeeding, the timing of introduction of solid food, the manner of its preparation, storage and dispensation may differ between depressed and non-depressed mothers. The educational status of the mothers and the presence of other skilled family members may modify this effect, and this needs further investigation.

Another possible mediating factor could be the difference in attributional styles of depressed and non-depressed mothers. Studies show that depressed mothers are more likely to have negative views of themselves as parents, seeing themselves as having less personal control over their child's development, and less able to positively influence their children (Goodman and Gotlib 1999). This may affect the way they cope with adversity such as poor infant health.

Development and evaluation of interventions

There is considerable potential for interventions aimed at promoting the mental health of mothers that couldnot only reduce the burden of disease in these mothers, but also improve the physical well-being and psychological development of their offspring. A number of individual and group interventions targeting maternal depression have been developed and tested, mostly in developed countries. Treatment trials have shown that non-directive counselling by health visitors, dynamic psychotherapy, cognitive behaviour counselling, and antidepressants are all effective (Sockol *et al.* 2011; Stuart *et al.* 2003). An interesting intervention that addresses not just maternal mood, but mother–infant relationship in a disadvantaged South African population found no impact on maternal mood but significant improvements in mother-infant relationship (Cooper *et al.* 2009).

Group-based approaches have usually been used to improve outcomes in children through parent-training programmes. A meta-analysis of such programmes shows that these can also be effective in improving psychosocial and mental health of the mothers (Barlow and Coren 2003).

However, a number of health system and cultural differences make it difficult for mental health interventions to be extrapolated from the developed to the developing world (Patel 2000). Treatments are unlikely to be adopted by professionals and policy makers unless they are shown to be efficacious, cost-effective, integrated in existing community health services, and linked to other health problems perceived to be higher in priority. Multimodal or combined interventions are more likely to fit these criteria. For example, a multimodal intervention for depressed mothers could include support for the mother, nutritional and practical child-care knowledge, and responsive parenting techniques, all delivered in a psychologically therapeutic manner. These could also have relatively lesser delivery costs, less duplication of services, and appropriate identification of those who are most likely to benefit; and families are more likely to be motivated to seek such services where outcomes such as infant growth are perceived to be more tangible (WHO 1999).

We have developed a psychosocial intervention along these lines for depressed mothers and their infants living in rural Pakistan. Called the 'Thinking Healthy Programme (THP)' (Rahman 2007), it is based on our findings that maternal depression probably affects infant development and growth through multiple processes. Disability due to depressive symptoms (such as fatigue, poor concentration, loss of interest) is likely to affect child-care abilities directly, while impaired social functioning is likely to have indirect consequences through lack of support in childcare. Disturbances in mother–infant relationship in depressed mothers would negatively influence the infant's development. THP is designed to target these processes and includes a supportive component (non-directive empathic listening), an educational component (nutritional and healthcare advice, delivered within a cognitive-behaviour framework), and a mother–infant relationship component (warmth, attentive listening, stimulation, and support for exploration and autonomy for the infant). The objective is to help mothers feel supported, empowered and confident about their parenting abilities, and through this process positively influence their mood. Rather than the directive approach of the medical model, health workers are trained to adopt a more patient-centred approach, tailoring the three components according to individual needs of the patient.

The Thinking Healthy Programme has been evaluated through a randomised controlled trial in Pakistan (Rahman *et al.* 2008). Using a community-based sample of mothers, 15 individual home-based counselling sessions based on cognitive behavioral therapy were delivered by community health workers to intervention participants and controls. When evaluated at 6 months postpartum only 23% of women in the intervention group, versus 53% in the control group had major depression, results which were sustained a year following the intervention. There were also a number of positive outcomes in the children, such as less frequent diarrhoea, higher rates of contraceptive use, and increased time that mothers engaged in play with their children (Rahman *et al.* 2008).

Further trials in this area are warranted. These can also provide information on moderators and mediators of treatment outcomes (Kraemer *et al.* 2002). Treatment moderators would specify for whom or under what circumstances the treatment works. They would also suggest to public health professionals which at-risk groups might be most responsive to intervention and for which groups other, more appropriate, treatments might be sought. Moderators may also identify subpopulations with possibly different causal mechanisms or course of illness.

Treatment mediators could identify possible mechanisms through which a treatment might achieve its effects. Thus, in testing a multimodal intervention, both health-seeking behaviour and mother–infant interaction could be studied for change with intervention.

The mediator that shows the most change in relation to improved outcome could help determine the focus of future interventions.

Implications for child health policy

Traditionally, child health programmes have focused on short-term, disease specific, technologically dependant strategies aimed at achieving a high rate of success in relatively short time (Claeson and Waldman 2000). An example is the successful smallpox eradication programme. Subsequently, however, the limited success of ambitious programmes such as the malaria eradication programme launched in the 1950s and abandoned in the 1970s, led to a change in strategy towards more people-centred rather than disease-specific programmes of health care. New programmes were launched under this strategy that were more primary-care and community based. These include provisions such as universal services for maternal and child health, family planning, improved sanitation and water supplies, the emphasis shifting from clinic-based curative interventions to prevention through a multisectoral approach and community involvement. These two types of strategies are not mutually exclusive, and recent programmes such as the Integrated Management of Childhood Illnesses (IMCI) initiative (WHO 2001) combine many aspects of both. The IMCI programme focuses on under-nutrition, diarrhoea, and acute respiratory infections as most important contributors to increased child mortality, but incorporates community participation and development of health systems, combined with medical technology as the major approach towards their eradication.

As child health strategies evolve further, focus is increasingly turning to the household as a centre of child health activity. As Claeson and Waldman (2000) state:

> In all cases, further improvements (in child health gains) will depend to a large extent on what happens in the household and community and to what extent the health system is responsive and will play a supportive part. The promotion of a limited set of household behaviours that have a direct link to the prevention and cure of common childhood illnesses needs to become the centrepiece of intensified activity.

These household behaviours, such as infant feeding practices, immunization, home-health, and care-seeking practices rely heavily on the mother, who is the primary care-provider in most developing societies. Implicit, therefore, in this approach to achieving good health outcomes in children is the recognition that this will need to depend not only on interventions in childhood, but also on the psychological health and receptivity of the mother.

One way to conceptualize the critical role of maternal depression in child survival is to see it as both a *marker* as well as a *mechanism* for poor infant health. This has implications for prevention as well as intervention. As a marker, depression can be identified with relative ease, using simple checklists that have excellent validity. The use of these instruments can help identify a group of mothers whose infants are at greater risk of poor health. Resources can then be targeted at this group. It might be feasible, for example, to include the assessment of maternal mental health, into the World Health Organization's

ICMI strategy. There is already advice to check mother's understanding of home based interventions, and observe her practice, but in the section on maternal health, mental state is not addressed (WHO 2001) Health workers could be taught simple mental health techniques to engage with these mothers, provide counselling, practical help, and advice on child health in a more effective way. Encouragement of positive mother–infant interaction with infants in depressed mothers is likely to benefit not only their physical, but also psychological and cognitive development. We have described above the Thinking Healthy Programme that utilizes this approach.

Implications for women's health policy

There is a widespread lack of awareness of mental health issues in developing countries, and mental illness carries a stigma that hinders treatment seeking (Claeson and Waldman 2000). Mental health remains low on the agenda of planners and policy-makers in the developing world. If maternal mental health and child physical health were shown to be linked, this could help bring maternal mental health up the healthcare agenda in a manner that could be culturally and socially acceptable.

Even if greater awareness towards mental health issues were achieved, what could be done about it? In the last two decades, significant developments have taken place in the pharmacological and psychosocial treatment of depression. At the same time, a number of innovative strategies that have led to the development of quality health services in even some of the poorest countries (Patel *et al.* 2007). Most approaches employ common principles, calling for services to be decentralized, multisectoral, culturally relevant, and sustainable.

An example of such a programme relevant to maternal depression is the Perinatal Mental Health Project, based at the Mowbray Maternity Hospital in the Western Cape Province of South Africa, which developed a stepped care intervention for maternal mental health that is integrated into antenatal care (Honikman *et al.* 2012). Mowbray Maternity Hospital is a secondary level maternity hospital, linked to the University of Cape Town, and located centrally within the city. The Perinatal Mental Health Project services are based at the hospital within the Midwife Obstetric Unit, which provides a primary level antenatal clinic. Midwives at the Midwife Obstetric Unit are trained to screen women routinely for maternal mood disorders during their antenatal visits. Those who screen positive are referred to on-site counsellors who also act as case managers. Where specialist intervention is indicated, women are referred to an on-site psychiatrist. The Perinatal Mental Health Project works directly with facility managers and health workers through collaborative partnerships, focusing on problem solving and capacity development in the primary health care system. Over a 3-year period, 90% of all women attending antenatal care in the maternity clinic were offered mental health screening with 95% uptake. Of those screened, 32% qualified for and received counselling through the programme.

A number of important lessons have been learned from this programme: (a) maternity health workers may be trained to screen for and refer mental distress in low-resource primary care settings; (b) training programmes that address and support the mental health needs of health workers may help staff to manage their workload and prevent compassion fatigue and 'burn out'; (c) on-site screening and counselling fosters the establishment of efficient referral mechanisms and access to mental health care often lacking in maternity settings in LAMIC; (d) on-site, integrated mental health services increase access for women who have scarce resources and competing health, family, and economic priorities; (e) coordinating mental health visits with subsequent antenatal visits further facilitates access for women with insufficient resources.

At the same time, epidemiologic and anthropologic data indicate that the origins of such high rates of depression in women can be traced to the social circumstances of their lives. As Desjarlais and colleagues point out (1995):

> Hopelessness, exhaustion, anger and fear grow out of hunger, overwork, violence, and economic dependence. Understanding the sources of ill health for women means understanding how cultural and economic forces interact to undermine their social status. If the goal of improving women's well-being from childhood through old age is to be achieved, healthy policies aimed at improving the social status of women are needed along with health policies targeting the entire spectrum of women's health needs.

But it is often hard to develop an impetus to change the direction of such culturally well-entrenched forces that undermine women's status. Once again, linking maternal well being to child health can provide a universally acceptable 'window of opportunity' for creating such an impetus, leading to policies aimed at uplifting the social status of women, and in the process, improving their and their children's physical and mental well-being.

The association between maternal depression and child health could also help the building of bridges between disciplines in healthcare. Healthy policy and research is often narrowly focused—mental health professionals focus on strategies for mental health care provision and child health professionals on strategies for reducing child morbidity and mortality. Interventions such as the Thinking Healthy Programme would, by necessity, derive their theoretical and practical framework from many disciplines including paediatrics, psychiatry, primary care, sociology, public health, epidemiology, and medical anthropology. We feel such a multidisciplinary and holistic approach to health care is more likely to succeed than a narrowly focused one.

Acknowledgement

This article was originally published in the *Harvard Health Policy Review* (2005 autumn issue) and this updated version has been reproduced with permission of the journal.

References

Anoop, S., Saravanan, B., Joseph, A., Cherian, A., and Jacob, K.S. (2004). Maternal depression and low maternal intelligence as risk factors for malnutrition in children: a community based case-control study from South India. Archives of Diseases of Childhood **89**(4): 325–9.

Barlow J, Coren E, Stewart-Brown S. Parent-training programmes for improving maternal psychosocial health. Cochrane Database of Systematic Reviews 2003, Issue 4. Art. No.: CD002020. DOI: 10.1002/14651858.CD002020.pub2.

Claeson, M. and Waldman, R.J. (2000). The evolution of child health programmes in developing countries: from targeting diseases to targeting people. Bulletin of the World Health Organization **78**(10): 1234–45.

Cooper, P.J, Tomlinson, M., Swartz, L., *et al.* (2009). Improving quality of mother-infant relationship and infant attachment in socioeconomically deprived community in South Africa: randomised controlled trial. BMJ **338**: b974.

Cooper, P.J., Tomlinson, M., Swartz, L., *et al.* (1999). Post-partum depression and the mother-infant relationship in a South African peri-urban settlement. British Journal of Psychiatry **175**: 554–8.

Copper, R.L., Goldenberg, R.L., Das, A., *et al.* (1996). The preterm prediction study: maternal stress is associated with spontaneous preterm birth at less than thirty-five weeks' gestation. National Institute of Child Health and Human Development Maternal-Fetal Medicine Units Network. American Journal of Obstetrics and Gynecology **175**(5): 1286–92.

Cox, J.L. (1979). Psychiatric morbidity and pregnancy: a controlled study of 263 semi-rural Ugandan women. British Journal of Psychiatry **134**: 401–5.

Desjarlais, R., Eisenberg, L., Good, B., and Kleinman, A. (1995). World Mental Health: problems and priorities in low income countries. Oxford, Oxford University Press.

Fisher, J., de Mello, M.C., Patel, V., *et al.* (2012) Prevalence and determinants of common perinatal mental disorders in women in low- and lower-middle-income countries: a systematic review. Bulletin of the World Health Organization **90**:139–149

Ghubash, R. and Abou-Saleh, M.T. (1997). Postpartum psychiatric illness in Arab culture: prevalence and psychosocial correlates. British Journal of Psychiatry **171**: 65–8.

Goodman, S.H. and Gotlib, I.H. (1999). Risk for psychopathology in the children of depressed mothers: a developmental model for understanding mechanisms of transmission. Psychological Reviews **106**(3): 458–90.

Grote, N.K., Bridge, J.A., Gavin, A.R., *et al.* (2010). A meta-analysis of depression during pregnancy and the risk of preterm birth, low birth weight, and intrauterine growth restriction. Archives of General Psychiatry **67**(10): 1012–24.

Hedegaard, M., Henriksen, T.B., Sabroe, S., and Secher, N.J. (1993). Psychological distress in pregnancy and preterm delivery. BMJ **307**(6898): 234–9.

Hoffman, S. and Hatch, M.C. (2000). Depressive symptomatology during pregnancy: evidence for an association with decreased fetal growth in pregnancies of lower social class women. Health Psychology **19**: 535–43.

Honikman, S., van Heyningen, T., Field, S., Baron, E., and Tomlinson, M. (2012). Stepped care for maternal mental health: a case study of the perinatal mental health project in South Africa. PLoS Med **9**(5): e1001222.

Inandi T, Elci OC, Ozturk A, Egri M, Polat A, Sahin TK (2002). Risk factors for depression in postnatal first year, in eastern Turkey. International Journal of Epidemiology **31**: 1201–7.

Kerr, M.A., Bogues, J.L., and Kerr, D.S. (1978). Psychosocial functioning of mothers of malnourished children. Pediatrics **62**(5): 778–84.

Kraemer, H.C., Wilson, G.T., Fairburn, C.G., and Agras, W.S. (2002). Mediators and moderators of treatment effects in randomized clinical trials. Archives of General Psychiatry **59**(10): 877–83.

Livingood, A.B., Daen, P., and Smith, B.D. (1983). The depressed mother as a source of stimulation for her infant. Journal of Clinical Psychology **39**(3): 369–75.

Milberger, S., Faraone, S.V., Biederman, J., Testa, M., and Tsuang, M.T. (1996). New phenotype definition of attention deficit hyperactivity disorder in relatives for genetic analyses. American Journal of Medical Genetics **67**(4): 369–77.

Montgomery, S.M., Bartley, M.J., and Wilkinson, R.G. (1997). Family conflict and slow growth. Archives of Diseases of Childhood **77**(4): 326–30.

O'Callaghan, M.J. and Hull, D. (1978). Failure to thrive or failure to rear? Archives of Diseases of Childhood **53**(10): 788–93.

O'Connor, T.G., Heron, J., Golding, J., Beveridge, M., and Glover, V. (2002). Maternal antenatal anxiety and children's behavioural/emotional problems at 4 years. Report from the Avon Longitudinal Study of Parents and Children. British Journal of Psychiatry **180**: 502–8.

O'Hara, M.W. and Swain, A.M. (1996). Rates and risk of postpartum depression: a meta-analysis. International Review of Psychiatry **8**: 37–54.

Pagel, M.D., Smilkstein, G., Regen, H., and Montano, D. (1990). Psychosocial influences on new born outcomes: a controlled prospective study. Social Science and Medicine **30**(5): 597–604.

Patel, V. (2000). The need for treatment evidence for common mental disorders in developing countries. Psychological Medicine **30**(4): 743–6.

Patel, V., Araya, R., Chatterjee, S., *et al.* (2007). Treatment and prevention of mental disorders in low-income and middle-income countries. Lancet **370**(9591): 991–1005.

Patel, V., Rodrigues, M., and DeSouza, N. (2002). Gender, poverty, and postnatal depression: a study of mothers in Goa, India. American Journal of Psychiatry **159**(1): 43–7.

Patel, V., DeSouza, N., and Rodrigues, M. (2003). Postnatal depression and infant growth and development in low income countries: a cohort study from Goa, India. Archives of Diseases of Childhood **88**(1): 34–7.

Patel, V., Rahman, A., Jacob, K.S., and Hughes, M. (2004). Effect of maternal mental health on infant growth in low income countries: new evidence from South Asia. BMJ **328**(7443): 820–3.

Prince, M., Patel, V., Saxena, S., *et al.* (2007). No health without mental health. Lancet **370**(9590): 859–77.

Rahman, A. (2007). Challenges and opportunities in developing a psychological intervention for perinatal depression in rural Pakistan—a multi-method study. Archives of Womens Mental Health **10**(5): 211–9.

Rahman, A. and Creed, F. (2007). Outcome of prenatal depression and risk factors associated with persistence in the first postnatal year: prospective study from Rawalpindi, Pakistan. Journal of Affective Disorders **100**(1–3): 115–21.

Rahman, A., Harrington, R., and Bunn, J. (2002). Can maternal depression increase infant risk of illness and growth impairment in developing countries? Child Care and Health Development **28**(1): 51–6.

Rahman, A., Iqbal, Z., and Harrington, R. (2003). Life events, social support and depression in childbirth: perspectives from a rural community in the developing world. Psychological Medicine **33**(7): 1161–7.

Rahman, A., Lovel, H., Bunn, J., Iqbal, Z., and Harrington, R. (2004a). Mothers' mental health and infant growth: a case-control study from Rawalpindi, Pakistan. Child Care and Health Development **30**(1): 21–7.

Rahman, A., Iqbal, Z., Bunn, J., Lovel, H., and Harrington, R. (2004b). Impact of maternal depression on infant nutritional status and illness: a cohort study. Archives of General Psychiatry **61**(9): 946–52.

Rahman, A., Malik, A., Sikander, S., Roberts, C., and Creed, F. (2008). Cognitive behaviour therapy-based intervention by community health workers for mothers with depression and their infants in rural Pakistan: a cluster-randomised controlled trial. Lancet **372**(9642): 902–9.

Rutter, M. (1966). Children of sick parents: an environmental and psychiatric study. London, Maudsley Monographs.

Sockol, L.E., Epperson, C.N., and Barber, J.P. (2011). A meta-analysis of treatments for perinatal depression. Clinical Psychology Reviews **31**(5): 839–49.

Stewart, R.C. (2009). Maternal depression and infant growth: a review of recent evidence. Maternal & Child Nutrition **3**(2): 94–107.

Stuart, S., O'Hara, M.W., and Gorman, L.L. (2003). The prevention and psychotherapeutic treatment of postpartum depression. Archives of Womens Mental Health **6**(Suppl 2): S57–S69.

Surkan, P.J., Kennedy, C.E., Hurley, K.M., and Black, M.M. (2011). Maternal depression and early childhood growth in developing countries: systematic review and meta-analysis. Bulletin of the World Health Organization **89**(8): 608–15.

Tomlinson, M. and Landman, M. (2007). 'It's not just about food': mother-infant interaction and the wider context of nutrition. Maternal and Child Nutrition **3**(4): 292–302.

Wachs, T.D., Black, M.M., and Engle, P.L. (2009). Maternal depression: a global threat to children's health, development, and behavior and to human rights. Child Development Perspectives **3**: 51–9.

Widdowson, E.M. (1951). Mental contentment and physical growth. Lancet **195**: 1316–8.

World Health Organization (1999). A critical link: Interventions for physical growth and psychological development—A review. Geneva, World Health Organisation.

World Health Organization (2001). IMCI Care for Development: For the healthy growth and development of children. Geneva, World Health Organization—Department of Child and Adolescent Health and Development.

Section 3

The effects of perinatal mental disorders on the mother–offspring dyad

Chapter 10

Maternal and offspring mental health
From bench to bedside

Susan Pawlby and Deborah Sharp

Introduction

Translational research has become one of the key concepts of medical science in the 21st century, with academics and clinicians coming together in a joint effort to bring findings from basic research into the clinical setting so that they can benefit patients. Channi Kumar may not have recognized this phrase, but his work was truly translational. Indeed his perinatal research programme was bi-directional in its translation. As a clinician and an academic, Channi's research was informed by his clinical work with mothers suffering from severe mental illness (SMI) following childbirth. He recognized the importance of treating a mother's mental illness, while at the same supporting her in the care of her baby. His clinical work on the Mother and Baby Unit at the Bethlem Royal Hospital gave rise to research into the understanding of antenatal and postnatal mental illness and its effects on the child as well as into improving services and treatment for women and their babies.

In this chapter we will show how two of Channi's flagship studies, the South London Child Development Study (SLCDS) and a video feedback intervention programme on the Mother and Baby Unit, continue to gather evidence and to inform perinatal guidelines in the 21st century.

The South London Child Development Study

The SLCDS is unique in that it is one of the first longitudinal studies of women's mental health and its impact on the children to begin during pregnancy. Specifically, families from two inner-city London General Practice sites were initially recruited into a longitudinal prospective study of emotional disorders related to childbirth when the women were pregnant between 1 January and 31 December 1986. It has followed the lives of 151 families through pregnancy and the index child's first year, with 86% participating when the index child was 4 years, 89% at 11 years, and 83% at 16 years. At the outset of the study, the mean age of the women was 25.9 years (range 16–43 years); 60% were married, 32% had a regular partner, and 8% were single; 78% were of white British origin; 86% were working class; 30%

had no educational qualifications. Seven phases of standardized interviews, assessments, and observations, with mothers, fathers, and the index children, as well as information from teachers, have enabled us to identify pathways to poor well-being, academic difficulties and adverse social outcomes, from fetal life into adolescence. Currently (2012–2013) we are interviewing the offspring as young adults, aged 25 years.

One of the most striking findings from the SLCDS was the high prevalence rate of maternal depression in pregnancy and throughout the offspring's childhood. The period prevalence of depression as ascertained by the Clinical Interview Schedule (CIS: Goldberg et al. 1970) was 33% during pregnancy and 32% in the first postnatal year; furthermore, the period prevalence of maternal depression, as ascertained by the Schedule for Affective Disorders and Schizophrenia—Lifetime version (SADS-L: Spitzer et al. 1978), was 35% between the child's first and fourth birthday, 25% between the child's fourth and eleventh birthday, and 29% between the child's 11th and 16th birthday. During the 17-year period of the study almost two-thirds of the women had been clinically depressed (Pawlby et al. 2009). Moreover we found that almost all (90.5%) of the women who were depressed in pregnancy had one or more further episodes of depression during the offspring's childhood. Indeed, compared to women who were not depressed in pregnancy, they were almost 10 times more likely to become depressed again and their offspring were exposed to three times as many periods of maternal depression.

Another striking finding was the 3-month rate of psychopathology among the study offspring, ascertained through interview with the Child and Adolescent Psychiatric Assessment (CAPA: Angold et al. 1995). At both 11 years and at 16 years 25% of the offspring had a psychiatric diagnosis (at both ages 9% had a diagnosis of an emotional disorder, 9% of a behavioural disorder and 7% were comorbid). We also found that the structure of the family in which the children were living changed over the period of study. At the 16-year assessment 49% of the children were living with their two biological parents, compared with 87% at the child's first birthday. Specifically, at age 16, 17% of children lived with the biological mother and her new partner, 25% with the biological mother only, 6% with their fathers; four children lived in other family arrangements and two lived independently. Furthermore 38% of the children gained no passes in the national examinations taken at the end of 12 years of full time education in England.

The initial findings of the SLCDS showed that psychosocial factors in pregnancy, such as marital conflict, insufficient social support, lower age at first birth, financial problems, unemployment, and past emotional health problems, were associated with maternal depression in pregnancy and post partum (Sharp 1993). At subsequent assessments, we have found that these factors are also associated with emotional, behavioural and cognitive outcomes in the children. However, our results have shown that the impact of these factors on the children is mediated by the mother's mental health problems (i.e. depression), either in pregnancy or in the postpartum period. For example, compared with children whose mothers are well, children of mothers with depression post partum have lower IQ scores at 4, 11, and 16 (Sharp et al. 1995; Hay et al. 2001; 2008), with boys being most affected. At 11 years they were also more likely to have problems with reading comprehension and mathematical reasoning tasks and to have a statement of educational need (Hay *et al.* 2001). In contrast, behavioural and emotional problems were associated with maternal depression in *pregnancy*. Maternal *antenatal* depression is a significant predictor of off-spring antisocial behaviour, especially acts of violence, in adolescence, even after control-ling for prior sociodemographic factors, the child's later exposure to maternal depression, the mother's smoking and drinking during pregnancy, and parents' antisocial behaviour (Hay *et al.* 2010). Without exception, all the children who suffered depression in adoles-cence had mothers who were depressed at some point during their lives, with 65% of such children being exposed to depression for the first time in utero, during their mother's pregnancy (Pawlby *et al.* 2009). Thus, one of the key findings to emerge from the SLCDS is that maternal depression in the perinatal period, either before or after the birth, is as-sociated with difficulties in the regulation of emotion in the children. This is supported by a number of on-going prospective, longitudinal research studies showing the adverse impact of exposure to mild-to-moderate anxiety or depression in the perinatal period on the offspring into childhood (O'Connor *et al.* 2002) and adolescence (Halligan *et al.* 2007; Murray *et al.* 2010; for a review, see Brand and Brennan 2009).

A further novel finding from the SLCDS is that maternal mental health in pregnancy contributes to the accumulating evidence of the association between maltreatment and psychopathology (Danese *et al.* 2008). We have shown (Pawlby *et al.* 2011) that the off-spring's exposure to both maternal depression in utero *and* the experience of maltreatment in childhood increases 12-fold the risk of depression and/or conduct disorder in adoles-cence. Furthermore we found that a woman's experience of maltreatment in her own child-hood increases the risk of her developing depression in pregnancy and their co-occurrence significantly increases offspring childhood maltreatment and adolescent antisocial behav-iour (Plant *et al.* 2012). We thus show that maternal depression in pregnancy plays an exac-erbating role in the intergenerational transmission of maltreatment and psychopathology.

A case history

The adolescent offspring of a mother diagnosed as depressed in pregnancy (this case is a composite and identifying information has been altered in order to protect confidentiality).

Renee was interviewed in the second trimester of pregnancy and diagnosed as being depressed. She regretted being pregnant and was worried that she wouldn't be a good mother, despite being a mother of two other children. Renee had no wish to breast feed or look after the baby. One year after the birth, Renee continued to be depressed and reported having frequent urges to throw the baby out of the window or put a pillow over her head. At the 11-year-old interview Renee described her daughter, Beatrice, as 'feeling hopeless when she was in my tummy. Nothing positive has ever come out of anything she has done. There was something different about this child'. Renee drew parallels between her relationship as a child with her own mother and that between Beatrice and herself. She had been physically and emotionally abused by her own mother. Renee reported that she didn't think Beatrice had any feelings, but qualified this by saying that Beatrice felt that she was an ugly, horrible person. Renee had never seen Beatrice having fun or enjoying herself.

At the 16-year-old interview Beatrice had dropped out of school and run away from home where she had been physically and emotionally abused. Drugs and alcohol were her life and she was constantly getting into fights and stealing money to buy drugs. She was frequently in trouble with the law and had become very depressed. She had already made two suicide attempts and felt that she would be dead by the time that she was 30. She said "I don't care about anything, nothing at all. I was being evil, spiteful, getting in a lot of trouble from the police and stuff. I just didn't care. I feel miserable and sad, deeper than when you watch something sad on television; you don't know why; you just feel like you want to cry. I'm sluggish, drag myself around. I think 'why are those people looking at me?' I feel paranoid and stuff. It's really strange'.

During her later adolescence Beatrice accepted support and at 25 years she was no longer taking drugs, her mental health was stable and she was employed.

Translating the research into policy

The two most important findings to emerge from the SLCDS are, first, that depression in pregnancy is as common as in the postnatal period, and second, that exposure to depression in utero or after birth is associated with long term difficulties for the child albeit by different pathways. Pregnancy is a period in a woman's life when she is likely to have frequent contact with health care professionals. Early detection of maternal depression may accelerate treatment and offer support for women who are vulnerable to further recurrent depressive episodes in the postnatal period and later in their child's lifetime. During the 20th century, research focused on the detection of maternal depression in the postnatal period and its effect on the child's development. Evidence from the SLCDS and other studies (Evans *et al.* 2001; Andersson *et al.* 2006) that depression in pregnancy is as common as in the post partum has already contributed to recommendations made in the NICE Antenatal and Postnatal Mental Health Guidelines (NICE 2007). Assessment of maternal mental health is now part of routine practice in antenatal clinics and appropriate support is offered. Furthermore the SLCDS has informed the NSPCC's All Babies Count campaign (NSPCC 2012), emphasizing the importance of identifying and monitoring mental illness in the antenatal period and offering support to families where the mother is depressed.

Findings from the SLCDS in childhood and adolescence also suggest that the *children* whose mothers suffer from depression in the perinatal period may be in special need of support. Teenage pregnancy, violence, crime and academic failure are at unacceptably high levels in the UK. Interpersonal violence is the third leading cause of death, and the leading cause of disability for 10–29-year-olds in the European region (WHO 2010). The SLCDS has the potential to inform interventions as proposed in The Good Childhood Inquiry (Children's Society 2009), The Foundation Years: Preventing Poor Children Becoming Poor Adults (Field 2010) and The Next Steps (Allen 2011). Each has emphasised the importance of family life and parental well-being in the foundation years, beginning in pregnancy, in determining each child's life-chances. Findings from the SLCDS are helping refine targeting of limited resources to those families in which the mother is depressed during pregnancy and in the period after the birth.

The Channi Kumar Mother and Baby Unit

It was Channi Kumar's vision that led to the setting up of the MBU. Research into the long-term effect of perinatal mental illness on the offspring has shown that early mother–infant interaction plays a significant role in the outcome for the child. Observational studies have shown that women with postnatal depression often have problems in relating to their new babies (Murray *et al.* 1996). They may appear indifferent and withdrawn, finding it difficult to smile and talk to their babies, or they may be intrusive, over-stimulating, and handle their babies roughly. The babies, in turn, may react by protesting and crying excessively or by becoming passive and avoidant (Weinberg and Tronick 1998). Most observational studies of mother-infant interaction in psychosis have been limited to carer-report (and therefore non-blind) rating scales such as the Bethlem Mother–Infant Rating Scale (BMIS; Kumar and Hipwell 1996). Thus, Snellen *et al.* (1999) found that the BMIS scores of mothers with schizophrenia spectrum disorders admitted to a MBU with their babies improved between admission and discharge. One exception (Riordan *et al.* 1999) compared the interaction of mothers with schizophrenia and mothers with an affective disorder on discharge from an MBU. Mothers with schizophrenia were more remote, insensitive, intrusive and self-absorbed and had babies who were more avoidant. The deficits in mother–infant interaction were not explained by measures of illness severity or factors relating to adverse social circumstances (Wan *et al.* 2007).

One important feature of mother–infant relationships is the security of the attachment relationship (Ainsworth *et al.* 1978). A handful of studies have looked at the impact of maternal SMI on the baby's later attachment to the mother, with differing results. Naslund (1984) and D'Angelo (1986) both found that infants of mothers with schizophrenia were more likely than healthy controls to receive insecure classifications in the Strange Situation (the standard laboratory assessment of attachment security in infancy). Jacobsen and Miller (1999) reported that, in a diagnostically diverse sample of 30 infant–mother pairs, only four demonstrated a secure attachment. In their study of 25 mothers (with a range of diagnoses) who had been inpatients at an MBU, Hipwell *et al.* (2000) found an association between depression, both psychotic and non-psychotic, and insecure attachment at 12 months. Findings such as these suggest that early experiences with mothers suffering from mental illness may interfere with the infant's regulation of emotion and attention (Hill 2004; Gerhardt 2004), with cognitive and memory function (Hay 1997) and with the ability to make self/other distinctions (Tronick and Weinberg 1997), and may continue to exert direct effects on children's lives over a decade later (Murray *et al.* 2002; Hay *et al.* 2001, 2003).

It was against this background that Channi Kumar proposed that treatment offered by perinatal services should include support for mothers in developing their relationship with their baby. He was responsible for ensuring that nursery nurses, specialist mother-baby nurses and developmental psychologists form part of the inpatient and community multidisciplinary teams so that the treatment of the mother's mental illness is combined with work to promote her relationship with her baby and develop caregiving skills.

One of the challenges of working with mothers with SMI is their psychological unavailability when they are very ill. The symptoms of their disorder may include flat affect, preoccupation with delusions or frequent auditory hallucinations, extreme negativism or mutism, disinhibition, grandiosity, repetitive rituals, irritability or aggression, disorganized speech or behaviour, all symptoms which make it difficult for the mother to engage with others. Mothers with SMI often lack insight into their disorder when they are acutely unwell and are unaware that their symptoms may make it difficult for them to give appropriate care to their infant. They are usually, however, totally committed to being a mother and providing for the infant. The threat of being separated from the baby (Kumar *et al.* 1995) makes the mother particularly anxious to show that she can care for and respond to her baby's needs.

The Channi Kumar Mother and Baby Unit, set up 30 years ago, is a 13-bedded in-patient unit at the Bethlem Royal Hospital, South London & Maudsley NHS Foundation Trust & King's Health Partners. Mothers with schizophrenia, bipolar disorder, psychosis, severe depression, and anxiety disorders who either relapse or become ill for the first time in pregnancy or following the birth can be admitted with their unborn or new baby. On admission mothers are not only acutely unwell but often overwhelmed by feelings of guilt that they are not providing adequate love and care for their baby. Some mothers describe feelings of emptiness while others blame the baby for their illness or have intrusive thoughts that they might harm the baby. Mothers may also be preoccupied with the knowledge that their illness might have an adverse effect on the development of the baby in utero or after birth, or worse, mean that they will be separated from the baby.

Several treatments that focus on the relationship between the mother and baby have been pioneered on the Mother and Baby Unit. One way of helping parents of newborns to get to know their baby is to show them his/her wonderful abilities, using the Neonatal Behavioral Assessment Scale (NBAS: Brazelton and Nugent 1995). Fathers are also invited to be part of these sessions. The NBAS is an interactive assessment focusing on the baby's strengths. It looks at how the baby responds to light and sound when asleep, (habituation) and faces and objects (orientation). It also looks at the baby's physical activity/reflexes (motor performance) and how the baby is able to regulate his/her states (from sleeping through to crying). By observing the baby and seeing how the newborn can focus on the face and turn to the sound of the voice, parents learn to understand the communicative skills of their baby and how they can respond to his/her cues, thus entering into a dialogue that is dynamic and reciprocal. They are helped to look at what their baby likes and dislikes and how they can understand his/her signals, in order to develop ways to handle and look after their baby. These skills are reinforced by the nursery nurses and occupational therapists in infant massage, rhyme time and mother-and-baby swimming.

We also support the mother in getting to know her baby by inviting them to play together while we make a 3-minute video-recording of the play session. This invitation is offered on admission, during the mother's stay on the MBU, and again on discharge. The mother is asked to place her baby in a baby seat or high chair with a mirror placed adjacent to the chair. The mother sits facing the baby on the opposite side to the mirror so that the camera captures a reflection of her face in the mirror and the baby is seen full on. Mothers are asked to play with or talk to their babies as they would normally, preferably without the use of toys. On a separate occasion the mother is invited to view the play session. The aim of the feedback session is to make the experience as positive as possible for the mother and to build on the skills and strengths that she already has. The package is designed to promote maternal sensitivity through the use of video-recordings of mother infant interaction, with individually-tailored feedback. The therapeutic work, with a professional trained in infant observation, centres on watching and learning about the baby's cues so that the mother becomes more sensitive to seeing her baby as a person and learning what works and what does not work in creating a smooth dialogue between them.

Discussion initially focuses on the most positive moments from the video. When was baby happiest? What did baby like best? What did mother like best? The mother can practise recognizing baby's cues: In what ways is the baby telling you things? What do you think baby is trying to say here? This may also include disengagement cues. The mother is encouraged to make links between her own behaviour and that of the baby: What did you do that baby liked/disliked? It may be helpful to count the number of occurrences of a particular cue, for example how often does the baby look towards the mother, or appear attentive and listening? The video may also form a basis for discussion about what the baby is like in terms of temperament.

Feedback addresses the different domains of communication used by both mother and infant: facial expression, body language, and verbal communication. Engagement cues in the baby include focused expression, calm attentiveness, relaxed posture, reaching towards the mother, smiles and vocalization. Disengagement cues include gaze aversion, yawning, arching, grimacing, anxious tongue poking, possetting, closing eyes, hiccoughing, sneezing, arms held in a defensive position, and legs held stiffly. It may be helpful to pay attention to the following aspects of the mother's behaviour: smiling, eye contact, touching, variation in her voice, commenting on the environment or on baby's experience, mirroring behaviours, responses to baby's vocalizations, the congruence of her facial expressions with those of the baby, the pacing of her interactions. Some mothers may tend to be over-intrusive, whilst others may under-stimulate the baby and fail to respond to the baby's cues.

Mothers are encouraged to identify something new that they would like to try (for example, mimicking sounds made by the baby, or using more or less physical contact) and to practise this outside of the session. Subsequent sessions then reflect on this process and on the impact it has had on the relationship with the baby.

In order to assess the progress made over the admission to the MBU, the mother–infant pattern of interaction is evaluated using the CARE-Index (Crittenden 2004) whereby both the mother and infant are evaluated on seven aspects of dyadic behaviour. The first four—facial expression, verbal expression, position and body contact, and affection—are assessments of affect within the dyad, while the final three—turn-taking contingencies, control, and choice of activity – refer to temporal contingencies. These ratings for the seven aspects of interactional behaviour contribute to one of seven specific scales, three for the mother—sensitive, controlling, unresponsive—and four for the child—co-operative, difficult, compulsive, passive. The central construct of sensitivity is a dyadic one. 'The adult's sensitivity in play is any pattern of behaviour that pleases the infant and increases the infant's comfort and attentiveness and reduces its distress and disengagement' (Crittenden 2004, p. 3).

After the intervention on the MBU, the CARE-Index shows that 73% of mothers responded, by becoming more sensitive and responsive to the baby's cues; moreover, babies were more co-operative and less passive, and at group-level there were no differences any longer when compared with well mothers and their babies. These improvements were observed in mother and babies across the different diagnostic groups—mothers with schizophrenia, psychotic disorders and mood disorders. Of note, these beneficial effects of our intervention were not simply due to concomitant symptomatic improvement in mothers, since mother–infant interaction after the intervention was also significantly better than in a group of women with SMI and their babies who had not received the treatment and had similar levels of psychopathology (Kenny *et al.*, 2013). These results are consistent with a recent meta-analysis of intervention studies (Bakermans-Kranenburg et al. 2003), which concludes that video feedback is the most successful technique in enhancing maternal sensitivity, and that a small number of sessions (less than 5) is optimal.

A case study

(Identifying information has been altered in order to protect confidentiality.)

Max was a much-wanted, planned first baby. His mother, Margaret, aged 29, and her husband, had made all the necessary preparations, attended antenatal classes, and were eagerly looking forward to parenthood. However, after a traumatic delivery Margaret became very depressed and suicidal with thoughts of harming the baby. She described how she felt oppressed by the baby and did not know what she would be capable of if left alone with him. Her husband, recognizing that something was wrong, sought help, and Margaret was admitted to the MBU with her baby when he was 5 weeks old. In the first few days on the ward, Margaret took no interest in Max, allowing her husband and the staff to care for him. Slowly Margaret was encouraged to watch her baby, while staff demonstrated the amazing capabilities of the newborn, using the Neonatal Behavioral Assessment Scale. At first, Margaret felt detached from Max, empty and with no feelings. She felt that she was inadequate as a mother, describing herself as a 'wimp'. Gradually she came to see that Max was listening to her, quietening to her voice; that he was looking at her and following her with his eyes. This was a turning point for Margaret and she began to experience warm feelings for Max.

Margaret and Max participated in four video-feedback sessions over the course of an 8-week admission to the MBU. During these sessions, Margaret was encouraged to observe the baby signals. She began to interpret what he might be thinking and feeling. As Max looks up at his mother they engage in mutual eye-contact and smiling. Margaret begins to imitate Max's sounds and vocalizations, pausing and allowing time for Max to respond. In this way they were beginning to have conversations. At 12 weeks they were enjoying communicating with one another. Margaret was becoming aware of Max's internal states, commenting 'You are in a good mood! Are you laughing?' as Max smiles and has eye-contact with his mother; 'What do you want to tell me?' as Max vocalizes; 'What are you trying to do? Do you want to sit up?' as he moves forward in the chair.

Margaret and Max are engrossed in a dialogue with one another. They are communicating. They are learning to understand one another. The process by which they do this is dynamic, reciprocal and important for the development of the child (see Figure 10.1).

Margaret and Max were soon discharged together from the ward at 13 weeks.

A novel treatment package for women with a severe mental illness following childbirth: Effects on mother-infant interaction.

Before: Mother has flat facial expression, baby is looking away, his arms are uncontained. They are not engaged.

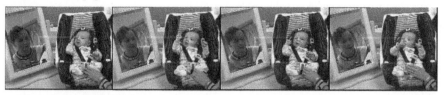

After: Mutual eye gaze and smiling, imitation of head movement, baby's arms are contained. They are having fun!

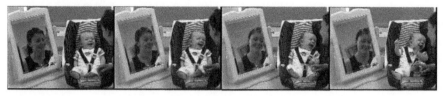

A woman aged 29, was admitted to the Channi Kumar Mother and Baby Unit (South London and Maudsley NHS Foundation Trust) with an episode of major depressive disorder. She was suicidal and had thoughts of harming her baby. The pictures show the video before and after the intervention. The baby was 5 and 12 weeks old, respectively. Pictures are presented with kind permission of the mother.

Fig. 10.1 Mother and baby at play.

Conclusion

In this chapter we have described two of Channi Kumar's research studies, one showing the long-term adverse effects for the children of exposure to untreated maternal depression in utero and after birth. The second study provides evidence for specific intervention programmes aimed at supporting parents experiencing severe mental health problems in developing their relationships with their infants and providing 'good-enough' care to ensure the improved mental health and academic performance of the next generation who are already genetically vulnerable. In response to patient wishes, the guidelines laid down by the National Institute for Health and Care Excellence (2007) recommend that perinatal services include support for mothers with SMI in developing their relationship with their baby as part of their treatment. Furthermore, in its recent 'All Babies Count' campaign, the NSPCC (2012) emphasize that it is not be enough to treat the women's mental illness in order to improve care of babies, but we also need to work explicitly with mothers and fathers to promote a secure attachment, positive relationships and good parenting. These are Channi's legacies and challenges for the 21st century.

References

Ainsworth, M., Blehar, M., Waters, E. and Wall, S. (1978). Patterns of Attachment. Hillsdale, NJ, Lawrence Erlbaum Associates.

Andersson, L., Sundström-Poromaa, I., Wulff, M., ⊠ström, M., and Bixo, M. (2006). Depression and anxiety during pregnancy and six months postpartum: a follow-up study. Acta Obstetrica Gynecologica Scandinavica **85**: 937–944.

Angold, A., Prendergast, M., Cox, A., *et al.* (1995). The Child and Adolescent Psychiatric Assessment (CAPA). Psychological Medicine **25**: 739–753.

Allen, G. (2011). Early Intervention: The Next Steps. An Independent Report to Her Majesty's Government. London: The Stationery Office. Available from http://www.dwp.gov.uk/docs/early-intervention-next-steps.pdf (accessed 13 September 2013).

Bakermans-Kranenburg, M. J., Van Ijzendoorn, M. H., and Juffer, F. (2003). Less is more: meta-analyses of sensitivity and attachment interventions in early childhood. Psychological Bulletin **129**(2): 195.

Brand, S.R. and Brennan, P.A. (2009). Impact of antenatal and postpartum maternal mental illness: how are the children? Clinical Obstetrics and Gynaecology **52**(3): 441–455.

Brazelton, T. and Nugent, J. (1995). Neonatal Behavioral Assessment Scale, 3rd Ed. London, MacKeith.

Children's Society (2009). The Good Childhood Enquiry. Avaialble from http://www.childrenssociety.org.uk/what-we-do/research/good-childhood-inquiry (accessed 13 September 2013).

Crittenden P.M. (2004). Care-Index; Manual. Miami, FL, Family Relations Institute.

D'Angelo, E.J. (1986). Security of attachment in infants with schizophrenic, depressed, and unaffected mothers. Journal of Genetic Psychology **147**: 421–2.

Danese, A., Moffitt, T.E., Pariante, C.M., Ambler, A., Poulton, R. and Caspi, A. (2008). Elevated inflammation levels in depressed adults with a history of childhood maltreatment. Archives of General Psychiatry **65**: 409–15.

Evans, J., Heron, J., Francomb, H., Oke, S., Golding, J. (2001). Cohort study of depressed mood during pregnancy and childbirth. BMJ. **323**: 257–60.

Field, F. (2010). The Foundation Years: Preventing Poor Children Becoming Poor Adults. Independent Review of Poverty and Life Chances. Available from http://webarchive.nationalarchives.gov.uk/20110120090128/http:/povertyreview.independent.gov.uk/news/101203-review-poverty-life-chances.aspx

Gerhardt, S. (2004). Why love matters. How affection shapes a baby's brain. London: Brunner-Routledge.

Goldberg, D., Cooper, B., Eastwood, M.T., Kedward, H.B., and Shepherd, M. (1970). A standardised psychiatric interview for use in community surveys. British Journal of Preventative Social Medicine **24**: 18–23.

Halligan, S. L., Murray, L., Martins, C., and Cooper, P.J. (2007). Maternal depression and psychiatric outcomes in adolescent offspring: a 13-year longitudinal study. Journal of Affective Disorders **97**(1): 145–54.

Hay, D.F. (1997). Postpartum depression and cognitive development. In Postpartum Depression and Child Development L. Murray and P. Cooper editors. New York, Guilford, pp. 85–110.

Hay, D.F., Pawlby, S., Sharp, D., Asten, P., Mills, A. and Kumar, R. (2001). Intellectual problems shown 11-year-old children whose mothers had postnatal depression. Journal of Child Psychology and Psychiatry **42**: 871–90.

Hay, D.F., Pawlby, S., Angold, A., Harold, G. and Sharp, D, (2003). Pathways to violence in the children of depressed mothers. Developmental Psychology **39**: 1083–1094.

Hay, D.F., Pawlby, S., Waters, C.S., and Sharp, D. (2008). Antepartum and postpartum exposure to maternal depression: different effects on different adolescent outcomes. Journal of Child Psychology and Psychiatry **49**(10): 1079–88.

Hay, D.F., Pawlby, S., Waters, C.S., Perra, O., and Sharp, D. (2010). Mothers' antenatal depression and their children's antisocial outcomes. Child Development **81**(1): 149–165.

Hill, J. (2004) Parental psychiatric disorder and the attachment relationship. In Parental Psychiatric Disorder: Distressed Parents and their Families, M. Gopfert, J. Webster and M.V. Seeman editors. Cambridge, Cambridge University Press, pp 50–61.

Hipwell, A. E., Goossens, F. A., Melhuish, E. C., and Kumar, R. (2000). Severe maternal psychopathology and infant—mother attachment. Development and Psychopathology **12**: 157–75.

Jacobsen, T., and Miller, L. J. (1999). Attachment quality in young children of mentally ill mothers. In Attachment Disorganization, J. Solomon and C. George editors. New York, Guilford Press, pp. 347–378.

Kenny, M., Conroy, S., Pariante, CM., Seneviratne, G. and Pawlby, S. (2013). Mother-infant interaction in Mother and Baby Unit patients: Before and after treatment. Journal of Psychiatric Research.

Kumar, R., Marks, M., Platz, C., and Yoshida, K. (1995). Clinical survey of a psychiatric mother and baby unit: Characteristics of 100 consecutive admissions. Journal of Affective Disorders **33**: 11–22.

Kumar, R. and Hipwell, A.E. (1996). Development of a clinical rating scale to assess mother—infant interaction in a psychiatric mother and baby unit. British Journal of Psychiatry **169**: 18–26.

Murray, L., Cooper, P. and Hipwell, A. (2002). Mental health of parents caring for infants. Archives of Women's Mental Health **6**(Suppl.2.): s71–s77.

Murray, L., Fiori-Cowley, A., Hooper, R. and Cooper, P.J. (1996). The impact of postnatal depression and associated adversity on early mother-infant interactions and later infant outcome. Child Development **67**: 2512–2526.

Murray, L., Arteche, A., Fearon, P., Halligan, S., Croudace, T., and Cooper, P. (2010). The effects of maternal postnatal depression and child sex on academic performance at age 16 years: a developmental approach. Journal of Child Psychology and Psychiatry **51**(10): 1150–9.

Naslund, B., Persson-Blennow, I., McNeil, T., Kaij, L. and Malmquist-Larsson, A. (1984). Offspring of women with non-organic psychosis: infant attachment to the mother at one year of age. Acta Psychiatrica Scandinavica **69**: 231–41.

National Institute for Health and Care Excellence (2007). Clinical Practice Guideline Number 45. Antenatal and Postnatal Mental Health. Available from http://publications.nice.org.uk/antenatal-and-postnatal-mental-health-cg45 (accessed 13 September 2013).

National Society for the Prevention of Cruelty to Children (2012). All babies count: prevention and protection for vulnerable babies. Available from http://www.nspcc.org.uk/inform/resourcesforprofessionals/underones/all_babies_count_pdf_wdf85569.pdf

O'Connor, T.G., Heron, J. and Glover V. (2002). Antenatal anxiety predicts child behavioural/emotional problems independently of postnatal depression. Journal of the American Academy of Child and Adolescent. Psychiatry **41**: 1470–7.

Pawlby, S., Hay, D.F., Sharp, D., Waters, C.S. and O'Keane, V. (2009). Antenatal depression predicts depression in adolescent offspring: prospective longitudinal community based study. Journal of Affective Disorders **113**: 236–43.

Pawlby, S., Hay, D.F., Sharp, D., Waters, C.S., and Pariante, C.M. (2011). Antenatal depression and offspring psychopathology: the influence of childhood maltreatment. British Journal of Psychiatry **199**: 106–12.

Plant, D.T., Barker, E.D., Waters, C.S., Pawlby, S., and Pariante, C.M. (2102). Intergenerational transmission of maltreatment and psychopathology: the role of antenatal depression. Psychological Medicine doi:10.1017/S0033291712001298.

Riordan, D., Appleby, L. and Faragher, B. (1999). Mother—infant interaction in post-partum women with schizophrenia and affective disorders. Psychological Medicine **29**: 991–5.

Sharp, D. (1993). Childbirth-related emotional disorders in primary care: A longitudinal prospective study. Unpublished PhD thesis, University of London.

Sharp, D.J., Hay, D.F., Pawlby, S.J., Schmücker, G., Allen, H., and Kumar, R. (1995). The impact of postnatal depression on boys' intellectual development. Journal of Child Psychology and Psychiatry **36**: 1315–36.

Snellen, M., Mack, K. and Trauer, T. (1999). Schizophrenia, mental state, and mother—infant interaction: Examining the relationship. Australian and New Zealand Journal of Psychiatry **33**: 902–911.

Spitzer, R.L., Endicott, J., and Robbins, E. (1978). The Schedule for Affective Disorders and Schizophrenia—Lifetime version (SADS-L), 3rd ed. New York, Biometric Research.

Tronick, E.Z. and Weinberg, M.K. (1997). Depressed mothers and infants: Failure to form dyadic states of consciousness. In Postpartum Depression and Child Development, L. Murray and P. Cooper editors. New York, Guilford, pp. 54–81.

Wan, M. W., Salmon, M.P., Riordan, D.M., Appleby, L., Webb, R. and Abel, K.M. (2007). What predicts poor mother-infant interaction in schizophrenia? Psychological Medicine 37: 537–46.

Weinberg, M.K. and Tronick, E.Z. (1998). The impact of maternal psychiatric illness on infant development. Journal of Clinical Psychiatry 59: 53–61.

World Health Organization (2010). European report on preventing violence and knife crime among young people. Copenhagen, World Health Organization Regional Office for Europe. http://www.euro.who

Chapter 11

Mother- and father-to-infant emotional involvement

Bárbara Figueiredo

When we become parents to a child powerful emotions are
evoked, emotions as strong as those which bind a young child
to his mother or lovers to one another
Bowlby, 1979/1982, p. 17.

Mother's emotional and hormonal specific state after childbirth

A mother's specific emotional and hormonal state after childbirth ensures her emotional
involvement and adequate parental behaviour.

Soon after delivery, or even in late pregnancy, the mother's emotional state—in particular, an increased sensitivity—becomes fully adapted to the identification and satisfaction
of the infant's physical and psychological needs. Winnicott (1956, 1960) was perhaps one
of the first authors to point out the presence of a particular emotional state in recently
delivered mothers—'primary maternal preoccupation', referring to the mother's correct
identification and immediate satisfaction of the infant's physical and psychological needs[1].
Winnicott (1990) later defined and described four main tasks to be fulfilled in the maternal
role, including the emotional involvement with the child, which he termed 'holding'. Holding tasks are: (1) to provide protection and care to the child, (2) to take into account the
child's limitations and dependency status, (3) to provide the necessary care for the child's
growth and development, and (4) to love the child.

In the meantime, Yalom *et al.* (1968) and Pitt (1973) both described the 'postpartum/
maternity blues—a transient state of emotional dysphoria, emerging within a few hours
to 2 weeks after childbirth, in about 50 to 70% of puerperal women, and characterized by
intermittent mild fatigue, tearfulness, worry, difficulty in thinking, and sleep disturbances.

Progesterone and oestrogen levels, which gradually increase during pregnancy, fall suddenly after delivery, returning to prepregnancy levels in just 3 days. This rapid decline, the
most severe threat to a women's hormonal and emotional balance, has been proposed as
the main cause of postpartum/maternity blues (e.g. Pitt 1973; Yalomand *et al.* 1968).

The mother's behavioural sensitivity to such a drop in reproductive hormones was later associated with higher reactivity to the infant's stimuli and greater proximity with the neonate (e.g. Barrett and Fleming 2011; Carter 2005; Fleming *et al.* 1997; Miller and Rukstalis 1999), and was proposed as serving the function of eliciting mother-to-infant involvement, to ensure that the infant receives the required care to survive (e.g. Carter 2005; Figueiredo 2003; Pedersen 1997)[2].

Parents' caregiving system ensures the proximity and survival of the child

The evolutionary point of view had its clearest proponent in John Bowlby (1969/1982, 1980) who proposed the presence of a behavioural system (that is, an organized set of behaviours) in parents—the 'caregiving system', to guarantee the proximity and protection of the child. The parent caregiving system, complementary and reciprocal to the child attachment system, ensures the protection of the child and the child/species survival.

Bowlby (1969/1982, 1988) provided a behavioural description of the attachment and caregiving systems. The attachment system is formed by attachment behaviors – actions that promote proximity between the child and the caregiver. Infants engage in three classes of behaviour, which establish or maintain proximity to the caregiver (Belsky and Cassidy, 1994). Signaling behaviours (such as smiling, non-nutritional sucking, babbling, calling) draw the caregiver toward the child, usually for positive interactions. Aversive behaviours (such as crying, screaming) bring the caregiver to the child, typically to terminate the aversive reactions. Active behaviours (such as approaching, following, and seeking) move the child toward the caregiver.

> Though different phenotypically, these behaviors all serve the same biological function: To keep vulnerable infants in close physical proximity to their caregivers, thereby increasing their chances of survival (Simpson and Belsky 2008, p. 137).

The caregiving system was also examined in an ethological framework, as 'observing and describing a set of behavioral patterns characteristic of parenting' (Bowlby 1988, p. 4). The author stated that the caregiving system is formed by caregiving behaviors, including nursing, nest-building, and retrieving. Maternal retrieval behavior is of special interest, but, in fact, the caregiving system refers to: 'any behavior of a parent a predictable outcome of which is that the young are brought either into the nest or close to mother, or both' (Bowlby, 1969/1982, p. 240).

Bowlby also offered a conceptualization of the purpose, way of functioning and determinants of the caregiving system. When activated, the caregiving system ensures 'that the infant remain close to the caregiver' (Bowlby 1969/1982, p. 194), therefore guaranteeing the survival of the child. When not activated, the child's exploration of the world is allowed. The central feature of the caregiving system is then 'the provision . . . of a secure base from which a child . . . can make sorties into the outside world and to which he can return . . . ' (Bowlby 1988, p. 11).

The caregiving system works in reciprocity with the child attachment system, and constant feedback is observed between them (Bowlby 1969/1982, 1988). The activation and deactivation of both systems—the attachment and the caregiving systems—are regulated by a feedback system, dependent on achieving goals and therefore guided and corrected by obtaining them. 'A shared dyadic programme' between the parent and the child occurs 'as the behavior of the one is the complement of the other' (Bowlby 1969/1982, p. 377). 'When mother is called away a child's attachment behavior is likely to be elicited and exploratory behavior inhibited; conversely, when a child explores too far, mother's care behavior is likely to be elicited' (Bowlby 1969/1982, p. 237). The caregiving system is enabled, disabled and guided by child attachment behaviours, and a wide range of behaviours and cues are put into action by the child, acting as true social triggers to the mother's caregiving responses.

Finally, with regard to its determinants, Bowlby stated that, as with the child's attachment system, the caregiving system 'is in some degree preprogrammed and therefore ready to develop along certain lines when conditions elicit it' (Bowlby 1988, p. 4). The caregiving system 'is certainly not the product of some unvarying parenting instinct, but nor is it reasonable to regard it simply as the product of learning' (Bowlby 1988, p. 5). It is because it serves a vital function that the caregiving system would be, to some extent, pre-programmed. The author argues that to leave caregiving 'solely to the caprices of individual learning would be the height of biological folly' (op. cit., p. 5).

In sum, Bowlby's (1969/1982) basic assumptions about the caregiving system are as follows. First, it is composed of a repertoire of behaviours coordinated to achieve the specific goal of protecting the child, and has an adaptive function, which is the survival of the child/species. Second, the caregiving system is complementary and reciprocal to the child attachment system. Third, the caregiving system is goal-corrected and guided by a feedback system. Fourth, it is activated, regulated and terminated by a feedback system that monitors internal (biological and representational) and external cues (particularly, the caregiver's evaluation of the child's attachment cues). Fifth, the caregiving system is organized and integrated by specific cognitive control systems (particularly, mental representations).

Although primarily focused on the behavioral dimension of the caregiving system, Bowlby also considered an emotional dimension, as he comments 'when we become parents to a child powerful emotions are evoked, emotions as strong as those which bind a young child to his mother or lovers to one another' (Bowlby 1979/1982, p. 17). Bowlby (1988) considers that the strong biological root of parenting behavior 'accounts for the very strong emotions associated with it' (p. 5).

Maternal–infant bonding at childbirth

As proposed by Klaus and Kennell (1976), 'maternal–infant bonding' is a unique and specific bond between the mother and the child, which begins at childbirth for the majority of mothers, and endures over time. Childbirth is a sensitive and critical period for the establishment of mother-to-infant bonding, depending on the mother's specific hormonal equipment, the infant's presence, and the articulation between the bio-behavioral equipment of the mother and the child.

In their book *Maternal-infant bonding: The impact of early separation or loss on family development*, Klaus and Kennell (1976) proposed that mother-to-infant bonding is an unique, specific and enduring bond between the mother and the child, normally established from the first contacts with the newborn after delivery, to ensure the proximity of mother and child. As defined by the authors, maternal-infant bonding refers to the mother's emotional involvement with her child:

> It is a process that builds and grows with repeated meaningful and pleasurable experiences. At the same time, another tie, usually referred as attachment, is developing in infants, toward their parents and others that help in their care. It is from this emotional connection that infants can begin to develop a sense of who they are and from which a child can evolve and be able to venture into the world. . . . When a parent feels this emotional connection or bond to the infant, it's much more than an interest in feeding or changing or tending the infant, it's caring—feeling oneself into the child's place, sensing and responding to the infant's needs, whether physical or emotional. The infant is powerfully influenced by this emotional investment (Klaus *et al.* 1996, p. 192).

Three main ideas characterize the contribution of Klaus and Kennell in understanding the establishment of maternal-infant bonding, generally observed in mothers: (1) the existence of a critical and sensitive period in the moments following childbirth; (2) the importance of the mother's hormonal equipment and of the infant's presence; and (3) the feedback between the bio-behavioural equipment of both the mother and the infant.

The moments following childbirth are both optimal/sensitive and critical to maternal–infant bonding. The early postpartum is an optimal/sensitive period, depending on the adequacy of the hormonal system of the mother and on the infant's presence. 'A cascade of reciprocal interactions begins between the mother and baby which locks them together and mediates the further development of attachment' (Sosa *et al.* 1976, p. 187). In their famous article published in 1972 in the *New England Journal of Medicine* entitled '*Maternal attachment—Importance of the first post-partum days*', Klaus and Kennell reported how mothers who were allowed more contact with their newborn after delivery showed the following more optimal maternal behaviour: They 'were more reluctant to leave their infants with someone else, usually stood and watched during the examination, showed greater soothing behavior, and engaged in significantly more eye-to-eye contact and fondling' (Klaus *et al.* 1972, p. 460). The early postpartum was seen as a critical period – that is, a crucial moment to establish maternal-infant bonding (Kennell *et al.* 1975). Therefore, in the absence of postpartum contact, maternal-infant bonding is compromised: 'Events may have lasting effects' . . . 'affectional ties can be easily disturbed and may be permanently altered during the immediate postpartum period' (Klaus and Kennell 1976, p. 50, 52). For example, 'early brief separation of the mother and infant during the first minutes and hours after delivery can alter the behavior of the mother with her child months and years later' (Sosa *et al.* 1976, p. 179). However, the authors later admitted that, although critical, the time immediately after delivery cannot be the unique moment for maternal-infant bonding to be established, because it would be too dangerous for the preservation of the species if it could happen only in the initial postpartum (Klaus *et al.* 1996).

Maternal–infant bonding would be established during the first contacts between mother and newborn following delivery, facilitated by the adequacy of the mother's hormonal system and elicited by the presence of the neonates (Klaus and Kennell 1976). With regard to hormones, the authors highlighted the role of oxytocin and stated that 'the attachment felt between the mother and infant may be biochemically modulated through oxytocin' (Klaus 1998, p. 1244). However, it is also necessary for neonates to respond to the mother by some signal, such as body movements or eye contact, so that bonding can be established (Klaus and Kennell 1976).

Feedback between the bio-behavioural equipment of both the mother and the infant is acknowledged: their behavior complements each other, serving to lock the pair together. 'The infant elicits behaviors from the mother which in turn are satisfying to him, and vice versa, the mother elicits behaviors in the infant which in turn are rewarding to her' (Klaus and Kennell 1976, p. 67). The authors gave the following examples of such complementary behaviour. Guided by odour, the newborn crawls toward the breast, finds the nipple, and initiates suckling; the mother, in response, offers a perfect complement, regulating the temperature of the newborn, keeping him warm (Klaus 1998). The sucking of the breast by the newborn, in turn, increases the mother's oxytocin, which in turn, results in closer proximity and stimulates maternal-infant bonding, an 'increased love for the infant' (Klaus 1998, p. 1246). The newborn also stimulates the production of prolactin, while touching the mother's nipples, and this increase in prolactin in turn stimulates the proximity of the mother, and therefore the protection and survival of the infant. The production of oxytocin and prolactin is a biological mechanism that effectively serves to promote the infant's survival (Klaus 1988; Klaus and Kennell 1976).

Mother's initial indifference to the infant is a frequent and normative response

Channi Kumar conceived 'maternal attachment' as a gradual process of mother-to-infant affection, which is stimulated by the infant's specific behaviours and is largely influenced by the mother's mental state. The author also pointed out that the mother's initial indifference to the infant is a frequent and normative response, and is distinct from the response which occurs in maternal bonding disorders (Kumar 1997; Robson and Kumar 1980). He emphasized that maternal attachment is critical to the relationship and parenting of the infant and to the child's well-being and development.

Kumar (1997) refers to 'maternal attachment' as the mother's affection toward the child. This is a gradual process, which is conceived as stimulated by specific behaviors of the infant and varies according to the characteristics of the mother. In the establishment of 'maternal attachment', Robson and Kumar (1980) valued, above all, the infant's interactive skills, including mutual eye-eye contact with the mother (Robson 1967).

The delivery is here only one possible moment for 'the beginning of growth reciprocal attachment . . . progressively developed along branching pathways' (Kumar 1997, p. 180). Questioning the idea that mothers are physiologically primed at birth to manifest specific maternal behaviours, because this did not fit with empirical data from many mothers whose initial reaction to their neonate is one of indifference, the author hypothesized that it nevertheless seemed plausible that some early human maternal and emotional responses to the newborn share characteristics and possibly underlying mechanisms with other mammals.

Kumar was interested in describing and distinguishing typical from atypical patterns of maternal emotional involvement with the infant (Kumar 1997; Robson and Kumar 1980; Robson and Moss 1970). Calling attention to the feature of a lack of immediate mother-to-infant emotional involvement, Robson and Kumar (1980) reported that for 40% of primiparous and 25% of multiparous mothers, the first reaction to the newborn following childbirth was indifference. In a retrospective study, a high proportion of mothers did not recall any affection, but rather 'their predominant emotional reaction when holding their babies for the very first time had been one of indifference' (Robson and Kumar 1980, p. 347). The authors reported that feelings of affection for the child were delayed in many mothers, particularly following a difficult or painful delivery. They considered such initial indifference as normal, since the mother subsequently developed an equal affection for the child, only more slowly over the weeks following childbirth. This reaction was also conceived as a normal variant with caregiving advantages, because maternal attachment would be delayed until the newborn's survival was assured.

This transient delay in the onset of maternal affection, lasting no more than a few days, is unlike what happens in maternal bonding disorders. Kumar (1997) later clarified that severe bonding disturbances are different from this initial reaction of indifference, being prolonged over time and associated with mental illness. Occasionally, a prolonged failure in maternal emotional involvement could occur beyond the immediate postpartum period. Some 'women reported absent affection, sometimes hate, rejection, neglect or impulse to harm . . . these feelings often began immediately or very shortly after the birth' (Kumar 1997 p. 175). Postnatal mental illness and recalled severe pain during labour, but not childhood experiences, were significantly associated with such maternal bonding disorders, 'which, in their severe forms, did not occur in the absence of postnatal mental illness' (Kumar 1997 p. 175).

The need to refine the distinction between early or acute disorders of maternal affection and the delayed normative process of mother-to-infant attachment, has since been repeatedly stressed (e.g. Brockington *et al.* 2006; Klier and Musick 2004; Wittkowski *et al.* 2007). Three types of distinct maternal bonding disorders were recently proposed: (1) delay, ambivalence, or lack of maternal response, (2) rejection, and (3) anger toward the infant (Klier and Musick 2004). Additionally, it has been proposed that different psychological disorders may be associated with different types of maternal bonding disorders (e.g. Brockington *et al.* 2006; Wittkowski *et al.* 2007).

Prenatal attachment and paternal attachment as evidence

Some conceptual and empirical evidence has been provided subsequently in the literature that emotional involvement with the infant is a fundamental developmental task of the transition to parenthood, existing from early pregnancy and in fathers, too.

In Reva Rubin's (1976, 1984) description, 'becoming a mother'—that is maternal identity and role acquisitions and the building of a relationship with the child—is a process established since pregnancy. The author stated that the transition to motherhood develops from pregnancy and implies the achievement of the following maternal tasks: (1) to ensure the infant's safety, (2) to ensure the infant's acceptance, (3) to create an idea of the real infant, and (4) to give of oneself. The developmental tasks of the transition to motherhood are mostly to ensure the infant's safety and acceptance and to develop the capacity to give and bond with the unborn child.

Greenberg and Morris (1974), in turn, described the impact of the newborn (which may already be present in pregnancy) on fathers—including, similarly to mothers, a high absorption, concern, and interest—using for this purpose the term 'engrossment'.

Galinsky (1981) proposed that the transition to parenthood begins in pregnancy in both women and men, and develops along several stages, combining specific developmental tasks. The first stage (the image-making stage) refers to pregnancy, and a major task is the formation of feelings towards the infant. In the next stage (the nurturing stage), corresponding to the first two years after childbirth, conflicts between expectations formed in pregnancy and the current reality of the child and parenting are normal. A major task is 'becoming attached to the baby', a process which often takes some time, as described by one of the participants in Galinsky's (1981) study: 'It took a couple of weeks until it wasn't like having an object in our home' (p. 74).

Although first defined as a crisis by some authors, the transition to parenthood was further considered, for both the mother and the father, as a developmental phase beginning in pregnancy, and associated with positive outcomes, with the emergence of psychopathology only in high-risk circumstances (e.g. Figueiredo and Conde 2011).

Transitions are:

> long term processes that result in a qualitative reorganization of both inner life and external behavior, . . . involving a qualitative shift from the inside looking out (how the individual understands and feels about the self and the world) and from the outside looking in (reorganization of the individual's or family's level of personal competence, role arrangements, and relationships with significant others)' (Cowan 1991, p. 5).

The psychological challenges of becoming a parent provide significant opportunities for growth and integration in women and men (e.g. Cowan *et al.* 1985; Demick 2002; Slade *et al.* 2006). The transition to parenthood, a major life developmental stage, has 'powerful potential for parents' reorganization across a number of spheres; reorganization of self . . . and of environment' (Demick 2002, p. 391). Accordingly, the 'very emotional turmoil of pregnancy and of the neonatal period can be seen as a positive force in the mother's (and father's) healthy adjustment, enabling her to provide a more individualizing flexible environment to the infant' (Brazelton and Nugent 1987, p. 221).

Developmental tasks have been defined for pregnancy, including mother and father-to-infant emotional involvement, each of which corresponds to a specific gestational timing. For the mother, these tasks would be: (1) to decide whether or not to have and be the mother of that child, (2) to consider the reality of and engage emotionally with the infant, (3) to prepare for childbirth. Progressively, the mother turns her attention from the external world to the world with her baby, the psychological transition accelerates this process—'not only is she becoming a mother physically, she is now evolving into one psychologically' (Slade *et al.* 2006, p. 23).

The caregiving system is activated over the course of pregnancy (Slade *et al.* 2006), and so the parents will be prepared to take care of the infant after childbirth.

Cranley (1981) and Condon (1993) reiterated that the relationship with the child starts during pregnancy and has an emotional dimension from the beginning, designated 'prenatal attachment'. They added that this emotional dimension is also present in fathers, designated 'paternal attachment'. These authors drew attention to two important circumstances that had been empirically demonstrated in their studies: Emotional involvement is already present during the gestational period and in both parents, because the father also establishes an affectionate relationship with the child.

For Condon (1993), mother and father prenatal attachment indicators are: desire to know the fetus, pleasure in interacting with the fetus, and desire to protect and to meet the fetus' needs. To support the view that the attachment process begins in pregnancy, the author gave, by way of example, the reactions of pain, sadness, and loss that mother and father expressed after fetal or neonatal death (e.g. Canário *et al.* 2011; Kennell *et al.* 1970).

Similar to that described in mothers, paternal attachment refers to feelings, cognitions and behaviors of fathers towards the child. Condon posits, 'the core of parental attachment is a feeling state ("affection") which gives rise to a series of goal directed needs or dispositions to action' (Condon *et al.* 2008, p. 198). 'Multiple and complex factors will determine whether these dispositions actually find expression in overt behavior (Condon *et al.* 2008, p. 198). The author also comments 'the nature of the relationship which female and male expectant parents develop during pregnancy with their unborn baby has both theoretical and clinical significance' (Condon 1993, p. 167).

Some criticism was made of the use of the term 'attachment' in referring to parent-to-infant behaviour, as this relationship does not conform to criteria established in the attachment literature, relating to the lack of complementarity in the parent-to-infant relationship.

Bowlby (1969/1982, 1980) had addressed this issue, warning that 'there is a tendency to extend the use of the word "attachment" to several relationships' (Bowlby 1969/1982, p. 376), but 'whatever the different types of affectional bond may have in common, they cannot be regarded as identical' (Bowlby 1980, p. 40). The author pointed out the need to differentiate and emphasize the uniqueness of child attachment to the caregiver, restricting the term attachment to child-to-parent behavior, and avoiding 'using it to describe the complementary behavior and behavioral system of the parent' (Bowlby 1969/1982, p. 377). Bowlby clarified: 'attachment is limited to behavior normally directed towards someone conceived as better able to cope with the current situation; whilst caregiving specifies the complementary behavior directed towards someone conceived as less able to do so' (Bowlby 1979/1982 p. 377).

More recently, Walsh (2010) also comments:

> since Cranley's conceptualization in 1981, which produced a useful measure to investigate the construct, maternal–fetal relationships have most often been referred to as maternal–fetal, antenatal or prenatal 'attachment'. However, critical analysis of the literature suggests that this relationship is not an attachment relationship at all, as Bowlby and Ainsworth first defined it, but a multi-faceted construct guided instead by the caregiving system, the reciprocal partner to the attachment system, which evolved to provide care and protection' (Walsh, 2010, p. 449).

Condon (2008) counter-argues with the fact that the term 'attachment' has many different meanings, although it traditionally refers to the child's attachment to the mother. Condon's term 'attachment' outside the established context is controversial, but appropriate, in that it meets the general criteria defined by Bowlby for an attachment relationship, 'enduring affective tie' and 'reciprocal' in nature (Condon *et al.* 2008, p. 70).

Parents' representations as determinants

The influence of parent's representations, namely of the caregiving representational system, on mother and father-to-infant emotional involvement and behaviour has been more recently valued in the literature.

Daniel Stern referred to the 'motherhood constellation' as a new and 'unique organization of mental life appropriate for and adapted to the reality of having an infant to care for' (Stern 1995, p. 3). The motherhood constellation is progressively constructed throughout pregnancy and prepares the expectant mother to be a mother, and is based on a mother's past relationships, especially with maternal figures, which are revisited during pregnancy. This constellation comes from a reinvolvement and 'reengagement with maternal figures' (Stern 1995, p. 178) and 'will determine a new set of actions tendencies, sensibilities, fantasies, fears and wishes' (Stern 1995, p. 171). The expectant mother produces a representation of herself, as mother, and a representation of the infant (the imaginary baby), as her child; and initiates a representational and emotional relationship with the child.

Ammaniti (1994) found that mothers' preparatory representations of the infant are founded on the characteristics of the infant's father. These representations become progressively better defined, following the perception of fetal movements, from the 4th to the 7th gestational month, and then become less limited in order to better incorporate the real characteristics of the child.

These representations (of self as mother and of child as son/daughter) are worked out throughout pregnancy, to prepare a mental space to receive the newborn and to perform all necessary actions for the care of the infant after the birth (Ammaniti 1994; Stern 1995, 1998). Over pregnancy the mother prepares herself to be a mother and to the relationship with her child—she creates a mother for the child. She begins to imagine herself as a mother, to hold the baby in mind, developing flexible and pleasurable representations of her baby and herself as the mother (Slade *et al.* 2006).

In the core of attachment theory, George and Solomon resumed and extended Bowlby's conceptions of the caregiving system (George and Solomon 1996, 1999, 2008; Solomon and George 1996). Like Bowlby, the authors appreciate the interdependence and reciprocity of the mother and infant behavioural system, but especially the importance of mental representations of attachment (internal working models) in guiding the behaviour of the parents with the child. As we saw earlier, Bowlby proposed that the caregiving system would be maintained and corrected by the parent's mental representations. George and Solomon (2008) take up this idea, but are alert to the fact that, although internal models tend to be conservative they are open to change as well, as they are tested and updated based on new relationship experiences, particularly in experiences of taking care of a child.

Similarly to Stern (1995, 1998) and Ammaniti (1994) in the psychoanalytic field, mental representations—here, 'mental representations of attachment' – were equally valued as determinants of parenting in attachment theory. Attachment theory conceives that the caregiving system is guided by internal representations (or working models) of caregiving, based on previous attachment experiences with the caregiver in childhood (Solomon and George 1996). Caregiving internal working models integrate evaluations of the self as caregiver—willingness to respond, effectiveness of caregiving strategies and ability to read and understand signals. These representational processes are today a main issue in attachment theory (George and Solomon 2008). Research within the framework of this theory has shown that parents who are able to mentally and emotionally explore – with balance and coherence – the meaning of their attachment histories are best able to meet their children's emotional needs (Steele and Steele 2005).

While considering, as did Bowlby, that the caregiving system is a behavioural system with an adaptive function—that is to provide protection to the child and thereby ultimately increase one's reproductive fitness, and is regulated by internal representations, George and Solomon (2008) added that the caregiving system is 'guided by a representation of the current parent–child relationship' (p. 834). Caregiving internal working models reflect caregiving experiences: 'Experiences of providing care for the child', which are distinct 'from the mother's own childhood experiences with her attachment figures' (George and Solomon 2005, p. 202). The caregiving representational system has its roots in the construction of working models of self and other, in the context of attachment relationships during childhood, '*but is a distinct model of relationship with its own developmental trajectory*' (Solomon and George 1996, p. 190). This is because the system undergoes changes during the transition to parenthood and as a function of the interaction with the child.

Conclusion

Mother- and father-to-infant emotional involvement has not been fully studied, although often referred to as a key ingredient in providing adequate caregiving. Several authors have, however, addressed this important and interesting issue, as we have seen throughout this chapter. A summary of the main contributions in the literature, as well as some future perspectives on the study of emotional involvement of mothers and fathers with the infant are described next.

Interest in parental emotional involvement was established following observations about a particular emotional state in mothers, which accompanies and is accompanied by a particular hormonal state, more recently also described in fathers. In the days after childbirth, mother's emotional and hormonal patterns become fully adapted to the identification and satisfaction of the infant's physical and psychological needs. Descriptions of 'primary maternal preoccupation' (Winnicott 1956) and 'postpartum/maternity blues' (Pitt 1973; Yalom *et al.* 1968) in mothers and of 'engrossment' (Greenberg and Morris 1974) in fathers were reported in the literature.

Several authors became interested in mother-to-infant emotional involvement as a normative process at birth, and then tried to conceptually define and to empirically investigate dimensions that constitute and determine this important aspect of parenting. Klaus and Kennell (1976) described an emotional involvement toward the neonate in most mothers, founded in the first contacts after childbirth, a time defined as an appropriate timing for maternal-infant bonding establishment. Bowlby (1969/1982) reported the presence of a repertoire of caring behaviors in most parents (the caregiving system), aiming to ensure the proximity and protection of the infant, with a view to the child's survival. Although primarily focused on the behavioural dimensions of the caregiving system, the author did not neglect the powerful emotions, which are evoked and the strong bond, which is established between the mother and the child (Bowlby 1979/1982).

Channi Kumar opposed the idea of the presence of a normative emotional involvement with the newborn immediately after childbirth; he reported that for many mothers indifference was the initial reaction to the newborn, and conceived maternal attachment as a gradual process, depending on the child reciprocal attachment signs. In an article from 1980 the author warned that 40% of first-time mothers took some time to feel emotionally involved with the newborn, particularly following a difficult or painful delivery (Robson and Kumar 1980). Kumar considered such initial emotional indifference an equally normative response—since no impact on the mother-to-infant relationship was observed; mothers subsequently developed a similar affection, but more slowly over the weeks following the birth. An equal evolutionary advantage was argued for this maternal response—to ensure that emotional involvement is established only when the survival of the newborn is guaranteed.

Kumar was mainly interested in non-normative processes associated with profound alterations in maternal emotional involvement. Later, the author clarified that the normal reaction described above has very different features from other more severe difficulties, as observed in maternal bonding disorders (Kumar 1997). Occasionally, a prolonged failure in maternal emotional involvement could take place: 'women reported absent affection, sometimes hate, rejection, neglect or impulse to harm . . . these feelings often began immediately or very shortly after the birth' of the child (Kumar 1997, p. 175). Adding as a differential element, such disorders 'did not occur in the absence of postnatal mental ill-ness' (Kumar 1997, p.175).

Following these studies, attention was rarely given to non-normative processes of mother and father-to-infant emotional involvement, and little is known about the preva-lence, emergence, association with mental health, or about the psychological and biologi-cal correlates of maternal bonding disorders (e.g. Brockington *et al.* 2006; Wittkowski *et al.* 2007).

The emotional involvement with the infant was conceptualized as a major developmen-tal task of the transition to parenthood, already initiated in pregnancy, and for both moth-ers (e.g. Rubin 1976, 1984; Slade *et al.* 2006) and fathers (e.g. Galinsky 1981; Parke 2002), in order to facilitate adequate parenting. Special interest was devoted to the mother's behav-ior and emotional state after childbirth, given its uniqueness. The gestational period (e.g., Rubin 1976) and the father (e.g. Condon 1993; Weaver and Cranley 1983) were studied only more recently. Empirical evidence regarding these two specific areas—antenatal and father-to-infant emotional involvement—gives less weight to the importance of biological conditions, and of childbirth, as determinants of the parent's emotional involvement with the infant.

Several other more recent approaches have brought empirical evidence that similarly warns of the need for a more integrative conceptual model to explain mother and father-to-infant emotional involvement. For example, evidence that parental behavior and in-volvement is influenced by representations of past experiences of care, which largely influence the (more or less adequate) way parents take care of the child (e.g. George and Solomon 1996, 1999, 2008; Stern 1995).

Various aspects were recently mentioned in empirical research as determinants of mother- and father-to-infant emotional involvement, from biological, to psycho-logical, and sociocultural factors. A conceptual formulation is urgently needed that integrates all empirical contributions on the factors that may determine and explain the emotional involvement of mothers and fathers with their infant. Such should in-clude the diversity of empirical evidence about normal or developmental processes, but also the profound deviations from non-normative processes of parental emotional involvement.

Parenting includes the behaviours, emotions, and cognitions or representations, that parents direct toward the child in order to promote an adequate context for child health and physical and psychological development. Emotional and hormonal states shortly after birth become adapted to fulfil the infant's physical and psychological needs (cor-rect identification and satisfaction). Stimulated by the neonate's presence and behaviours, mother-to-infant emotional involvement is enhanced, and several caregiving behaviours are put in action to ensure the infant's protection and survival. This important develop-mental task of the transition to parenthood—to implement an emotional involvement with the infant—begins for both mothers and fathers in pregnancy, and the caregiving system is then activated over the course of pregnancy (Slade *et al.* 2006). Furthermore, mother- and father-to-infant emotional involvement is largely influenced by mental representations, formed during childhood experiences, but determined by biological and sociocultural aspects, as well.

Maternal/paternal bonding, attachment, and love were some of the words proposed to name an important emotional dimension of parenting. We proposed here the term 'mother- and father-to-infant emotional involvement' (Figueiredo and Costa 2009), considering the operationalization of what, in fact, parental bonding, attachment and love is, and to avoid confusion with other designations proposed in the literature, as reviewed in this chapter.

In summary, three main issues are suggested to improve the study of mother- and father-to-infant emotional involvement: (1) agreement on the operationalization of the concept; (2) development of a more integrative conceptual model, taking into account biological, psychological, and sociocultural determinants and normative and non-normative variants; (3) an increasing area of interest should also be the father, since most empirical research has so far been with mothers.

Notes

1 A similar emotional state–designated "Engrossment" – was more recently described also in recent fathers (e.g. Greenberg andand Morris 1974).

2 A similar hormonal state has been described in recent years and perceived as performing the same function in men (e.g. Berg and Wynne-Edwards 2001; Carter 2005; Conde and Figueiredo 2013; Storey *et al.* 2000).

References

Ammaniti, M. (1994). Maternal representations during pregnancy and early infant-mother interaction. In Psychoanalysis and development: Representations and narratives, M. Ammaniti, and D.S. Stern, editors. New York, New York University Press, pp. 79–96.

Barrett J. and Fleming, A.S. (2011). All mothers are not created equal: Neural and psychobiological perspectives on mothering and the importance of individual differences. Journal of Child Psychology and Psychiatry **52**(4): 368–97.

Belsky, J. and Cassidy, J. (1994). Attachment: Theory and evidence. In Development through life: A handbook for clinicians, M. Rutter, and D. Hay editors. Oxford, UK, Blackwell, pp. 373–402.

Berg, S. and Wynne-Edwards, K. (2001). Changes in testosterone, cortisol, and estradiol levels in men becoming fathers. Mayo Foundation for Medical Education and Research **76**: 582–92.

Bowlby, J. (1979/1982). Attachment and loss: Vol. 1. Attachment, 2nd Ed. New York, Basic Books.

Bowlby, J. (1980). Attachment and loss: Vol. 3. Loss: Sadness and depression. New York, Basic Books.

Bowlby, J. (1988). A secure base. New York, Basic Books.

Brazelton, T. B. and Nugent, J.K. (1987). Neonatal assessment as an intervention. In Advances in Psychology vol 46, H. Rauh and H.-C. Steinhausen, ed. Amsterdam, North-Holland, pp. 215–29.

Brockington I. F., Aucamp H.M., and Fraser, C. (2006). Severe disorders of the mother-infant relationship: Definitions and frequency. Archives of Women's Mental Health **9**(5): 243–51.

Canário, C., Figueiredo, B., and Ricou, M. (2011). Women and men's psychological adjustment after abortion: A 6-months prospective pilot study. Journal of Reproductive and Infant Psychology **29**(3): 262–75.

Carter, C.S. (2005). Biological perspectives on social attachment and bonding. In Attachment and bonding: A new synthesis, C.S. Carter, K.E. Ahnert, K.E. Grossman, *et al.*, editors. Cambridge, MA, MIT Press, pp. 85–100.

Conde, A. and Figueiredo, B. (2013). 24-hour urinary free cortisol from mid-pregnancy to 3-months postpartum: gender and parity differences and effects. Psychoneuroendocrinology, submitted.

Condon, J.T. (1993). The assessment of antenatal emotional attachment: Development of a questionnaire instrument. British Journal of Medical Psychology 66(2): 167–83.

Condon, J.T., Corkindale, C.J., and Boyce, P. (2008). The assessment of postnatal paternal-infant attachment: Development of a questionnaire instrument. Journal of Reproductive and Infant Psychology 26(3): 195–210.

Cowan, P.A. (1991). Individual and family life transitions: A proposal for a new definition. In Family transitions. P.A. Cowan and M. Hetherington, editors. Hillsdale, NJ, Lawrence Erlbaum Associates, pp. 3–30.

Cowan, C.P., Cowan, P.A., Heming, G., *et al.* (1985). Transitions to parenthood: His, hers, and theirs. Journal of Family Issues 6: 451–481.

Cranley, M.S. (1981). Development of a tool for the measurement of maternal attachment during pregnancy. Nursing Research 30: 281–4.

Demick, J. (2002). Stages of parental development. In Handbook of parenting: Vol 3. Being and becoming a parent, M.H. Bornstein, editor. Mahwah, NJ, Lawrence Erlbaum Publisher, pp. 389–413.

Figueiredo, B. (2003). Bonding: Understanding dimensions involved in the initial mother-to-infant bonding. International Journal of Clinical and Health Psychology 3(3): 521–39.

Figueiredo, B. and Conde, A. (2011). Anxiety and depression symptoms in women and men from early pregnancy to 3-months postpartum: Parity differences and effects. Journal of Affective Disorders 132: 146–57.

Figueiredo, B. and Costa, R. (2009). Mother's stress, mood and emotional involvement with the infant: 3 months before and 3 months after childbirth. Archives of Women's Mental Health 12(3): 143–53.

Fleming, A.S., Ruble, D., Krieger, H., and Wong, P.Y. (1997). Hormonal and experiential correlates of maternal responsiveness during pregnancy and the puerperium in human mothers. Hormones and Behavior 31: 145–58.

Galinsky, E. (1981). Between generations: The six stages of parenthood. New York, Berkeley.

George, C. and Solomon, J. (1996). Representational models of relationships: Links between caregiving and attachment. Infant Mental Health Journal 17: 198–216.

George, C. and Solomon, J. (1999). Attachment and caregiving: The caregiving behavioral system. In Handbook of attachment: Theory, research, and clinical applications, J. Cassidy, and P. R. Shaver editors. New York, Guilford Press, pp. 649–70.

George, C. and Solomon, J. (2008). The caregiving system: A behavioral systems approach to parenting. In Handbook of attachment: Theory, research, and clinical applications, 2nd ed., J. Cassidy, and P. R. Shaver, editors. New York, Guilford Press, pp. 833–56.

Greenberg, M. and Morris, N. (1974) Engrossment: The newborn's impact upon the father. American Journal of Orthopsychiatry 44(4): 520–31.

Kennell, J.H., Slyter, H., and Klaus, M.H. (1970). The mourning response of parents to the death of a newborn infant. New England Journal of Medicine 283(7): 344–9.

Kennell, J.H., Trause, M.A., and Klaus, M.H. (1975). Evidence for a sensitive period in the human mother. Ciba Foundation Symposium 33: 87–102.

Klaus, M. (1998). Mother and infant: Early emotional ties. Pediatrics 102(5): 1244–6.

Klaus, M. and Kennell, J. (1976). Maternal—infant bonding: The impact of early separation or loss on family development. Saint Louis, The C.V. Mosby Company.

Klaus, M.H., Jerauld, R., Wolfe, H., *et al.* (1972). Maternal attachment—importance of the first post-partum days. New England Journal of Medicine **286**: 460–3.

Klaus, M.H., Kennell, J.H., and Klaus, P.H. (1996). Bonding: Building the foundations of secure attachment and independence. Cambridge, MA, Da Capo Press.

Klier, C.M. and Muzik, M. (2004). Mother—infant bonding disorders and use of Parental Bonding Questionnaire in clinical practice. World Psychiatry **3**(2): 102–103.

Kumar, R.C. (1997). 'Anybody's child': Severe disorders of mother-to-infant bonding. British Journal of Psychiatry **171**(8): 175–181.

Miller, L. and Rukstalis, M. (1999). Beyond the 'blues': Hypotheses about postpartum reactivity. In Postpartum mood disorders, L. Miller, editor. Washington DC, American Psychiatry Press, pp. 3–20.

Parke, R. (2002). Fathers and families. In Handbook of parenting: Vol. 3: Being and becoming a parent (2nd ed.), Parke, R.D. and Bornstein, M.H., editors., Mahwah, NJ, Lawrence Erlbaum Associates Publishers, pp. 27–73.

Pedersen, C.A. (1997). Oxytocin control of maternal behavior: Regulation by sex steroids and offspring stimuli. Annals of the New York Academy of Sciences **807**: 126–45.

Pitt, B. (1973). Maternity blues. British Journal of Psychiatry **122**: 431–5.

Robson, K.S. (1967). The role of eye-to-eye contact in maternal-infant attachment. Journal of Child Psychology and Psychiatry **8**(1): 13–25.

Robson, K.S. and Kumar, R. (1980). Delayed onset of maternal affection after childbirth. British Journal of Psychiatry **136**: 347–53.

Robson, K. S., and Moss, H. (1970). Patterns and determinants of maternal attachment. Journal of Pediatrics **77**: 976–85.

Rubin, R. (1976). Maternal tasks in pregnancy. Journal of Advance Nursing **1**(5): 367–76.

Rubin, R. (1984). Maternal identity and the maternal experience. New York, Springer.

Simpson, J.A. and Belsky, J. (2008). Attachment theory within a modern evolutionary framework. In Handbook of attachment: Theory, research, and clinical applications, 2nd ed., J. **Cassidy** and **P.R. Shaver**, editors. New York, Guilford Press, pp. 131–57.

Slade, A., Cohen, L.J., Sadler, L.S., and Miller, M. (2006). The psychology and psychopathology of pregnancy: Reorganization and transformation. In Handbook of infant mental health, 3rd ed., C.H. Zeanah, editor. New York, Guilford Press, pp. 22–38.

Solomon, J. and George, C. (1996). Defining the caregiving system: Toward a theory of caregiving. Infant Mental Health Journal **17**: 183–197.

Sosa R., Kennell J.H., Klaus M., and Urrutia J.J. (1976). The effect of early mother-infant contact on breastfeeding, infection and growth. Ciba Foundation Symposium **45**: 179–93.

Steele, H. and Steele, M. (2005). Understanding and resolving emotional conflict: The London Parent-Child Project. In Attachment from infancy to adulthood: The major longitudinal studies, K.E. Grossmann, K. Grossmann, and E. Waters, editors. New York, Guilford Press, pp. 137–164.

Stern, D. (1995). The motherhood constellation. New York, Harper Collins.

Stern, D. (1998). Mothers' Emotional Needs. Pediatrics **102**(5): 1250–2.

Storey, A.E., Walsh, C.J., Quinton, R.L., and Wynne-Edwards, K. (2000). Hormonal correlates of paternal responsiveness in new and expectant father. Evolution and Human Behavior **21**: 79–95.

Walsh, J. (2010). Definitions matter: If maternal-fetal relationships are not attachment, what are they? Archives of Women's Mental Health **13**(5): 449–51.

Weaver R.H. and Cranley, M.S. (1983). An exploration of paternal-fetal attachment behavior. Nursing Research **32**(2): 68–72.

Winnicott, D.W (1956). Primary maternal preoccupation. Collected papers. New York, Basic Books.

Winnicott, D.W (1960). The theory of the parent–infant relationship. International Journal of Psycho-analysis **41**: 585–595.

Winnicott, D.W. (1990). The maturation process and the facilitating environment. Exeter, UK, Wheatons.

Wittkowski, A., Wieck, A., and Mann, S. (2007). An evaluation of two bonding questionnaires: A comparison of the Mother-to-Infant Bonding Scale with the Postpartum Bonding Questionnaire in a sample of primiparous mothers. Archives of Women's Mental Health **10**(4): 171–5.

Yalom, I., Lunde, D., Moos, R., and Hamburg, D. (1968). Postpartum blues syndrome. Archives of General Psychiatry **18**: 16–27.

Chapter 12

Specificity of effects in the association between maternal postnatal depression and child development: evidence from the Cambridge longitudinal study

Lynne Murray

Personal note

From 1985, when I first met Channi Kumar, he played a seminal role in the research I have conducted with my colleagues on the effects of postnatal depression on child development. At the time I was a very junior researcher, struggling to get my work underway, and his enthusiasm and encouragement were invaluable. Channi played a particularly important role from 1989 when, with the support of the Tedworth Charitable Trust and the Winnicott Trust, the Winnicott Research Unit was established in Cambridge, under the joint Directorship of myself and Peter Cooper, together with Alan Stein. Channi became a key member of the Unit's advisory committee and, right up until the time of his death, he regularly, and very kindly, provided the wisest counsel and support, and he is still very sorely missed. He was an inspiring friend and colleague, with the deepest compassion and humanity for the plight of the families he helped, and boundless enthusiasm for new perspectives and ideas that could advance understanding and clinical treatment, and I am greatly indebted to him for all his support.

This chapter describes research on a prospective longitudinal study of the development of children of depressed and well mothers conducted in the Winnicott Research Unit; much of it took place under Channi's watch. The work has involved a large number of colleagues, aside from the contributions of Peter Cooper and Alan Stein, and I am particularly grateful to Alison Hipwell, Matt Woolgar, Sheelah Seeley, Janet Edwards, Sarah Halligan, Adriane Arteche, Ian Goodyer, and Joe Herbert for their involvement and support.

Introduction

A diagnosis of 'postnatal depression' includes a wide range of possible symptoms, and therefore this unitary term can mask considerable variation in the nature of its presentation.

For example, one mother could be slowed down, sleeping excessively, and barely eating, while in another, the episode may manifest itself in restlessness and agitation, with the mother being hardly able to concentrate and feeling constantly irritable. Not surprisingly, then, studies of the effects of postnatal depression on mother-infant interactions have also identified striking variability. From the seminal work of Field and Tronick and their colleagues in the 1980s, researchers have consistently identified distinct patterns of maternal responsiveness in the context of postnatal depression (Cohn *et al.* 1986; Field *et al.* 1990). Thus, although difficulty in noticing the baby's signals and responding appropriately is common to many who suffer from postnatal depression, the manner in which this general difficulty impinges on the mother's interactions with her baby can vary markedly. The main patterns that have been described in the literature fall into two main groups: on the one hand, some mothers appear remote and withdrawn, and they interact little with their infants, while on the other, mothers can be overly stimulating, intrusive, and even hostile in their contacts with their baby. It is important to note, too, that a further subgroup of mothers who experience depression nevertheless function well in their interactions with their baby, being warm, responsive, and playful. Indeed, one study, conducted in a deprived multi-problem community in Melbourne, noted that, for some depressed mothers, the baby could be the one ray of sunshine in an otherwise sad, drab life, with the mother's care for her infant remaining relatively encapsulated from her wider concerns (Williams and Carmichael 1985).

As well as differences in the mother's interactions with her baby that maybe influenced by which particular depressive symptoms are present, other factors are also influential. The severity and chronicity of the disorder are of obvious importance, but so is the level of background adversity: where families live under social and economic hardship, the more likely it is that maternal difficulties in responding sensitively to her baby will be marked, whereas in low risk communities more subtle problems are prevalent (Cohn *et al.* 1990; Murray *et al.* 1996a), or may be elucidated only where some provocation to the interaction occurs (Tronick and Gianino 1986). (Notably, even in the absence of depression, marked adversity increases the risk of mother-infant interaction problems, in all probability because the mother's worries and preoccupations with her difficult circumstances interfere with her capacity to respond to her baby (Murray *et al.* 1996a)).

In parallel with the diversity of difficulties in mothers' interactions with their baby that can occur in the context of postnatal depression, the wide range of problematic developmental outcomes for children of mothers who were postnatally depressed is also striking. These include elevated rates of insecure attachments, behaviour problems in childhood of both externalising and internalizing kinds, poorer cognitive performance, and elevated rates of psychiatric disorder in adolescence. Such findings of poorer outcome are, like the difficulties in maternal responsiveness, far more likely to occur in populations where the mother's depression is severe and chronic, as well as in those with high levels of socioeconomic adversity (see Murray *et al.* 2010a for a review). Aside from the *prevalence* of poor outcomes, background adversity also appears to influence the *nature* of the child's problems, with increased antisocial and aggressive child behaviour being more strongly linked to postnatal depression in high vs. low risk communities (see for example, the findings of Hay *et al.* 2008, vs. those of Murray *et al.* 2011). The child's sex also appears to make a difference to child risk, especially for cognitive problems, with boys appearing to be more affected than girls (Murray *et al.* 2010a).

Given infants' total dependency on other people in the postnatal months, and their considerable sensitivity, even at this early stage, to the quality of engagement with others, together with the fact that, for many, their primary environment is constituted by their mother at this time, a key question is whether it is by virtue of the disturbances in the mother-infant relationship associated with postnatal depression that the poor child outcomes described above develop. Certainly, a large volume of research in developmental psychology with non-clinical populations has shown the considerable influence of a child's social relationships in the early years on their subsequent functioning (Murray 2014). Studies of mother–infant interactions in the context of postnatal depression have indeed shown the infant's behaviour during the interaction to be affected and, in large measure, these effects parallel the disturbances seen in maternal behaviour. Infants of depressed mothers, are, therefore, more likely than are those of non-depressed mothers to show avoidant and distressed behaviour while interacting with their mother, and this is particularly likely in high risk samples (Cohn *et al.* 1986; Field *et al.* 1990); further, there is a significant association between the degree to which the mother's behaviour is impaired and the extent of these signs of infant difficulty (Murray *et al.* 1996a). One striking aspect of the effects of disturbances in maternal interactions on infant behaviour is that they gradually begin to extend to the way the infant behaves with *other* people so that, by 4–6 months, but not before, babies of depressed mothers start to show rather difficult behaviour with other, unfamiliar, non-depressed, adults (Field *et al.* 1988; Morrell and Murray 2003).

An important feature of the findings from developmental psychology on the effects of social interactions on child psychological functioning, is that different aspects of parenting are associated with different kinds of child outcome, that is, there is considerable *specificity of effects* in the associations between parenting style and child development. Understanding the nature of these associations may be of considerable benefit in marshalling the most beneficial support to depressed mothers and their infants in the postnatal months, since interventions can then be focussed more precisely on specific aspects of a mother's relationship with her infant, according to the nature of the developmental difficulty concerned.

Key domains of child development that have been shown to be affected by the occurrence of postnatal depression, along with an account of the critical features of parent child relationships that are known to be associated with each domain, now follow. Where available, evidence concerning the operation of these mechanisms in the context of postnatal depression is presented. In particular, data are presented from the Cambridge longitudinal study, which compared the development of offspring of a community sample of depressed and non-depressed mothers, with mother–infant interactions being observed from 2 months. Throughout the conduct of this study, for each child outcome measure, theoretically based predictions have been made concerning the relevant maternal interaction characteristics that might affect such outcomes. Thus, while by no means complete, this has enabled a number of precisely targeted developmental hypotheses to be tested concerning key processes mediating any effects of postnatal depression on child development.

The social interaction mechanisms mediating effects of postnatal depression on child outcome

Child cognitive functioning

General responsiveness

A large body of evidence with normal populations has shown that parents' overall level of *child-centred responsiveness*, or *contingency*, during social interactions is of major importance for their child's child cognitive development (Eshel *et al.* 2006), and this is a dimension of others' communication, to which babies of even 2 months are sensitive (Murray and Trevarthen 1985; Nadel *et al.* 1999; Bigelow, 1998). 'Contingency' entails two key components: first, there needs to be a close association in time between what the baby does and the parent's response; second, the *proportion* of the parent's behaviours that show this close association in time with the baby's actions needs to be relatively high, so that the contingent responses stand out clearly, and are not swamped by a large number of maternal behaviours that are unrelated to what the baby does. If babies experience a high degree of such contingency in their caretaker's response, this appears to facilitate their making connections between events, and therefore helps fundamental learning processes (Lewis and Goldberg 1969; Dunham et al. 1989). The fact it is often difficult for depressed mothers to notice and respond to their baby's cues makes it likely that contingency levels in their interactions will be relatively low, and this may thereby contribute to poor cognitive functioning in their children. This possibility has been investigated in a number of studies: Stanley et al. (2004) found at least short-term effects of this kind, with reduced contingent responsiveness on the part of depressed mothers during face-to-face interactions in the first 2–3 postnatal months, predicting poorer infant performance in an operant learning task. In the Cambridge longitudinal study, the reduction found in depressed mothers' responsiveness to their infant accounted for the adverse effects of the postnatal episode on boys' performance on the Bayley Scales at 18 months (Murray *et al.* 1993). Furthermore, at 5-year follow up (Murray *et al.* 1996b), children whose mothers had shown a marked reduction in responsiveness postnatally were found to continue on a trajectory of poor cognitive functioning; indeed, where Bayley scores had been low at 18 months (an effect that was marked for boys of depressed mothers), children were found to perform significantly worse on public exams at age 16 (GCSEs), with boys of postnatally depressed scoring, on average, one grade lower on each of seven GCSE subjects (Murray *et al.* 2010b). Low contingent responsiveness in the early postnatal months appeared, therefore, to set the infant on a trajectory of poorer cognitive functioning that persisted right through childhood.

Evidence consistent with these findings also comes from the 1999 NICHD study, where variability in the interactions of depressed mothers was also highlighted and, in cases where interactions were particularly poor, with low levels of sensitive responsiveness, the risk for poor child cognitive outcome was substantial. In contrast, children whose mothers maintained good interactions, despite their depression, were buffered from the potentially negative effects of the maternal disorder on cognitive functioning. Finally, in a clinic-based Australian sample, Milgrom and colleagues (2004) found that low maternal responsiveness at six months mediated the adverse effect of maternal depression on boys' IQ at 42 months.

Attention regulation

Aside from overall contingency, difficulties in depressed mothers' interactions that concern infant attention regulation are also likely to contribute to poorer infant cognitive performance, since the infant's ability to sustain attention is a particularly robust predictor of childhood IQ (Slater 1995). The way in which parents modulate their vocalizations when engaging with their baby appear particularly important for gaining and maintaining infant attention (Stern *et al.* 1982). Thus, Kaplan et al. (1999) found that segments of infant-directed speech that had been recorded from postnatally depressed mothers failed to promote associative learning in infants of non-depressed mothers in a conditioned attention task. By contrast, speech samples from non-depressed mothers *did* promote infant learning. In the same study Kaplan and colleagues (1999) noted that the fundamental frequency of the final portion of the speech segments of mothers with more depressive symptoms was less modulated than that of other mothers, and they suggested that this reduced modulation may have failed to make the infants sufficiently aroused, and so they were less able to attend to, and efficiently process, the information required.

Book sharing

Sharing of picture books with infants is significantly associated with good infant language development and, indeed, this practice has been referred to as a 'language acquisition device', with around three quarters of all labeling of objects and events occurring in this particular context during home-based interactions between mothers and their young infants and children (Ninio 1983). Strikingly, these associations between picture book sharing and enhanced child language occur even when parental social class and other relevant variables are taken into account. This is particularly so when the style of book-sharing is 'dialogic', that is, it is sensitive to the infant's interests and initiatives, and pitched according to their language abilities. Importantly, recent research suggests that such picture book sharing, or rather its absence, may be a relevant dimension of parenting contributing to poorer cognitive outcomes among infants of postnatally depressed mothers.

Child emotional–behavioural regulation problems

Much research shows that parenting plays a significant role in the development of good child emotional and behavioural regulation, that is, their ability to modulate their responses to stimulation from both internal as well as external sources, in order to achieve a well-regulated state (Fox 1998). The capacity for self-regulation starts to develop from the earliest weeks, and is important because it is predictive of later child adjustment. A key aspect of parenting that helps promote these skills is a kind of '*emotional scaffolding*'. Early in development, this often takes the form of soothing, or giving comfort to the distressed infant, but it rapidly shifts to help support the infant's own self-regulation capacities, and such supportive processes can be seen even during face-to-face interactions in the first 3 months in normal populations, as well as in the development of capacities such as sleep regulation through the first year and beyond.

Repairing miscoordinations

In social interactions in non-clinical populations, mother and infant typically shift from miscoordinated to coordinated states; such normal, minor, miscoordinations may occur, for example, if some physiological event, like infant hiccoughing, occurs that momentarily disrupts the organization of the infant's behaviour. Alternatively, they may occur if the parent misjudges the baby's signals, perhaps briefly responding with greater intensity than the infant can manage to handle. Such miscoordinations are common and, indeed, some researchers have argued that, if mild, they serve the important purpose of providing opportunities for the infant to gain experience of recovery from destabilized states, and thereby develop capacities for self-regulation. Nevertheless, in early infancy when infants are still unable to regulate their behaviour and affect, such moments are quite likely to require parental support in order to foster the infant's own capacities (Tronick and Gianino 1986; Tronick 1989; Jaffe *et al.* 2001). Indeed, studies in which maternal behaviour is experimentally disrupted by means of the 'still-face' procedure (where the mother abruptly ceases to respond to her infant and instead looks at him with a still, blank, expression) show that where mothers do provide such support during normal interactions, infants appear better able to cope with the Still Face disruption (Gunning et al. 2013). Importantly, the studies of Tronick and colleagues suggest that postnatally depressed mothers may have difficulties in providing such 'emotional scaffolding' or support for the infant's developing self-regulation skills (Tronick and Weinburg 1997; Weinburg *et al.* 2006), as is the case for depressed mothers of older children (Jameson *et al.* 1997). To date, the mediating effects of such specific maternal difficulties on the behaviour problems experienced by children of postnatally depressed mothers have not been directly investigated. Nevertheless, evidence from normal populations concerning the longer term beneficial effects of parental strategies to promote infant self-regulation, as assessed by secure attachment (Isabella andand Belsky 1991; Jaffe *et al.* 2001) and in particular good sleep outcomes (Murray and Ramchandani 2007), suggests this is a highly plausible postnatal mechanism that may mediate effects of postnatal depression.

Maternal hostility and coercion

The hostile and intrusive, or coercive, behaviour that is characteristic of some depressed mothers (and especially those who experience marked background adversity) may directly cause infant distress and emotional–behavioural dysregulation. Indeed, a microanalysis of face-to-face interactions between depressed and well mothers and their infants in the Cambridge longitudinal study showed that episodes of infant behavioural dysregulation were immediately preceded by the mother's 'negating' the infant's experience, often through intrusive or hostile actions (Murray *et al.* 1996a). Long-term associations were also found in this sample, with early maternal hostility predicting poorer child capacities to cope with a mild challenge (Murray *et al.* 2001). Such an association was similarly identified in the study of Maughan *et al.* (2007). A path analysis of mother–infant/child interactions and child behaviour assessed in the Cambridge study over 8 years showed that infant emotional and behavioural dysregulation at 2 months, assessed in an interaction with a researcher, independently of the mother, was unrelated to depressed mothers' hostile and coercive interactions at this time, but that by 4 months an association was evident. Notably, from this point onwards, the infant's dysregulated behaviour began to show continuity over time and, in turn, it precipitated further maternal negativity and coerciveness, with the ensuing vicious cycle culminating in raised rates of child conduct problems and attention deficit hyperactivity disorder symptoms by age 5–8 years (Morrell and Murray 2003). Such findings are consistent with more general research with older children, showing the occurrence of disruptive behaviour disorders to be associated with parental hostility and coercive control (see review by Hill 2002).

Adolescent depression

It is well-established that parental depression in general is a risk factor for offspring disorder (Beardslee *et al.* 1998), and this risk appears to be environmentally mediated (Silberg *et al.* 2010). Although few studies have followed up *postnatal* samples for long enough to track the emergence of adolescent disorder, three have found exposure to maternal depression before two years to be associated with increased offspring depression (Hammen and Brennan 2003; Hay *et al.* 2008; Murray *et al.* 2011). While the study of Hay and colleagues showed overall duration of maternal depression to be more important than a postnatal episode, those of Hammen and colleagues and Murray and colleagues showed exposure to maternal postnatal depression to be sufficient, albeit not necessary, to raise adolescent risk; in the Cambridge longitudinal study, for example, the rate of life-time depression in 16 year olds of postnatally depressed mothers was 41.5%, vs. 12.5% in the control group, an odds ratio (OR) of 4.99. Since this sample had involved direct observations of interactions throughout the study, possible mechanisms of transmission involving the mother-infant/child relationship could be examined. These investigations focused on a number of key processes that, while differing in nature, are certainly not incompatible with each other but, rather, may operate in concert.

Emotion contagion

In Field's seminal work on postnatal depression (1984), an important suggestion was that the mother's sad affect might be transmitted to the infant by a process of emotional contagion. One of the most sensitive markers of affect is voice quality, and this was therefore investigated in the Cambridge longitudinal study (Marwick and Murray 2008). Analyses of maternal utterances showed, in common with other studies, that the usual intuitive adaptations parents make when talking to young infants occurred less often when the mother was depressed. Instead, depressed mothers' speech to their infants was characterized by low pitch and a greater preponderance of repeated falling contours. Together, these features give speech a flat and monotonous quality, similar to that associated with the perception of sorrow or sadness in non-depressed individuals. Notably, the prosodic qualities of infant-directed speech that signal emotion share features with vocalizations between non-human primates that serve important relational, social-affective functions. Together with the recent evidence for a 'mirror neuron system' that connects *observed* behaviour, including emotional displays, to activation of brain circuits involved in its *production* (Ferrari and Fogassi 2012), these findings are consistent with the idea that exposure to such 'sad speech' in the postnatal months may attune, or sensitize, the infant to specific emotions during a sensitive developmental period when selective responsiveness to the particular characteristics of the language environment emerges (Kuhl 2008). Indeed, analyses showed a significant association between these early maternal speech features signalling sadness, and the occurrence of affective disorder in offspring by age 13, an association that, notably, partially mediated the effect of postnatal depression on this adolescent outcome (Murray *et al.* 2010c).

Hypothalamus–pituitary–adrenal axis functioning

Research with rodents and non-human primates shows that early experience may determine adult functioning of the hypothalamus–pituitary–adrenal (HPA) axis, and associated stress responding (i.e. cortisol reactivity) (e.g. Champagne and Meaney 2001; Suomi 1997). This is an important area for investigation in the context of effects of maternal depression on offspring disorder, since elevations in cortisol are known to predict subsequent episodes of depression. Further, in human populations, elevated morning or daytime cortisol levels have been found in children adopted from very deprived institutional environments, and maltreated children (see review by Tarullo and Gunnar 2006). While these latter findings are consistent with the animal models, until recently their interpretation has been limited by a lack of evidence concerning the details of the rearing experience and, in many cases, by the presence of concurrent psychopathology (Tarullo and Gunnar 2006).

The question of the longer-term impact on the developing child's physiological functioning of early exposure to maternal depression and the associated parenting difficulties was addressed in the Cambridge sample: basal morning cortisol levels, measured on 10 consecutive days in the offspring at age 13 years, were found to be elevated in children of postnatally depressed mothers; importantly, this association was not accounted for by exposure to maternal depression beyond infancy, suggesting that maternal depression occurring *early* in offspring development was particularly relevant (Halligan *et al.* 2004). Indeed, when early parenting was examined in this sample, with a particular focus on the nearest possible equivalent to the absence of active licking and grooming found in rat models to be associated with offspring cortisol elevations (i.e. withdrawn, disengaged maternal behaviour), it was found that this feature of maternal interactions with the infant in the *first 9 months* (something that was significantly more common in the depressed group) was a significant predictor of the children's 13-year cortisol elevations, whereas *later* parenting on the same dimension (5 years) was unrelated to adolescent HPA axis functioning

(Murray *et al.* 2010d). Of further note was that, even when controlling for child symptoms at 13 years, elevations in cortisol levels at this time predicted depressive symptomatology at 16 years (Halligan *et al.* 2007a), suggesting a clear physiological route, via parenting, for the intergenerational transmission of disorder.

Psychological pathways: insecure attachment and low child resilience

In addition to the two processes outlined above concerning emotional sensitization and physiological functioning, more psychological processes were also investigated in the Cambridge study. A considerable body of research with diverse populations suggests that *insecure attachment* to the mother in infancy, an adverse outcome that is well-established as being associated with postnatal depression (Martins and Gaffan 2000), might confer early psychological vulnerability to depression. Attachment aspects of relationships concern the child's need for sensitive care, particularly in conditions of vulnerability, such as when feeling ill, fearful, or in the context of separations from a caretaker, and these needs need to be met if the child is to feel secure. In Bowlby's theory of attachment, someone with an *avoidant insecure attachment* is likely to have experienced parental emotional coldness or rejection, and will therefore deny their own needs and attempt to live without others' support, but nevertheless carry an underlying sense of themselves as being unworthy of love, and of others as rejecting; such individuals may, therefore, have low self-esteem and fail to develop the kinds of close supportive relationships that can be protective against depression. Similarly, the *insecure ambivalently attached* individual, who is likely to have had more inconsistent and possibly intrusive care, is liable to experience anxiety, especially about separation and the reliability of others' care, and is prone to be anxious about exploring the world, with the result that their capacity to cope with difficulties is impaired (Bowlby 1988). Both these main types of attachment insecurity, then, may mean that the individual develops low personal resilience, and poor support networks; indeed, prospective studies have confirmed this suggestion, with a constellation of cognitive, affective, and behavioural processes in school-aged children, that can be characterized as reflecting low 'ego-resiliency', being found in those who were insecure as infants. This constellation is shown in inflexibility in the face of changing and stressful circumstances, and difficulty in recovering from challenge or failure, and it shares certain core features with a profile of cognitive vulnerability for depression (e.g., negative affect, feelings of unworthiness, low self-aspirations) (Arend *et al.* 1979).

In the Cambridge sample, consistent with other studies, maternal postnatal depression was found to increase the odds of insecure attachment in late infancy by a factor of nearly 4 (OR 3.8) (Murray *et al.* 1996a), with the great majority of insecure attachments being of the avoidant type. Subsequently, difficulties in the mother–child relationship persisted in the postnatally depressed group, with direct observations of social interactions at 5 years showing that these children remained unresponsive to their mothers' bids to engage with them, despite their mothers having generally recovered and no longer being insensitive to their child, and this association was entirely mediated by the child's earlier insecure infant attachment (Murray *et al.* 1999a). Peer relationship difficulties were also apparent at this age: direct observations at school showed postnatally depressed mothers' children to be unresponsive to positive social approaches by other children (Murray *et al.* 1999a), and in the home they were more aggressive in peer play (Hipwell *et al.* 2005).

The Cambridge study also included assessments of child depressive cognitions and resilience. At the five and eight-year follow-ups, the children were observed as they played a specially designed competitive card game with a friend. The order of playing cards dealt by the researcher was predetermined, such that both children received winning hands, as well as the mild threat of being dealt losing cards. The children's responses revealed wide variations in their capacity to cope with the stress of a losing deal. Some quickly slipped into feeling that the outcome would be negative ('I know she's going to win'), or showed clear signs of general low self-worth ('I never win at games'). Others showed impressive resilience, for example, managing to reflect on positive personal attributes ('I can run faster than the big boys'), could rationalize the situation ('it's only a game, isn't it'), or imagine positive outcomes ('the winner just might be me, it might be me') (Murray *et al.* 2001). Analyses of such responses in this ecologically valid mildly challenging context, where the children's emotions were engaged, showed postnatally depressed mothers' children to be substantially more likely to have difficulties in coping (Murray *et al.* 2011) and to evince clear signs of depressive cognitions (Murray *et al.* 2001), and this latter effect was particularly likely where the mother had shown high levels of hostility in her interactions with the child.

The study also assessed the children's cognitions regarding their family via doll play at 5 years (Murray *et al.* 1999b; Woolgar and Murray 2010). Using a furnished doll's house, with doll characters of the child's own choosing, a relatively open-ended methodology was used, in which the child was invited to show a researcher what happened at home in a range of universal family contexts, i.e., meal time, bed time, a bad time, and a favourite time. Ratings of the children's representations of their family relationships (e.g. parental care and neglect, and the child in a caring role) showed recent, as well as postnatal depression to be influential, as well as the occurrence of parental conflict. Particularly noteworthy was the fact that key aspects of these family representations in early childhood were reflected in the way close friendship experiences were represented in adolescence (Murray *et al.* 2006). By this age, episodes of depression in the sample had started to emerge, often following on earlier experience of anxiety disorder (Halligan *et al.* 2007b). When the adolescents were asked to describe a recent experience with friends that had been difficult, the 13-year-old girls of postnatally depressed mothers, who had earlier appeared (especially where the mother continued to be depressed) to be highly sensitive to interpersonal relationships in their doll play (for example, giving extended accounts, and enacting how they and their mother cared for each other), showed the same kind of heightened sensitivity to their own and others' emotional experience. For example, they would dwell in detail on the subtleties of feelings experienced during recent interpersonal encounters. This pattern was particularly likely to occur in girls who had been insecurely attached as infants, whereas, as in early childhood, the insecure adolescent sons of postnatally depressed mothers often struggled to give an account of friendship difficulties. Of particular note in these adolescent assessments was that, when relationship representations were examined in relation to mood, it was found that the emotional sensitivity of the daughters of depressed mothers, especially in the context of infant insecurity, was significantly associated with high levels of their own depressive symptoms. Thus, high interpersonal sensitivity in the context of infant insecurity and a mother with depression, was a combined risk factor for girls' adolescent depressive symptoms, whereas in the context of a secure attachment, and without exposure to maternal depression, such heightened sensitivity was *not* associated with risk. Similar associations have also been reported by Hammen and Brennan (2003), whose follow up study found social relationship difficulties among adolescents of depressed mothers, together with insecure child-parent attachment, as assessed by self-report questionnaire.

When the main results concerning earlier child vulnerability were considered together in relation to the experience of depressive disorder by age 16, it was found that insecure attachment to the mother in infancy did indeed predict depression in adolescence; further, this association arose largely *via* lower child resilience, as expressed in the social challenge of the competitive card game, some years before first onset of depression. Notably, however, continuing family adversity (poor maternal support, marital conflict and prolonged maternal depression) was also important, and indeed added substantially to offspring risk. In particular, the occurrence of marital conflict, which was often present in the postnatally depressed group, and further maternal depression were partial mediators of the effects of postnatal depression on adolescent depression. With regard to the latter, however, only maternal depression that accumulated for more than 17 months beyond the postnatal period added significantly to offspring risk, and even such prolonged subsequent maternal depression did not entirely eliminate the association between the postnatal episode and offspring depression. In this sample, therefore, the presence of postnatal depression did seem to be of particular importance for offspring outcome, not least in part because of a trajectory of psychological vulnerability, starting with insecure mother-infant attachment, which the occurrence of postnatal depression set in place.

Conclusion

Postnatal depression is associated with a range of difficulties in the mother–infant relationship and, in turn, with a diversity of adverse child outcomes. Longitudinal data including direct observations of the mother–child relationship demonstrate that different kinds of interaction difficulty are associated with different kinds of poor child outcome. Thus, while there is inevitably some overlap between the various forms of problem that depressed mothers may experience in their parenting role, there is also some specificity of effects. Given that the treatment of postnatal depression as such does not appear to confer benefits for the mother–child relationship or child outcome (Nylen *et al.* 2006), such evidence linking particular parenting difficulties to particular kinds of adverse child outcome offers a promising approach for intervention, where treatment can be precisely targeted to particular profiles of impairment in the parent–infant/child relationship.

References

Arend, R., Gove, F. L., and Sroufe, A.L. (1979). Continuity of individual adaptation from infancy to kindergarten: a predictive study of ego-resilience and curiosity in preschoolers. Child Development **50**(4): 950–9.

Beardslee, W.R., Versage, E.M., and Gladstone, T.R.G. (1998). Children of affectively ill parents: a review of the past 10 years. Journal of the American Academy of Child and Adolescent Psychiatry **37**(11): 1134–41.

Bigelow, A. (1998) Infants' sensitivity to familiar imperfect contingencies in social interaction. Infant Behavior and Development **21**(1): 149–162

Bowlby, J. (1988). Lecture 7: The role of attachment in personality development. In A secure base: clinical applications of attachment theory. Routledge, London.

Cohn, J.F., Matias, R., Tronick, E.Z., Connell, D., and Lyons-Ruth, K. (1986). Face-to-face interactions of depressed mothers and their infants. In Maternal depression and infant disturbance, Z. Tribucjm and E.T. Field, editors. Jossey-Bass, San-Francisco, pp. 31–46.

Cohn, J.F., Campbell, S.B., Matias, R., and Hopkins, J. (1990). Face-to-face interactions of postpartum depressed and nondepressed mother-infant pairs at 2 months. Developmental Psychology **26**(1): 15–23.

Champagne, F. and Meaney, M.J., (2001). Like mother, like daughter: evidence for non-genomic transmission of parental behavior and stress responsivity. Progress in Brain Research **133**: 287–302.

Dunham, P., Dunham, F., Hurshman, A., and Alexander, T (1989), Social contingency effects on subsequent perceptual-cognitive tasks in young infants. Child Development **60**: 1486–96.

Eshel, N., Daelmans, B., Cabral De Mello, M., and MartinesJ. (2006). Responsive parenting: Interventions and outcomes. Bulletin of the World Health Organization **84**(12): 992–8.

Ferrari, P. and Fogassi, L. (2012). The mirror neuron system in monkeys and its implications for social cognitive functions. In The Primate Mind: built to connect with other minds, F. de Waal and P. F. Ferrari, editors. (13–31) London, Harvard University Press,

Field, T.M. (1984). Early interactions between infants and their postpartum depressed mothers. Infant Behaviour and Development **7**: 517–22.

Field, T., Healy, B., Goldstein, S., *et al.* (1988). Infants of depressed mothers show "depressed" behavior even with nondepressed adults. Child Development **59**: 1569–79.

Field, T., Healy, B., Goldstein, S., and Guthertz, M. (1990). Behavior state matching and synchrony in mother—infant interactions of nondepressed versus 'depressed' dyads. Developmental Psychology **26**: 7–14.

Fox, N.A. (1998). Temperament and regulation of emotion in the first years of life. In New perspectives in early emotional development, Johnson & Johnson Pediatric Round Table Series, Vol 1., J.G. Warhol, editor. New Brunswick, New Jersey, USA. Johnson & Johnson Pediatric Institute Ltd.

Gunning, M., Halligan, S.L., Murray L., (2013) Contributions of maternal and infant factors to infant responding to the Still Face paradigm: A longitudinal study. Infant Behavior and Development, **36** (3), 319–328

Halligan, S.L., Herbert, J., Goodyer, I., and Murray, L. (2004). Exposure to postnatal depression predicts elevated cortisol in adolescent offspring. Biological Psychiatry **55**: 376–81.

Halligan, S.L., Herbert, J., Goodyer, I. and Murray, L. (2007a). Disturbances in morning cortisol secretion in association with maternal postnatal depression predict subsequent depressive symptomatology in adolescents. Biological Psychiatry **62**: 40–6.

Halligan, S.L., Murray, L., Martins, C., and Cooper, P.J. (2007b). Maternal depression and psychiatric outcomes in adolescent offspring. Journal of Affective Disorders **97**: 145–54.

Hammen, C. and Brennan, P. (2003). Severity, chronicity, and timing of maternal depression and risk for adolescent offspring diagnoses in a community sample. Archives of General Psychiatry **60**(3): 253–60.

Hay, D.F., Pawlby, S., Waters, C.S., and Sharp, D. (2008). Antepartum and post partum depression: different effects on different adolescent outcomes. Journal of Child Psychology and Psychiatry **49**(10): 1079–88.

Hill, J. (2002). Biological, psychological and social processes in the conduct disorders. Journal of Child Psychology and Psychiatry and Allied Disciplines **43**(1): 133–64.

Hipwell, A.E., Murray, L., Ducournau, P. and Stein, A. (2005). The effects of maternal depression and parental conflict on children's peer play. Child: Care, Health and Development **31**(1): 11–23.

Isabella, R.A. and Belsky, J. (1991) Interactional synchrony and the origins of infant—mother attachment: a replication study. child development. *Child Development* **62**(2): 373–84.

Jaffe, J., Beebe, B., Feldstein, S., Crown, C.L., and Jasnow, M. D. (2001). Rhythms of dialogue in infancy. In W.D. Overton, editor, Monographs of the Society for Research in Child Development 66 (2).

Jameson, P.B., Gekfand, D.M., Kulcsar, E., and Teti, D.M. (1997). Mother—toddler interaction patterns associated with maternal depression. Development and Psychopathology **9**: 537–50.

Kaplan, P.S., Bachorowski, J., and Zarlengo-Strouse, P. (1999). Child-directed speech produced by mothers with symptoms of depression fails to promote associative learning in 4-month-old infants. Child Development **70**(3): 560–70.

Kuhl, P. (2004). Early language acquisition: cracking the speech code. *Nature Neuroscience* **5**: 831–43.

Lewis, M. and Goldberg, S. (1969). Perceptual-cognitive development in infancy: A generalized expectancy model as a function of the mother-infant interaction. Merrill-Palmer Quarterly **15**(1): 81–100.

Martins, C. and Gaffan, E. (2000). Effects of early maternal depression on patterns of infant-mother attachment: a meta-analytic investigation. Journal of Child Psychology and Psychiatry **41** (6): 737–46.

Marwick, H. and Murray, L. (2008). The effects of maternal depression on the 'musicality' of infant directed speech and conversational engagement. In Communicative musicality, S. Malloch and C Trevarthen, editors. (281–304) Oxford, Oxford University Press.

Maughan, A., Cicchetti, D., Toth, S.L., and Rogosch, F.A. (2007). Early-occurring maternal depression and maternal negativity in predicting young children's emotion regulation and socioemotional difficulties. Journal of Abnormal Child Psychology **35**(5): 685–703.

Milgrom, J., Westley, D.T., and Gemmill, A.W. (2004). The mediating role of maternal responsiveness in some longer term effects of postnatal depression on infant development. Infant Behavior and Development **4**: 443–54.

Morrell, J. and Murray, L. (2003). Parenting and the development of conduct disorder and hyperactive symptoms in childhood: a prospective longitudinal study from 2 months to 8 years. Journal of Child Psychology and Psychiatry and Allied Disciplines **44**(4): 489–508.

Murray, L. and Trevarthen, C. (1985). Emotional regulation of interactions between two month olds and their mothers. In Social perception in infants, T.M. Field and N. Fox, editors. New Jersey, Ablex.

Murray, L., Kempton, C., Woolgar, M and Hooper, R. (1993). Depressed mothers' speech to their infants and its relation to infant gender and cognitive development. Journal of Child Psychology and Psychiatry **34**: 1083–101.

Murray, L., Fiori-Cowley, A., Hooper, R., and Cooper, P. (1996a). The impact of postnatal depression and associated adversity on early mother—infant interactions and later infant outcome. Child Development **67**: 2512–26.

Murray, L., Hipwell, A., Hooper, R., Stein, A., and Cooper, P. (1996b). The cognitive development of 5-year-old children of postnatally depressed mothers. Journal of Child Psychology and Psychiatry **37**: 927–35.

Murray, L., Sinclair, D., Cooper, P., *et al.* (1999a). The socio-emotional development of five year old children of postnatally depressed mothers. Journal of Child Psychology and Psychiatry **40**(8): 1259–72.

Murray, L., Woolgar, M., Briers, S. and Hipwell A (1999b). The representation of family life of children of depressed and well mothers. Social Development **8**(2): 179–200.

Murray, L., Woolgar, M., Cooper, P.J. and Hipwell, A. (2001) Cognitive vulnerability in five year old children of depressed mothers. Journal of Child Psychology and Psychiatry **42** (7): 891–9.

Murray, L., Halligan, S.L., Adams, G.C., Patterson, P. and Goodyer, I. (2006). Socioemotional development in adolescents at risk for depression: the role of maternal depression and attachment style. Development and Psychopathology **18**: 489–516.

Murray, L. and Ramchandani, P. (2007) Might prevention be better than cure? A perspective on Improving Infant Sleep and Maternal mental Health: a Cluster Randomized Trial, Archives of Disease in Childhood **92**: 943–4.

Murray, L., Halligan, S.L., and Cooper, P.J. (2010a). Effects of postnatal depression on mother-infant interactions, and child development. In Applied and Policy Issues, Vol. 2, T. Wachs and G. Bremner, editors. (192–220). Oxford, UK, Wiley-Blackwell.

Murray, L., Arteche, A., Fearon, P., Halligan, S., Croudace, T. and Cooper, P. (2010b). The effects of maternal postnatal depression and child sex on academic performance at age 16 years: a developmental approach. Journal of Child Psychology and Psychiatry **51**: 1150–9.

Murray, L., Marwick, H. and Arteche, A. (2010c). Sadness in mothers' 'baby-talk' predicts affective disorder in adolescent offspring. Infant Behavior and Development **33**: 361–4.

Murray, L., Halligan, S.L., Goodyer, I., and Herbert, J. (2010d). Disturbances in early parenting of depressed mothers and cortisol secretion in offspring: a preliminary study. Journal of Affective Disorders **122**: 218–23.

Murray, L., Arteche, A., Fearon, P., Halligan, S., Goodyer, I. and Cooper, P. (2011). Maternal postnatal depression and the development of depression in offspring up to 16 years of age. Journal of the American Academy of Child and Adolescent Psychiatry **50**: 460–70.

Murray, L. (2014). The Psychology of Babies: How Relationships Support Development Zero-to-two. London, Constable & Robinson, in press.

Nadel, J., Carchon, I., Kervella, C., Marcelli, D., and Reserbat_Plantey, D. (1999). Expectancies for social contingency in 2-month-olds. Developmental Science **2**: 164–73.

NICHD Early Child Care Research Network (1999), Chronicity of maternal depressive symptoms, maternal sensitivity, and child functioning at 36 months. Dev Psychol **35**:1297–1310

Ninio, A. (1983). Joint book reading as a multiple vocabulary acquisition device. Developmental Psychology **19**: 445–51.

Nylen, K., Moran, T., Franklin, C., and O'Hara, M. (2006). Maternal depression: a review of relevant treatment approaches for mothers and infants. Infant Mental Health Journal **27**(4): 327–43.

Silberg, J.L., Maes, H., and Eaves, L.J. (2010).Genetic and environmental influences on the transmission of parental depression to children's depression and conduct disturbance: an extended Children of Twins study. Journal of Child Psychology and Psychiatry **51**(6): 734–44.

Slater, A. (1995). Individual differences in infancy and later IQ. Journal of Child Psychology and Psychiatry **36**(1): 69–112.

Stanley, C., Murray, L., and Stein, A. (2004). The effect of postnatal depression on mother-infant interaction, infant response to the Still-face perturbation and performance on an Instrumental Learning task. Development and Psychopathology **16**: 1–18.

Stern, D.N., Spieker, S., and MacKain, K. (1982). Intonation contours as signals in maternal speech to prelinguistic infants. Developmental Psychology **18**: 727–35.

Suomi, S. (1997). Early determinants of behaviour: evidence from primate studies. British Medical Bulletin **53**: 170–84.

Tarullo, A.R. and Gunnar, M.R., (2006). Child maltreatment and the developing HPA axis. Hormones and Behavior **50**: 632–9.

Tronick, E.Z. (1989). Emotions and emotional communication in infants. American Psychologist **44**(2): 112–19.

Tronick, E.Z. and Gianino, A.F. (1986). The transmission of maternal disturbance to the infant. New Directions for Child and Adolescent Development **34**: 5–11.

Tronick, E.Z. and Weinberg, M.K. (1997). Depressed mothers and infants: Failure to form dyadic states of consciousness. In Postpartum Depression and Child Development, L. Murray and P. Cooper, editors. (54–84), Guilford, New York.

Weinberg, M.K., Olson, K.L., Beeghly, M., and Tronick, E.Z. (2006). Making up is hard to do, especially for mothers with high levels of depressive symptoms and their infant sons. Journal of Child Psychology and Psychiatry **47**(7): 670–83.

Williams, H. and Carmichael, A. (1985). Depression in mothers in a multi-ethnic urban industrial municipality: aetiological factors and effects on infants and preschool children. Journal of Child Psychology and Psychiatry **26**(2): 277–88.

Woolgar, M., and Murray, L. (2010). The representation of fathers by children of depressed mothers: refining the meaning of parentification in high-risk samples. Journal of Child Psychology and Psychiatry **51**: 621–9.

Chapter 13

Neurobiological outcomes in the offspring of postnatally depressed mothers

Causes and consequences

Sarah L. Halligan

Introduction

Postnatal depression (PND) is the most common psychological disorder to affect women in the postpartum period, with an estimated prevalence of 13% in high-income countries (Gavin *et al.* 2005; O'Hara and Swain 1996). In low and middle income countries, the available evidence suggests that rates of PND may be substantially higher, with prevalence estimates ranging from 15 to 57% (Wachs *et al.* 2009). In terms of clinical presentation, depression occurring in the postnatal period appears to be indistinguishable from depression occurring at other times (Cooper *et al.*, 2007), with persistent low mood and/or a profound loss of interest and enjoyment being defining characteristics. Other symptoms are mood-related disturbances in sleep, altered appetite, concentration impairment, retardation, agitation, feelings of guilt and hopelessness, and suicidal thoughts or impulses. The duration of episodes varies, but the majority of postpartum depressive episodes resolve spontaneously within 6 months to a year (Cooper and Murray 1995; Cox *et al.* 1993).

Although PND may not be unique in terms of the symptom profile, the fact that this disorder occurs in the postpartum period is a particular concern. Specifically, PND affects the mother–infant dyad at a time when the infant is particularly reliant on his or her caregiver to meet their physical, social, and cognitive needs. The postpartum period is also a time when the family unit as a whole is likely to experience additional stress, and is therefore particularly vulnerable. Given these considerations, and the relatively high prevalence of PND, the potential for adverse impact is significant. One area of research focus, reviewed here, has examined the possibility the disturbances in the mother–child relationship occurring in the context of maternal PND result in fundamental alterations in key psychobiological systems in the infant, with persistent consequences. Notably, as PND typically resolves within the first year postpartum, and therefore is particularly relevant to early development, observations deriving from the study of PND in this area offer potentially broad insights into the relevance of *early* environmental factors to child neurobiological functioning.

Interactive impairments associated with maternal depression in the postnatal period

Given that depressive disorder is characterized by profound impairments in mood, energy levels, motivation, and feelings of self-worth, and has established detrimental effects on interpersonal functioning, it is perhaps unsurprising that mothers with PND have been found to show disturbances in the quality of care that they provide for their infant (for a review, see Murray *et al.* 2010a). In particular, PND has been linked to impairments in maternal capacity to respond sensitively to infant cues during face-to-face interactions, and with withdrawn and unresponsive maternal behaviour (Cohn *et al.* 1986; Field 1984; Murray *et al.* 1996). In addition, some studies also identify hostile/intrusive maternal behaviour to be characteristic of maternal depression, a pattern that has more typically been reported in low versus high income samples (Murray *et al.* 2010a). Disturbances in the quality of mother–infant interactions that occur in the context of PND may, to some extent, resolve over time as maternal depression remits. For example, in the Cambridge Longitudinal Study, when mother–infant interactions were examined at 2 and 4 months postpartum, mothers with PND were found to be significantly less sensitive and more withdrawn than control group mothers (Murray *et al.* 2010b). However, by 6 months postpartum many cases of maternal depression had remitted and significant group differences in observed maternal behaviour were no longer present (Murray *et al.*, 2010b). Nonetheless, there is evidence that early impairments in the quality of mother–infant interactions continue to affect the mother–child relationship. Elevated rates of insecure attachments were found in PND group infants at 18 months in the Cambridge Longitudinal Study, consistent with other research in the field (Martins and Gaffan 2000).

The occurrence of interactive impairments in the context of PND (and other parental mental health problems) is a concern, as these disturbances in parenting behaviour occur at a time of profound biological, cognitive, and social development for the infant. At the same time, the infant is highly dependent on the caregiver to meet his or her needs. Mother–infant interactions not only form the foundations of the mother–child relationship and provide crucial exposure to language and social experience, they also influence the infant's emotional state and may assist the infant in maintaining an appropriate level of arousal, facilitating the development of self-regulatory capacities (Tronick and Gianino 1986; Rothbart *et al.* 2011; Gunnar 1998). Experimental manipulation has demonstrated that perturbations in maternal responsiveness are associated with negative affect in the infant, and may trigger physiological responses that are consistent with the experience of stress, including increases in heart rate, skin conductance and cortisol secretion (Mesman *et al.* 2009). While brief disruptions in the synchrony of mother–infant interactions are a normal component of the early dyadic relationship and may support the development of infant self-regulation (Tronick and Gianino 1986), persistent impairments in maternal responding may be experienced as chronically stressful by the infant (Gunnar and Quevedo 2008). Such observations are pertinent in the light of animal models that indicate that early maternal input is critical to the development of biological stress response systems in offspring, and thereby influences offspring behaviour in the long term (Meaney 2010).

Animal models and sensitive periods for development

The hypothalamic–pituitary–adrenal (HPA) axis has become a model for examining the potential role of environmental input during early development in determining the functioning of the adult organism, particularly considering the organization of physiological and behavioural responses to stress. Glucocorticoids, the neurohormonal products of the HPA axis, are a core component of the endocrine stress response, and influence a diversity of critical processes, including cardiovascular activity, appetite, immune response, and also neural functioning and behaviour (de Kloet *et al.* 2009; Walker 2007; Huang and Herbert 2006; Dallman *et al.* 2007).

Research in rats has established that natural variation in early maternal behaviour influences the functioning of the HPA axis and associated behavioural responding in offspring as adults. Specifically, rats exposed to high levels of maternal licking and grooming as pups (including as a consequence of experimental manipulation) show more moderate HPA responses to stress and correspondingly reduced behavioural fearfulness than those exposed to low levels of licking and grooming (Champagne and Meaney 2001; Caldji *et al.* 2000; Francis *et al.* 1999). Ground-breaking research has provided insight into the biological pathways through which this effect of maternal behaviour is achieved (Meaney 2010). The HPA axis is regulated via negative feedback, occurring through the action of circulating glucocorticoids on glucocorticoid receptors (GR) in corticolimbic structures. Rats exposed to high levels of maternal licking and grooming as pups show significantly increased GR receptor expression in the hippocampus, and correspondingly enhanced glucocorticoid negative-feedback sensitivity and reduced HPA reactivity (Liu *et al.* 1997). The mechanism by which GR expression is altered is, at least in part, epigenetic. In brief, maternal licking and grooming triggers alterations in the neuronal environment in key brain regions in the pup, including increased turnover of 5-hydroxytryptamine (5-HT) in the hippocampus. Such changes, in turn, directly modify epigenetic markers on DNA regions that regulate GR transcription and expression (Weaver *et al.* 2004). As these epigenetic markers are stable, they provide a molecular basis for a persistent effect of early maternal behaviour on the offspring phenotype (Meaney 2010).

The above described observations from the preclinical literature have stimulated substantial interest in whether similar effects might operate in humans. HPA dysfunction is of particular significance, as stress is a crucial trigger for numerous psychological disorders, most notably the affective disorders (Hammen 2005). In addition, altered HPA axis activity has also been observed in association with numerous forms of psychopathology, and HPA dysregulation is hypothesized to be an aetiological agent in the development of depression (for reviews, see Gold *et al.* 2002; Southwick *et al.* 2005). If the human HPA axis is sensitive to early environmental input, this suggests one pathway via which aspects of early care may influence later adjustment. The study of maternal PND represents a particularly interesting context in which to examine this possibility, as it is associated with impairments in *early* parenting behaviour, and research has linked the presence of PND to a number of adverse outcomes in offspring, including elevated rates of affective disorder (Halligan *et al.* 2007). These observations have led to the hypothesis that postnatal maternal depression may lead to altered HPA-axis functioning in offspring, and the establishment of a corresponding vulnerability to stress and depression (Gunnar and Quevedo 2008; Essex *et al.* 2002; Halligan *et al.* 2004).

Maternal depression and offspring HPA development: associations, potential mechanisms, and consequences

Altered offspring cortisol secretion in the context of early maternal depression

The examination of HPA activity in relation to maternal PND has focused exclusively on the secretion of cortisol, the end product of the human HPA axis. In an initial investigation of this issue, Field and colleagues examined cortisol levels in 3–6-month-old infants following face to face interactions with their mothers and with a stranger (Field *et al.* 1988). Higher salivary cortisol levels were found in the infants of mothers who had elevated depressive symptom levels relative to control group infants. Whether or not this group difference represented altered basal cortisol secretion or elevated reactivity could not be determined in this study, as a pre-interaction cortisol sample was not obtained. Nonetheless, the potential for maternal depression to be an influence on offspring salivary cortisol was demonstrated (Field *et al.* 1988). Subsequent, cross-sectional research has tended to confirm the possibility of elevated basal cortisol and/or greater cortisol reactivity to a stressor in the young infants of depressed mothers (Brennan *et al.* 2008; Diego *et al.* 2004; Feldman *et al.* 2009). Thus, Brennan and colleagues identified increased cortisol reactivity to a mild laboratory stressor in association with peripartum maternal depression in 6-month-old infants (Brennan *et al.* 2008); and both basal cortisol and cortisol reactivity were found to be elevated in the 9-month-old offspring of depressed (or anxious) mothers relative to control group infants (Feldman *et al.* 2009).

Importantly, longitudinal studies have also demonstrated persistent associations between postpartum depression and offspring cortisol secretion, consistent with an early programming hypothesis. Thus, maternal depressive symptoms at 1-year have been found to predict basal cortisol levels in infants at 18 months (Bugental *et al.* 2003). Three-year-old children exposed to maternal depression in the postnatal period have been found to show higher salivary cortisol levels than non-exposed children (Hessl *et al.* 1998), although this effect was not replicated when the sample was reassessed at 7 years (Ashman *et al.* 2002). Salivary cortisol was elevated in 4.5-year-old children whose mothers were concurrently depressed only if maternal depression had also been present in the first 12 months postpartum (Essex *et al.* 2002). Finally, in the Cambridge Longitudinal Study, we found higher and more variable morning cortisol secretion in the offspring of PND versus control group mothers at 13 years (Halligan *et al.* 2004), controlling for possible confounds, including adolescent depression.

The consistency in these observations is encouraging, particularly given the significant variability in assessment methods across studies. However, it is currently unclear whether the effects reported can be directly attributed to aspects of the early environment. Both depression and aspects of HPA activity show a degree of heritability, meaning that genetic influences versus environmental exposures may explain the observed associations (Bartels *et al.* 2003; Sullivan *et al.* 2000). Moreover, mothers with PND are also substantially more likely to experience depression both prior to and subsequent to the postnatal period, meaning that offspring exposure is typically not isolated to early development (Halligan *et al.* 2007; Heron *et al.* 2004). As such, longitudinal studies have attempted to tease out timing effects in their analyses in order to establish whether early maternal depression shows an association with offspring cortisol that occurs over and above depression occurring at other times. Essex *et al.* (2002) were able to demonstrate that the children of currently depressed mothers showed elevations in afternoon salivary cortisol only if mothers also had early depression. In the Cambridge Longitudinal Study, we controlled for the total number of months of maternal depression throughout the course of offspring development, and found that PND associations with offspring cortisol were present over and above any effects of that index of overall maternal depression (Halligan *et al.* 2004). Such observations are consistent with a unique effect of early maternal depression on offspring HPA functioning.

Nonetheless, there is also evidence to indicate that *any* parental history of depression may also be associated with elevations in offspring basal cortisol (Mannie *et al.* 2007; Young *et al.* 2006; Ellenbogen *et al.* 2004) and/or cortisol reactivity (Azar *et al.* 2007). Intriguingly, Brennan and colleagues, in a study of 6-month-old infants, found that elevated basal cortisol secretion was associated with lifetime history of maternal depression, whereas increased cortisol reactivity to a stressor was specifically linked to peripartum maternal depression (Brennan *et al.* 2008). The authors propose that elevations in basal cortisol secretion may be predominantly explained by genetic influences (Bartels *et al.* 2003), whereas cortisol reactivity may be shaped via environmental exposures, consistent with the preclinical literature. This general hypothesis warrants further investigation (Gunnar and Quevedo 2008). Our own observations of elevated morning cortisol secretion in PND offspring were partially a consequence of increased day-to-day variability in cortisol levels across the 10 days of collection, which may indicate greater HPA reactivity to every day stressors (Halligan *et al.* 2004).

In sum, research has identified associations between maternal depression occurring early in development and both elevated basal cortisol secretion and cortisol reactivity in offspring, including longitudinal influences that persist as far as adolescence. Constraints that naturally arise in the study of infants and children mean that, to date, investigation of the HPA axis has been limited to the study of peripheral cortisol levels. Potentially key underlying biological processes, such as altered GR activity, have not been examined. With regards to the causes of the observed effects, multiple influences on human HPA axis reactivity are, of course, likely, with contributing factors including ongoing or concurrent stress (Ostiguy *et al.* 2011; Steptoe *et al.* 2005; Pruessner *et al.* 2003; Ockenfels *et al.*, 1995;

Schulz *et al.* 1998), antenatal exposures to maternal stress or depression (see Chapter 17 for a review), and genetic influences (Bartels *et al.* 2003). Nonetheless, there are some findings that are consistent with a unique effect of early *exposure* to maternal depression (Halligan *et al.* 2004; Essex *et al.* 2002; Brennan *et al.* 2008; Diego *et al.* 2004), in line with the hypothesis that the human HPA axis may be particularly sensitive to developmental influences.

The role of parenting behaviour

Following on from animal models that highlight early maternal behaviour as an influence on HPA axis functioning, research has been accumulating linking aspects of the early parent–child relationship to offspring cortisol secretion in humans (Gunnar and Quevedo 2008). This research has identified caregiver behaviour as an immediate modulator of infant cortisol reactivity in response to challenge, consistent with the assumption that parents can have direct input into biological and behavioural stress responses in their infant (Spangler *et al.* 1994; Gunnar *et al.* 1992). Notably, Gunnar and colleagues found that manipulating the behaviour of a randomly provided 'surrogate' caregiver modulates infant cortisol reactivity to maternal separation, indicating an influence of the quality of care that is independent of any genetic or pre-established relationship between infant and caregiver (Gunnar *et al.* 1992). The quality of early parenting has also been linked to offspring HPA activity outside of the actual parenting context. For example, in a study of more than 1,000 infants, Blair and colleagues reported that greater maternal engagement was cross-sectionally associated with lower infant basal cortisol at 7 months as well as greater cortisol reactivity (Blair *et al.* 2008). Moreover, 7-month maternal engagement scores also predicted lower child cortisol at 15 months, whereas there was no equivalent cross-sectional association at 15 months (Blair *et al.* 2008), consistent with a potentially unique influence of maternal behaviour in the first year of life on offspring HPA functioning.

Direct evidence that similar processes might explain cortisol disturbances in the offspring of depressed parents is extremely limited, but a small number of studies have investigated the possible intervening role of parenting behaviour. Feldman and colleagues examined infant cortisol responses to stress in relation to concurrent maternal sensitivity and affective disorder, in a sample that included mothers with anxiety disorders as well as depression (Feldman *et al.* 2009). Elevated cortisol reactivity in 9-month-old infants was associated with both the presence of maternal affective disorder and with lower observed maternal sensitivity. The possibility of an indirect pathway to from maternal affective disorder to infant cortisol reactivity, via maternal insensitivity, was not formally tested in this study. However, it was certainly *not* the case that elevated offspring cortisol reactivity in relation maternal disorder was explained by maternal sensitivity in this study, as independent effects of affective disorder and parenting behaviour were found (Feldman *et al.* 2009).

In the Cambridge Longitudinal Study, detailed observations of mother–infant interactions were completed in the first year postpartum (at 2, 4, 6, and 9 months infant age) for a subset of the sample, as well as a follow-up assessment of parenting behaviour at 5 years; mothers with PND were found to be significantly less sensitive and more withdrawn in interacting with their infants in early development relative to control group mothers

(Murray *et al.* 2010b). When we examined maternal parenting behaviour as a longitudinal influence on adolescent cortisol secretion, we found greater maternal withdrawal in the first 9 months and to predict higher offspring morning cortisol secretion at 13 years. By contrast, maternal withdrawal at 5 years was unrelated to later offspring cortisol (Murray *et al.*, 2010b). Tentatively, these findings suggest that early maternal behaviour influences offspring HPA functioning in a sustained way. However, *mediation* of the association between maternal depression and offspring cortisol by maternal behaviour was again not demonstrated in this study.

Other findings consistent with the above observations have been reported. For example, Bugental and colleagues reported that maternal 'emotional unavailability' was associated with elevated basal cortisol levels in toddlers, where unavailability was a composite of self-reported depressive symptoms and strategic withdrawal during conflict (Bugental *et al.* 2003). In a small-scale perinatal study, Kaplan and colleagues found that postnatal maternal sensitivity moderated the influence of *antenatal* maternal depression/anxiety on infant cortisol reactivity following mother–infant interaction. Specifically, higher infant cortisol levels were found in association with insensitive versus sensitive maternal behaviour only for mothers who had an antenatal diagnosis. Maternal sensitivity was unrelated to infant cortisol in the control group (Kaplan *et al.* 2008). The authors conclude that HPA alterations may occur in the context of antenatal maternal depression that are subsequently modifiable by the quality of postnatal care. Postnatal maternal disorder was not assessed in this study (Kaplan *et al.* 2008).

In sum, the available evidence suggests that maternal care, and perhaps withdrawn/insensitive maternal behaviour in particular, is an influence on offspring cortisol secretion. Findings are consistent with a broader literature that has documented associations between aspects of early care and child HPA axis activity. However, research to date is extremely limited, and there is no evidence to support the assumption that associations between maternal PND and child cortisol are mediated by the quality of maternal care. The availability of further longitudinal data would provide important information regarding the development cortisol alterations observed in association with maternal depression, and could specifically address the hypothesis that they initially arise in the context of unsupportive or stressful mother–infant interactions (Gunnar and Quevedo 2008).

HPA activity and offspring adjustment

The presence of increased cortisol secretion and/or greater HPA reactivity in association with maternal PND has potential consequences for offspring adjustment. Thus, the pattern of higher and more variable morning cortisol levels that we observed in association with PND in the Cambridge Longitudinal Study was of particular interest in the context of research demonstrating that elevated morning cortisol secretion can predict the subsequent onset of depressive disorder, including in adolescents (Goodyer *et al.* 2000; Harris *et al.* 2000; Adam *et al.* 2010).

We examined longitudinal associations between offspring cortisol secretion and depression in the Cambridge study and found that higher 13-year morning cortisol secretion predicted higher levels of depressive symptoms at 16 years, even controlling for 13-year depressive symptoms and intervening life events (Halligan *et al.* 2007). Moreover, a significant indirect pathway from maternal PND status to 16-year offspring symptoms via 13-year morning cortisol was identified, consistent with mediation.

Our observations suggest a possible mechanism whereby disturbances in the early maternal environment contribute to risk for depressive disorder in offspring via alterations in the functioning of the HPA-axis (Halligan *et al.* 2004). However, further studies examining the longitudinal consequences of altered salivary cortisol secretion for offspring adjustment are essential before conclusions can be drawn regarding their potential significance. Notably, a recent longitudinal study demonstrated that the presence of 'early life stress' (a composite which included maternal depressive symptoms) was linked to altered functionality in the neural circuitry of emotion regulation in adolescent offspring, as indexed by reduced coupling of activity between the prefrontal cortex and the amygdala (Burghy *et al.* 2012). This association was present only for girls, and was explained by intervening elevated cortisol levels, consistent with the key role of HPA-axis activity in the neural regulation of emotion. Altered neural activity was, in turn, a correlate of concurrent depressive symptoms in girls. Although this research did not focus specifically on maternal depression, it highlights the power of longitudinal studies beginning in early development to elucidate biological pathways to offspring psychopathology, and the need to integrate observations from multiple biological systems (Burghy *et al.* 2012).

Neural functioning in the context of early maternal depression

The possibility of alterations in neural functioning in association with maternal PND has been subject to considerable scrutiny, with a focus on neural systems implicated in the generation and regulation of emotional responding. Altered activity in the prefrontal cortex has been linked to depressive disorder across a variety of paradigms (Davidson *et al.* 2002), and is hypothesised to play an important role in the regulation of emotional states, with broad implications for adjustment (Davidson *et al.* 2007; Gross 2002). Moreover, rapid maturation of prefrontal regions occurs in early childhood, commensurate with marked advances in the ability to self-regulate emotional responses, and both behavioural and neural developments are assumed to be subject to environmental influence (Rothbart *et al.* 2011). As such, activity in the frontal cortex represents a logical target for studies examining the potential consequences of PND for infant neural development.

Numerous studies have linked the occurrence of early maternal depression with altered frontal activity in offspring, focusing particularly on left / right asymmetries in frontal cortical activity. EEG recordings taken from children of postnatally depressed mothers have shown reduced left frontal activation from the age of one to three months (Jones *et al.* 1997a), through to six (Field *et al.* 1995) and 15 months (Dawson *et al.* 1997; Dawson *et al.* 1999a).

Although the majority of studies have been cross-sectional, there is also some evidence of stability through to the early childhood years (Jones et al. 1997b). This pattern of activation has been observed in infants of depressed mothers from both low and high risk samples, and has been found to remain even after possible influences of prenatal maternal depression have been taken account of (Dawson et al., 1997). The findings have been interpreted in the light of research examining EEG responding in relation to basic emotions, which has robustly indicated that the expression of positive or 'approach' emotions (e.g. happiness) is associated with relative left frontal cortex activation, whereas negative or 'withdrawal' emotions (e.g., fear, disgust) are associated with relative right frontal activity (Davidson and Fox 1989; Tomarken et al. 1990; Davidson et al. 1990; Dawson 1994). Greater relative right versus left frontal EEG activation has been associated with negative affect, poor emotion regulation and depressive disorder and may therefore constitute a marker of risk for psychopathology (Davidson 1996; Fox 1994; Gotlib 1998).

Few longitudinal studies have examined longer-term offspring neural outcomes in association with early maternal depression, and consequently there is limited evidence that effects may persist beyond infancy (Jones et al. 1997b). Notably, there is also little available data to address the issue of the specificity of effects to early exposure. In this regard, one study that examined the timing of maternal depression over the first years of life, found evidence that maternal depression occurring *after* versus before 2 years child age was the strongest predictor of child EEG activity (Dawson et al. 2003). Thus, at present, conclusions regarding potentially unique effects of PND due to the timing in early development are premature.

The role of maternal behaviour

A lack of contingent and responsive maternal behaviour in depressed mothers is assumed to result in a corresponding lack of positive emotional experience and/or poor support for the development of emotion regulatory capacities in the infant, including at the neural level (Dawson et al. 2003). As such, researchers have examined maternal behaviour as a potential intervening variable underlying the observed link between infant EEG and early maternal depression. Diego and colleagues differentiated depressed mothers who showed intrusive parenting behaviour from those showing withdrawn behaviour, and found that reduced infant left frontal activation was particularly present in the infants of withdrawn versus intrusive mothers, a pattern that strengthened from shortly following birth to follow-up at 3–6 months (Diego et al. 2006). In their study of 3½-year-old children, Dawson and colleagues found overall reductions in frontal EEG activity in association with maternal depression occurring in the first years of life, rather than the asymmetric pattern observed in younger children (Dawson et al. 2003). Withdrawn maternal behaviour was a significant correlate of atypical frontal EEG activity in the child, although the association between maternal depression and child EEG activity was not wholly explained by maternal withdrawal. Thus, although at an early stage, evidence supports a potential role for maternal behaviour in development of the neural profile in the infants of depressed mothers. Longitudinal studies that chart the emergence, stability and generalizability of reduced left frontal activity are required.

Potential consequences for offspring functioning

The presence of atypical frontal EEG activity in the infants and children of depressed mothers has been interpreted as reflecting deficits in the development of the neural systems supporting emotion regulation, which, in turn, place the child at risk for adverse outcomes (Dawson *et al.* 2003), including depressive disorder (Gotlib 1998; Davidson 1996). The available evidence is consistent with this possibility. Reduced left frontal activation occurring in the context of early maternal depression has been cross-sectionally associated with a variety of adverse emotional consequences in infants and young children, including fewer approach behaviours, higher levels of behavioural inhibition and greater expression of negative affect (temper tantrums) (Dawson *et al.* 1999b; Diego *et al.* 2001). Moreover, Dawson *et al.* (2003) found that reduced frontal EEG activity mediated associations between maternal depression and behavioural problems in 3½-year-old children. However, as research to date has focused on cross-sectional associations between atypical frontal EEG and infant/child adjustment, the direction of effects is difficult to ascertain. Given the parallels between EEG responses in infants of depressed mothers and those of adults experiencing depression, it is important that follow-up studies of the infant populations be conducted to establish whether there are indeed direct links between early EEG functioning and subsequent disorder.

Summary and conclusions

The study of neurobiological outcomes in the offspring of postnatally depressed mothers has focused on two main outcomes: cortisol secretion as an index of HPA activity, and frontal cortex EEG asymmetry as an indicator of neural emotion regulation. In both areas, research has demonstrated a profile of disturbance in association with maternal PND. With regards to cortisol, cross-sectional studies have indicated elevated basal cortisol secretion and/or greater reactivity, and longitudinal research has demonstrated effects that persist through to adolescence. Moreover, altered cortisol secretion in the adolescent offspring of PND mothers has been found to predict later depressive symptoms, suggesting that the observed effects have significant consequences for adjustment. With respect to EEG abnormalities, reduced relative left frontal cortex activity has been demonstrated in the presence of early maternal depression, primarily based on cross-sectional studies. More longitudinal evidence is needed regarding the persistence of such effects, and their consequences for emotional and behavioural functioning.

Neurobiological alterations occurring in the context of maternal PND have broadly been interpreted as providing support for an early programming hypothesis, whereby aspects of early environmental experience shape developing biological systems in a persistent way. However, such interpretation is complicated by the genetic underpinnings of depression and the fact that postnatal disorder is typically associated with the presence of prior and subsequent maternal depression. Given the complexities of differentiating such influences, no study has definitively demonstrated an early programming effect of maternal PND exposure on offspring neurobiological functioning. However, there are two sets of observations that speak to this issue. First, some studies have attempted to disentangle influences PND from antenatal and/or later maternal depression, and have provided evidence for early maternal depression effects on offspring cortisol that occur over and above other exposures. Second, researchers have identified direct associations between early maternal behaviour and offspring neurobiological functioning, which is perhaps remarkable given the problems inherent in trying to index something as rich and complex as human maternal behaviour through the brief assessments afforded to psychological researchers.

To date, limited longitudinal studies have been conducted, and research that charts the emergence and persistence of neurobiological alterations in offspring alongside alterations in maternal disorder and behaviour is required. In addition, it is essential that we develop a better understanding of the biological underpinnings of the peripheral alterations observed. Although probing neurobiological systems represents a particular challenge in paediatric populations, such work is critical to the identification of biological targets for intervention. Finally, intervention studies that examine the neurobiological consequences of treating maternal depression or associated interactive disturbances are required to advance the field. Evidence that offspring biological outcomes can be modulated by changes in maternal behaviour would not only provide key evidence for the hypothesised role of environmental exposure, it would also further highlight the paramount importance of effective intervention for perinatal mental health problems.

References

Adam, E.K., Doane, L.D., Zinbarg, R.E., *et al.* (2010). Prospective prediction of major depressive disorder from cortisol awakening responses in adolescence. Psychoneuroendocrinology 35: 921–1.

Ashman, S.B., Dawson, G., Panagiotides, H., Yamada, E., and Wilkins, C.W. (2002). Stress hormone levels of children of depressed mothers. Development and Psychopathology 14: 333–49.

Azar, R., Paquette, D., Zoccolillo, M., Baltzer, F., and Tremblay, R.E. (2007). The association of major depression, conduct disorder, and maternal overcontrol with a failure to show a cortisol buffered response in 4-month-old infants of teenage mothers. Biological Psychiatry 62: 573–9.

Bartels, M., Van den, B.M., Sluyter, F., Boomsma, D.I., and deGeus, E.J. (2003). Heritability of cortisol levels: review and simultaneous analysis of twin studies. Psychoneuroendocrinology 28: 121–37.

Blair, C., Granger, D.A., Kivlighan, K.T., *et al.* (2008). Maternal and child contributions to cortisol response to emotional arousal in young children from low-income, rural communities. Developmental Psychology 44: 1095–109.

Brennan, P.A., Pargas, R., Walker, E.F., *et al.* (2008). Maternal depression and infant cortisol: influences of timing, comorbidity and treatment. Journal of Child Psychology and Psychiatry 49: 1099–107.

Bugental, D.B., Martorell, G.A., and Barraza, V. (2003). The hormonal costs of subtle forms of infant maltreatment. Hormones and Behavior 43: 237–44.

Burghy, C.A., Stodola, D.E., Ruttle, P.L., *et al.* (2012). Developmental pathways to amygdala-prefrontal function and internalizing symptoms in adolescence. Nature Neuroscience 15(12): 1736–41.

Caldji, C., Diorio, J., and Meaney, M.J. (2000). Variations in maternal care in infancy regulate the development of stress reactivity. Biological Psychiatry 48: 1164–74.

Champagne, F. and Meaney, M.J. (2001). Like mother, like daughter: evidence for non-genomic transmission of parental behavior and stress responsivity. Progress in Brain Research 133: 287–302.

Cohn, J.F., Matias, R., Tronick, E.Z., Connel, D., and Lyons-Ruth, K. (1986). Face-to-face interactions of depressed mothers and their infants. In Maternal Depression and Infant Disturbance, E.Z. Tronick, and T. Field, editors. San Francisco, Jossey-Bass, pp. 31–45.

Cooper, C., Jones, L., Dunn, E., *et al.* (2007). Clinical presentation of postnatal and non-postnatal depressive episodes. Psychological Medicine **37**: 1273–80.

Cooper, P.J. and Murray, L. (1995). Course and recurrence of postnatal depression. Evidence for the specificity of the diagnostic concept. British Journal of Psychiatry **166**: 191–5.

Cox, J.L., Murray, D., and Chapman, G. (1993). A controlled study of the onset, duration and prevalence of postnatal depression. British Journal of Psychiatry **163**: 27–31.

Dallman, M.F., Akana, S.F., Pecoraro, N.C., *et al.* (2007). Glucocorticoids, the etiology of obesity and the metabolic syndrome. Current Alzheimer Research **4**: 199–204.

Davidson, R.J. (1996). Cerebral assymetry, emotion and affective style. In Brain Assymetry, Davidson, R.J. and Hugdahl, K., editors. Cambridge, MA, MIT Press, pp. 361–87.

Davidson, R.J. and Fox, N.A. (1989). Frontal brain asymmetry predicts infants' response to maternal separation. Journal of Abnormal Psychology **98**: 127–31.

Davidson, R.J., Ekman, P., Saron, C.D., Senulis, J.A., and Friesen, W.V. (1990). Approach-withdrawal and cerebral asymmetry: emotional expression and brain physiology. I. Journal of Personality and Social Psychology **58**: 330–41.

Davidson, R.J., Pizzagalli, D., Nitschke, J.B., and Putnam, K. (2002). Depression: perspectives from affective neuroscience. Annual Review of Psychology **53**: 545–74.

Davidson, R.J., Fox, A., and Kalin, N.H. (2007). Neural bases of emotion regulation in non-human primates and humans. In Handbook of Emotion Regulation, J.J. Gross, editor. New York, Guilford Press, pp. 47–68.

Dawson, G. (1994). Frontal electroencephalographic correlates of individual differences in emotion expression in infants: a brain systems perspective on emotion. Monographs of the Society for Research in Child Development **59**: 135–51.

Dawson, G., Frey, K., Panagiotides, H., Osterling, J., and Hessl, D. (1997). Infants of depressed mothers exhibit atypical frontal brain activity: a replication and extension of previous findings. Journal of Child Psychology and Psychiatry **38**: 179–86.

Dawson, G., Frey, K., Panagiotides, H., Yamada, E., Hessl, D., and Osterling, J. (1999a). Infants of depressed mothers exhibit atypical frontal electrical brain activity during interactions with mother and with a familiar, nondepressed adult. Child Development **70**: 1058–66.

Dawson, G., Frey, K., Self, J., *et al.* (1999b). Frontal brain electrical activity in infants of depressed and nondepressed mothers: relation to variations in infant behavior. Development and Psychopathology **11**: 589–605.

Dawson, G., Ashman, S.B., Panagiotides, H., *et al.* (2003). Preschool outcomes of children of depressed mothers: role of maternal behavior, contextual risk, and children's brain activity. Child Development **74**: 1158–75.

de Kloet, E.R., Fitzsimons, C.P., Datson, N.A., Meijer, O.C., and Vreugdenhil, E. (2009). Glucocorticoid signaling and stress-related limbic susceptibility pathway: about receptors, transcription machinery and microRNA. Brain Research **1293**: 129–41.

Diego, M.A., Field, T., and Hernandez-Reif, M. (2001). BIS/BAS scores are correlated with frontal EEG asymmetry in intrusive and withdrawn depressed mothers. Infant Mental Health Journal **22**: 665–75.

Diego, M.A., Field, T., Hernandez-Reif, M., *et al.* (2004). Prepartum, postpartum, and chronic depression effects on newborns. Psychiatry **67**: 63–80.

Diego, M.A., Field, T., Jones, N.A., and Hernandez-Reif, M. (2006). Withdrawn and intrusive maternal interaction style and infant frontal EEG asymmetry shifts in infants of depressed and non-depressed mothers. Infant Behavior and Development **29**: 220–9.

Ellenbogen, M.A., Hodgins, S., and Walker, C.D. (2004). High levels of cortisol among adolescent offspring of parents with bipolar disorder: a pilot study. Psychoneuroendocrinology **29**: 99–106.

Essex, M.J., Klein, M.H., Cho, E., and Kalin, N.H. (2002). Maternal stress beginning in infancy may sensitize children to later stress exposure: effects on cortisol and behavior. Biological Psychiatry **52**: 776–84.

Feldman, R., Granat, A., Pariante, C., et al. (2009). Maternal depression and anxiety across the postpartum year and infant social engagement, fear regulation, and stress reactivity. Journal of the American Academy of Child and Adolescent Psychiatry **48**: 919–27.

Field, T. (1984). Early interactions between infants and their postpartum depressed mothers. Infant Behavior and Development **7**: 537–40.

Field, T., Healy, B., Goldstein, S., et al. (1988). Infants of depressed mothers show "depressed" behavior even with nondepressed adults. Child Development **59**: 1569–79.

Field, T., Fox, N.A., Pickens, J., and Nawrocki, T. (1995). Relative right frontal EEG activation in 3- to 6-month-old infants of 'depressed' mothers. Developmental Psychology **31**: 358–363.

Fox, N.A. (1994). Dynamic cerebral processes underlying emotion regulation. Monographs of the Society for Research in Child Development **59**: 152–166.

Francis, D.D., Caldji, C., Champagne, F., Plotsky, P.M., and Meaney, M.J. (1999). The role of corticotropin-releasing factor—norepinephrine systems in mediating the effects of early experience on the development of behavioral and endocrine responses to stress. Biological Psychiatry **46**: 1153–66.

Gavin, N.I., Gaynes, B.N., Lohr, K.N., et al. (2005). Perinatal depression: a systematic review of prevalence and incidence. Obstetrics and Gynecology **106**: 1071–83.

Gold, P.W., Drevets, W.C., and Charney, D.S. (2002). New insights into the role of cortisol and the glucocorticoid receptor in severe depression. Biological Psychiatry **52**: 381–385.

Goodyer, I.M., Tamplin, A., Herbert, J., and Altham, P.M. (2000). Recent life events, cortisol, dehydroepiandrosterone and the onset of major depression in high-risk adolescents. British Journal of Psychiatry **177**: 499–504.

Gotlib, I.H. (1998). EEG alpha asymmetry, depression, and cognitive functioning. Cognition and Emotion **12**: 449–78.

Gross, J.J. (2002). Emotion regulation: affective, cognitive, and social consequences. Psychophysiology **39**: 281–91.

Gunnar, M.R. (1998). Quality of early care and buffering of neuroendocrine stress reactions: potential effects on the developing human brain. Preventive Medicine **27**: 208–11.

Gunnar, M.R. and Quevedo, K.M. (2008). Early care experiences and HPA axis regulation in children: a mechanism for later trauma vulnerability. Progress in Brain Research **167**: 137–49.

Gunnar, M.R., Larson, M.C., Hertsgaard, L., Harris, M.L., and Brodersen, L. (1992). The stressfulness of separation among nine-month-old infants: effects of social context variables and infant temperament. Child Development **63**: 290–303.

Halligan, S.L., Herbert, J., Goodyer, I.M., and Murray, L. (2004). Exposure to postnatal depression predicts elevated cortisol in adolescent offspring. Biological Psychiatry **55**: 376–81.

Halligan, S.L., Herbert, J., Goodyer, I, Murray, L. (2007). Disturbances in morning cortisol secretion in association with maternal postnatal depression predict subsequent depressive symptomatology in adolescents. *Biological Psychiatry*, **62**, 40–46.

Halligan, S.L., Murray, L., Martins, C., and Cooper, P.J. (2007). Maternal depression and psychiatric outcomes in adolescent offspring: A 13-year longitudinal study. Journal of Affective Disorders **97**: 145–54.

Hammen, C. (2005). Stress and depression. Annual Reviews in Clinical Psychology **1**: 293–319.

Harris, T.O., Borsanyi, S., Messari, S., *et al.* (2000). Morning cortisol as a risk factor for subsequent major depressive disorder in adult women. British Journal of Psychiatry **177**: 505–10.

Heron, J., O'Connor, T.G., Evans, J., Golding, J., and Glover, V. (2004). The course of anxiety and depression through pregnancy and the postpartum in a community sample. Journal of Affective Disorders **80**: 65–73.

Hessl, D., Dawson, G., Frey, K., *et al.* (1998). A longitudinal study of children of depressed mothers: Psychobiological findings related to stress. In Advancing Research on Developmental Plasticity: Integrating the Behavioral Sciences and the Neurosciences of Mental Health, D.M. Hann, L. C. Huffman, K. K. Lederhendler, and D. Minecke, editors. Bethseda, MD, National Institutes of Mental Health, p. 256.

Huang, G.J. and Herbert, J. (2006). Stimulation of neurogenesis in the hippocampus of the adult rat by fluoxetine requires rhythmic change in corticosterone. Biological Psychiatry **59**: 619–24.

Jones, N.A., Field, T., Fox, N.A., Lundy, B., and Davalos, M. (1997a). EEG activation in 1-month-old infants of depressed mothers. Development and Psychopathology **9**: 491–505.

Jones, N.A., Field, T., Davalos, M., and Pickens, J. (1997b). EEG stability in infants/children of depressed mothers. Child Psychiatry Human Development **28**: 59–70.

Kaplan, L.A., Evans, L., and Monk, C. (2008). Effects of mothers' prenatal psychiatric status and postnatal caregiving on infant biobehavioral regulation: can prenatal programming be modified? Early Human Development **84**: 249–56.

Liu, D., Diorio, J., Tannenbaum, B., *et al.* (1997). Maternal care, hippocampal glucocorticoid receptors, and hypothalamic- pituitary-adrenal responses to stress. Science **277**: 1659–62.

Mannie, Z.N., Harmer, C.J., and Cowen, P.J. (2007). Increased waking salivary cortisol levels in young people at familial risk of depression. American Journal of Psychiatry **164**: 617–21.

Martins, C. and Gaffan, E.A. (2000). Effects of early maternal depression on patterns of infant-mother attachment: a meta-analytic investigation. Journal of Child Psychology and Psychiatry **41**: 737–46.

Meaney, M.J. (2010). Epigenetics and the biological definition of gene x environment interactions. Child Development **81**: 41–79.

Mesman, J., van IJzendoorn, M.H., and Bakermans-Kranenburg, M.J. (2009). The many faces of the still-face paradigm: a review and meta-analysis. Developmental Review **29**: 120–62.

Murray, L., FioriCowley, A., Hooper, R., and Cooper, P. (1996). The impact of postnatal depression and associated adversity on early mother—infant interactions and later infant outcome. Child Development **67**: 2512–26.

Murray, L., Halligan, S., and Cooper, P. (2010a). Effects of postnatal depression on mother—infant interactions and child development. In Handbook of Infant Development, 2nd ed., J.G. Bremner and T.D. Wachs, editors. Chichester, UK, Wiley-Blackwell, pp. 192–220.

Murray, L., Halligan, S.L., Goodyer, I., and Herbert, J. (2010b). Disturbances in early parenting of depressed mothers and cortisol secretion in offspring: a preliminary study. Journal of Affective Disorders **122**: 218–23.

O'Hara, M.W. and Swain, A.M. (1996). Rates and risk of postpartum depressionГÇöa meta-analysis. International Review of Psychiatry **8**: 37–54.

Ockenfels, M.C., Porter, L., Smyth, J., *et al.* (1995). Effect of chronic stress associated with unemployment on salivary cortisol: overall cortisol levels, diurnal rhythm, and acute stress reactivity. Psychosomatic Medicine **57**: 460–67.

Ostiguy, C.S., Ellenbogen, M.A., Walker, C.D., Walker, E.F., and Hodgins, S. (2011). Sensitivity to stress among the offspring of parents with bipolar disorder: a study of daytime cortisol levels. Psychological Medicine **41**: 2447–57.

Pruessner, M., Hellhammer, D.H., Pruessner, J.C., and Lupien, S.J. (2003). Self-reported depressive symptoms and stress levels in healthy young men: associations with the cortisol response to awakening. Psychosomatic Medicine **65**: 92–9.

Rothbart, M.K., Sheese, B.E., Rueda, M.R., and Posner, M.I. (2011). Developing mechanisms of self-regulation in early life. Emotions Reviews **3**: 207–13.

Schulz, P., Kirschbaum, C., Pruessner, J., and Hellhammer, D. (1998). Increased free cortisol secretion after awakening in chronically stress individuals due to work overload. Stress Medicine **14**: 91–7.

Southwick, S.M., Vythilingam, M., and Charney, D.S. (2005). The psychobiology of depression and resilience to stress: implications for prevention and treatment. Annual Reviews in Clinical Psychology **1**: 255–91.

Spangler, G., Schieche, M., Ilg, U., Maier, U., and Ackermann, C. (1994). Maternal sensitivity as an external organizer for biobehavioral regulation in infancy. Developmental Psychobiology **27**: 425–37.

Steptoe, A., Brydon, L., and Kunz-Ebrecht, S. (2005). Changes in financial strain over three years, ambulatory blood pressure, and cortisol responses to awakening. Psychosomatic Medicine **67**: 281–7.

Sullivan, P.F., Neale, M.C., and Kendler, K.S. (2000). Genetic epidemiology of major depression: review and meta-analysis. American Journal of Psychiatry **157**: 1552–62.

Tomarken, A.J., Davidson, R.J., and Henriques, J.B. (1990). Resting frontal brain asymmetry predicts affective responses to films. Journal of Personality and Social Psychology **59**: 791–801.

Tronick, E.Z. and Gianino, A. (1986). Interactive mismatch and repair: Challenges to the coping infant. Zero to Three: Bulletin of the National Center for Clinical Infant Programs **6**: 1–6.

Wachs, T.D., Black, M.M., and Engle, P.L. (2009). Maternal depression: a global threat to children's health, development, and behavior and to human rights. Child Development Perspectives **3**: 51–9.

Walker, B.R. (2007). Glucocorticoids and cardiovascular disease. European Journal of Endocrinology **157**: 545–59.

Weaver, I.C., Cervoni, N., Champagne, F.A., *et al.* (2004). Epigenetic programming by maternal behavior. Nature Neuroscience **7**: 847–54.

Young, E.A., Vazquez, D.M., Jiang, H., and Pfeffer, C.R. (2006). Saliva cortisol and response to dexamethasone in children of depressed parents. Biological Psychiatry **60**, 831–6.

Chapter 14

Young motherhood, perinatal depression, and children's development

Cerith S. Waters, Susan Pawlby, Stephanie H. M. van Goozen, and Dale F. Hay

Introduction

The aim of this chapter is to examine young women's experience of mental health problems during the perinatal period. We shall argue that women who were young at the time of their transition to parenthood are at elevated risk for perinatal depression, in their first and subsequent pregnancies. Evidence for the impact of perinatal depression on children's development will be outlined, and we propose that the elevated rates of mental health problems among young mothers may partly account for the increased prevalence of adverse outcomes often seen among their children. However, for these young women and their offspring, the impact of perinatal depression may be compounded by many other social, psychological, and biological risk factors, and young women's circumstances may exacerbate their own and their children's difficulties. Therefore any clinical strategies regarding the identification and treatment of depression during the antenatal and postnatal months may need to take into account the age of women, with women bearing children earlier and later than the average presenting different challenges for health professionals.

Demographic trends in the age of childbearing

Across the industrialized nations the demographics of parenthood are changing, with both men and women first becoming parents at increasingly older ages (Bosch 1998; Martin *et al.* 2005; Ventura *et al.* 2001). In the UK for example, the average maternal age at first birth in 1971 was 23.7 years, compared to the present figure of 29.5 years (ONS 2012). Correspondingly, over the last four decades, birth rates for women aged 30 and over have increased extensively, whilst those for women in their teenage years and early twenties have declined (ONS 2012, 2007). Since the 1970s, the proportion of children born to women aged 20–24 in the UK has been decreasing, with women aged 30–34 years now displaying the highest birth rates (ONS 2010). These changes in the demography of parenthood are not confined to the UK with similar trends toward delayed first births observed across

Western Europe (Ventura *et al.* 2001), the United States (Mirowsky 2002), New Zealand (Woodward *et al.* 2006) and Australia (Barnes 2003). Thus, a transition to parenthood during adolescence and the early 20s is non-normative for Western women, and the implications of this '*off-time*' transition (Elder 1997, 1998) for the mother's and the child's mental health warrants attention.

Paradoxically, whilst the rates of teenage childbearing have declined during the last four decades with small oscillations in the absolute numbers from year to year (Botting *et al.* 1998; Kiernan 1997; ONS 2012), governmental and media interest into teenage parenthood has intensified. In view of the rising age of first birth, teenage motherhood is now even more statistically deviant from population means than in previous decades, and findings suggest that an early transition to parenthood may now be more disadvantageous than in decades past (Maughan and Lindelow 1997; Moffitt *et al.* 2002). This might imply that services provided to childbearing women, such as childbirth classes, are even less appropriate for young mothers, who will be considerably younger than other members of the target population, but more at risk of perinatal mental health problems due to their generally disadvantaged environments and developmental histories.

Furthermore, women who give birth for the first time in their early 20s are also making the transition to parenthood much earlier than is currently the norm, and may similarly be at risk for mental health problems during the perinatal period. The prevalence of several types of risk behaviours that impact upon mental health, such as illegal substance misuse, unprotected sex, and binge drinking, have been found to peak in late adolescence and the early 20s (Arnett 1992; Bachman *et al.* 1996), and many psychiatric disorders have been found to onset by or during these years (Kessler *et al.* 2005). Thus, it is possible that the correlates and consequences of an 'off-time-early' transition to parenthood in the early 20s are similar to those of adolescent parenthood. Yet women in their early 20s are not traditionally seen as an 'at risk' group and thus their problems, as well as their children's, may be less well recognized. It is certainly the case that most of the relevant literature focuses on teenage motherhood and its association with a variety of adverse outcomes for children.

Mothers' early entry into parenthood conveys risk for their children

The offspring of teenage mothers have higher mortality rates and lower birth weights (Elfenbein and Felice 2003; Kirchengast and Hartmann 2003; Pevalin 2003). They suffer more health-related problems as neonates, and are at a greater risk of physical neglect and abuse (Stevens-Simon, Nelligan and Kelly, 2001; Rodgers *et al.* 1996). As development progresses, infants born to adolescent mothers obtain lower scores on the mental development index of the Bayley Scales at 6 months of age (Pomerleau *et al.* 2003), and their attachment relationships in the second year of life are often described as avoidant or insecure (Lamb *et al.* 1987; Spieker and Bensley 1994). However, adverse health related outcomes and sub-optimal attachment relationships are not always found (Andreozzi *et al.* 2002; Pardo *et al.* 2003), and many infants born to young mothers follow typical patterns of development. In addition, within age group variability has been reported; babies born to girls in their early to mid adolescent years are at greater risk of adverse outcomes than the infants of older adolescents (Cooper *et al.* 1995; Furstenberg 1992; Kirchengast and Hartmann 2003).

When compared to the offspring of older parents, children born to adolescent mothers score lower on standardized tests of cognitive ability (Cornelius *et al.* 2009; Manlove 1997; Moffitt *et al.* 2002; Moore and Synder 1991; Sommer *et al.* 2000) and they are significantly more likely to be referred to special educational services (Gueorguieva *et al.* 2001; Moffitt *et al.* 2002). Similarly, longitudinal and cross-sectional studies have found the offspring of adolescent parents to display elevated rates of behavioural problems (Black *et al.* 2002a, b; Leadbeater *et al.* 1996; Moffitt *et al.* 2002; Sommer *et al.* 2000), as well as increased difficulties in the socio-emotional domain of functioning (Black *et al.* 2002a, b; Miller *et al.* 1996; Moffitt *et al.* 2002; Sommer *et al.* 2000). What is more, whilst few studies have followed the offspring of young mothers into adolescence and early adulthood, those that have report a persistence in the risk of adverse outcomes, with the childhood difficulties being shown to translate into higher rates of educational under-achievement, unemployment, criminal convictions, and mental health problems (Coley and Chase-Lansdale 1998; Fergusson and Woodward 1999; Jaffee *et al.* 2001; Shaw *et al.* 2006).

In evaluating the literature on the risks of early motherhood, it is important to keep two key findings in mind. First, women who enter into parenthood in their teenage years are likely to confer risk to their children, irrespective of whether they are actually teenagers at the time of subsequent births (Berrington *et al.* 2005; Jaffee *et al.* 2001; Moffitt *et al.* 2002). Thus, first born and non-first born children are at elevated risk. Second, even though the offspring of teenage mothers are at elevated risk, adverse outcomes are not inevitable. Heterogeneity in functioning among the offspring of adolescent mothers has been noted, and many children and adolescents show adaptive patterns of adjustment (Furstenberg *et al.* 1993; Jaffee *et al.*, 2001).

Studies of perinatal depression: younger mothers are under-represented

Many of the adverse outcomes associated with young motherhood are also associated with maternal depression, regardless of the mother's age. Professor Kumar's pioneering work did much to draw attention to the impact of perinatal depression for women's lives and the lives of their children (Sharp *et al.* 1995; Hay *et al.* 2001). Over the past three decades, much attention has been paid to depressive illness following childbirth (e.g. Murray and Cooper 1997). More recently, academic and clinical interest has been drawn to depressive and anxious symptomatology during pregnancy (O'Keane 2006; O'Connor *et al.* 2002). However, in neither literature has much attention been given to the mental health of younger mothers (Bennett *et al.* 2004). Similarly, in studies that have investigated the association between the mother's mental state and the child's development, young maternal age at entry into parenthood has often been used as a sample exclusion criterion (e.g. Murray 1992).

The antenatal depression literature

Prevalence

Traditionally, pregnancy has been thought of as a period of emotional well-being and satisfaction for the expectant mother (Bonari *et al.* 2004), frequently described as a time period during a woman's life course where the risk of mental health problems is decreased (Bonari *et al.* 2004; Buist 2000; Nonacs and Cohen 2003). As a consequence of this perspective, research and clinical focus in perinatal psychiatry has largely centred upon the months following childbirth (O'Keane 2006), and the *Diagnostic and Statistical Manual of Mental Disorders* (DSM-IV-TR) gives special emphasis to postnatal but not to antenatal mood disorders (American Psychiatric Association 2000).

However, research over the last decade has documented higher levels of depressive and anxious symptomatology in the antenatal relative to the postnatal period (Evans *et al.* 2001; Heron *et al.* 2004; Rubertsson *et al.* 2005). Prevalence estimates for antenatal depression vary widely between studies, depending on the measurement technique, the population of interest, and the trimester of pregnancy in which the results were recorded. In general, questionnaire methods produce higher prevalence rates than semi-structured diagnostic interviews (see Bennett *et al.* 2004), and cohort studies that canvass the emotions and feelings of women from a broad range of socioeconomic groups find greater frequencies of depressive symptoms than studies that have more selected samples, such as married women, mothers of mid to high socio-economic status, and women aged 18 and over (Evans *et al.* 2001; Marcus *et al.* 2003; Affonso *et al.* 1990; O'Hara *et al.* 1990).

The literature search for this chapter identified two meta-analyses into the prevalence of antenatal depression. Bennett and colleagues (2004) included 21 studies in their analysis, 7 of which used a standardized psychiatric interview to identify cases of antenatal depression, with the other 14 studies using self-report questionnaires. Studies on samples of teenage mothers were excluded from this meta-analysis and prevalence rates for antenatal depression were reported by the trimester of pregnancy: 7.4% of women were estimated to be depressed in the first trimester, 12.8% in the second, and 12% in the third. The second meta-analysis conducted by Gavin and colleagues (2005) included only studies that had used a diagnostic interview ($N = 12$) to ascertain the presence of antenatal depression. In this study, 11% of women were estimated to be depressed in the first trimester of pregnancy, and 8.5% in the second and third trimesters. Additionally, Gavin and colleagues (2005) reported the prevalence of antenatal depression for the entire pregnancy period which was reported at 18.4%.

Whilst providing important information, there are many caveats to the results of both meta-analyses. First, the confidence intervals for the prevalence data were often wide, largely due to the small number of studies pooled together to derive the statistics. For example, the trimester estimates reported by Gavin and colleagues were derived from a minimum of two and a maximum of five studies. Second, some of the studies included in both meta-analyses excluded women with a recent history of mental health problems, while others excluded women of low socio-economic status—both known risk factors for antenatal depression (Nonacs and Cohen 2003; Kumar and Robson 1984; O'Keane 2006). Thus, the exclusion of these two groups of women along with the omission of studies of young mothers would ultimately produce a downward bias in the pooled prevalence estimates. Indeed, when Bennett and co-authors repeated their analyses on studies of women of low socio-economic status only, the estimates for the 2nd and 3rd trimesters were 47% and 39% for questionnaire assessments, and 28% and 25% for diagnostic interview studies.

Outcomes for children

Depressive and anxiety symptoms during pregnancy are associated with sub-optimal infant outcomes on the Brazelton Neonatal Behaviour Assessment Scale (Field *et al.* 2004), the Bayley Scales of Infant Development (Huizink *et al.* 2003), and parental and observers' ratings of an infant's emotional state (Davis *et al.* 2005; Huizink *et al.* 2002). Importantly in these studies, associations between antenatal mood and infant outcome remained significant after postnatal anxiety and depressive symptoms were accounted for (Davis *et al.* 2005; Huizink *et al.* 2002 *et al*, 2003). Longer-term follow-up studies have found antenatal depression (along with perceived stress and anxiety in pregnancy) to be associated with children's later disruptive behaviour, including attention deficit hyperactivity disorder symptoms and conduct problems, as well as violence in adolescence (Hay *et al.* 2010; Maki *et al.* 2003; O'Connor *et al.* 2002). The link between antenatal depression and disruptive behaviour is already evident in infancy. Our own work has shown that depression in pregnancy is associated with infants' elevated tendencies to express anger and use physical aggression against parents and peers (Hay *et al.*, 2011 Hay *et al.*, in press).

The postnatal depression literature

Prevalence

There has been much academic and clinical interest into postnatal depression (PND) during the last three decades with prevalence estimates ranging between 8% and 15% (O'Hara 1997). Similar to the antenatal depression literature, prevalence estimates of PND vary widely between studies, depending on the definition of PND, the measurement technique, and the population of interest. In general, questionnaire methods produce higher prevalence rates than diagnostic interviews, and, in contrast to the antenatal depression literature, a greater number of studies that include young mothers have been published (Table 14.1).

Outcomes for children

Maternal depression is a well-known risk factor for children's development (Cummings and Davies 1994; Goodman and Gotlib 1999). In infancy, the offspring of mothers suffering from postnatal depression show cognitive and regulatory disturbances (Field *et al.* 1995, Galler *et al.* 2000; Murray 1992). In childhood and adolescence, cognitive impairments persist (Hay and Kumar 1995; Hay *et al.* 2008), and socio-emotional deficits have

Table 14.1 Studies of the prevalence of depression in samples of young mothers at various points during the perinatal period

Reference	Design and assessments	Measures	Parity	Sample Comparison group/age	Results
Beards lee et al. (1988)	Cross sectional design; 3–6 months postpartum. Life-time prevalence and incidence of depression	SADS Interview	2	Young mothers (N = 18; 18–21 years) who had all given birth as teenagers. No comparison group	Life-time prevalence of depression 44% and incidence 33%. Majority of episodes onset in pregnancy
Troutman and Cutrona (1990)	Longitudinal design; 3rd trimester of pregnancy and 6 and 52 weeks postpartum	SADS Interview	1	Pregnant teenagers (N = 128; 14–18 years) vs. non-parent friends (N = 114)	No diagnostic differences at each assessment however the parents reported significantly more symptoms of depression
Leadbeater and Linares (1992)	Longitudinal design; assessments at 1, 6, 12, and 28–36 months postpartum	BDI ≥16	2	Teenage mothers (N = 89–120; 13–19 years). Puerto Rican vs. Black mothers	No differences between ethnic groups. Proportion scoring in the clinical range at 1, 6, 12, and 28–36 months was 31%, 31%, 22%, and 18%
Prodromidis et al. (1994)	Cross sectional design; assessment at 1–3 days postpartum	BDI ≥16	2	Young mothers (N = 154; 14–21 years). No comparison group	Prevalence data for depression not reported. Depressed mothers experienced more psychosocial stress
Barnet et al. (1996)	Longitudinal design; assessments during the third trimester of pregnancy and 2 and 4 months postpartum	CES-D ≥21	2	Teenage mothers (N = 104; 12–18 years. No comparison group	Prevalence of antenatal depression was 42%. Prevalence at 2 and 4 months post-partum was 36% and 32%
Caldwell et al. (1998)	Cross sectional design; assessment at 3 months postpartum	CES-D No cut-score	1	Teenage mothers (N = 48; 14–19 years. Comparisons made between racial groups	Prevalence data for depression not reported. No significant differences between black and white mothers

Table 14.1 (continued) Studies of the prevalence of depression in samples of young mothers at various points during the perinatal period

Reference	Design and assessments	Measures	Parity	Sample Comparison group/age	Results
Caldwell et al. (1997)	Cross-sectional design; assessment at 3 months postpartum	CES-D No cut-score	1	Teenage mothers (N = 83; ≤19 years. Comparisons made between racial groups	Prevalence data for depression not reported. No significant differences between black and white mothers
Hudson et al. (2000)	Cross-sectional design; assessment at 3 months postpartum	CES-D ≥16	1	Teenage mothers (N = 21; 15–19 years). No comparison group	At the postnatal assessment 53% of the sample scored above the cut-score. Depression was found to be negatively related to social support
Quinlivian et al. (2004)	Cross-sectional design; assessment during pregnancy, gestational age not reported	GHQ-28 No cut-score	1	Teenage mothers (N = 50; ≤19 years) vs. older mothers (N = 50, ≥20 years	Teenage mothers had significantly higher depression, anxiety and total scale scores. The % above the cut-score not reported
Rich-Edwards et al. (2005)	Longitudinal design; assessments during pregnancy and at 6 months postpartum	EPDS ≥13	2	Young mothers (N = 74; ≤22 years) vs. mothers aged 23–29 (N = 376) and mothers aged 30 and older	The young mother group had the highest depression scores at each assessment, with 23% scoring above the cut-score during pregnancy and 22% postpartum
Hand et al. (2006)	Cross-sectional design; assessment at 5 days postpartum	PSI No cut-score	2	Teenage mothers (15–19 years) vs. adult mothers (≥20 years). Total N = 52	Adult mothers had significantly higher mean depression scores
Schmidt et al. (2006)	Longitudinal design; assessments at 3, 12, 24, and 28 months postpartum	BDI ≥8	2	Teenage mothers (N = 623; 13–18 years). Comparisons between White, Black, and Mexican American mothers	The highest proportion of the sample to score above the cut-score was at 3 months postpartum; 57% scored above the cut-score at one or more assessment
Caputo and Bordin (2007)	Cross-sectional; assessment during pregnancy, gestational age not reported	YSR ≥64	1	Teenage mothers (N = 207; 13–17 years) vs. non-pregnant teens (N = 308; 13–17 years)	Pregnant women had higher depression and anxiety scores with 24% scoring above the cut-score

Table 14.1 (continued) Studies of the prevalence of depression in samples of young mothers at various points during the perinatal period

Reference	Design and assessments	Measures	Parity	Sample Comparison group/age	Results
Figueiredo et al. (2007)	Longitudinal; assessments during the third trimester of pregnancy and 2–3 months postpartum	EPDS ≥13	2	Young mothers (N = 54; ≤18 years) versus adult mothers (N = 54; 19–40 years)	A greater number of young mothers scored above the cut-score during pregnancy (26% vs. 11%) and postpartum (26% vs. 9%)
Secco et al. (2007)	Cross-sectional assessment at 4 weeks post-partum	BDI ≥10	2	Young mothers (N = 69; 15–19 years) no comparison group	At the post-partum assessment 44% scored above the cut-score
Lanzi et al. (2009)	Longitudinal design; assessments during pregnancy and at 6 months postpartum	BDI No cut-score	1	Teenage mothers (N = 396; 14–19 years) vs. adult mothers (N = 286; ≥20 years)	Teenage mothers displayed significantly higher symptom scores for depression during pregnancy and at 6 months postpartum
Ramos-Marcuse et al. (2010)	Longitudinal design; assessments at 3 weeks, 6 months, and 24 months postpartum	BDI ≥9	1	Teenage mothers (N = 148; ≤19 years). No comparison group. Mothers all of African American origin	Almost half of the teenage mothers (49%) scored above the cut-score at 3 weeks post-partum, with 37% and 36% scoring above the cut-score at 6 and 24 months postpartum

Parity: 1 = Primiparous; 2 = Multiparous; EPDS = Edinburgh Postnatal Depression Scale; BDI = Beck Depression Inventory; CES-D = Centre for Epidemiological Studies of Depression Instrument; YSR = Youth Self Report Questionnaire; PSI = Psychiatric Symptom Index; GHQ-28 = General Health Questionnaire-28 item; EPDS = Edinburgh Postnatal Depression Scale; SADS = Schedule for Affective Disorders and Schizophrenia.

been documented (Essex *et al.* 2001; Halligan *et al.* 2007; Murray *et al.* 1999). Thus, children exposed to PND show similar patterns of maladjustment as the offspring of teenage mothers. PND has been found to disrupt the quality of the caregiving environment (Campbell *et al.* 1992; Murray *et al.* 1993), and such disturbances are believed to have long lasting effects via their impact upon the developmental tasks of infancy. For example, PND is thought to disrupt attachment formation and infants' ability to learn to regulate their attention and emotions (Goodman and Gotlib 1999; Hay 1997).

The exclusion of young mothers from the literature on perinatal depression

Underestimating the prevalence of perinatal illness

A major source of bias inherent in the literature on perinatal depression, and one that is illustrated clearly in both meta-analyses of the prevalence of antenatal depression, is the omission of studies that have a focus on young mothers (Bennett *et al.* 2004; Gavin *et al.* 2005). Neither study justified the exclusion of this population from their meta-analysis, though one can hypothesize that the authors assumed that young mothers would be more likely to suffer from depression during the pregnancy period and as such, did not want to produce an 'upward bias' in their prevalence estimates. However, this may not be the only basis for exclusion. Individual studies in the antenatal and postnatal depression literatures often cite 'medical complications' as the reason for excluding mothers under 18 from their sample (e.g. Hobfoll *et al.* 1995). Evidently, the omission of this age group from such analyses renders it difficult to decipher whether or not young mothers are at a heightened risk of depression in the perinatal period. What is more, the exclusion of this segment of the population from many studies can only add to the uncertainty surrounding the true prevalence of perinatal mental health problems.

Young mothers and perinatal depression: a summary of the existing literature

Relevant studies of young mothers' experience of depression during the perinatal period are summarized in Table 14.1[1]. As is the case with the wider literature, rather than reporting rates of clinically significant mental health problems, the vast majority of studies have focused on the prevalence of depressive symptoms. During the literature search, no study that focused exclusively on anxiety symptoms or clinically significant anxiety disorders among young mothers was identified. As is the case with the adult literature, the majority of studies that have assessed the mental state of young mothers during the perinatal period have focused on the months following childbirth. For example, of the 17 identified studies, 15 assessed the mother's mental state during the postnatal period, with five of these studies beginning their assessments during pregnancy (see Table 14.1). Two studies assessed the mother's mental state during the pregnancy only (Caputo and Bordin 2007; Quinlivan *et al.* 2004. Thus, seven studies assessed the mother's mental state during pregnancy.

Antenatal depression

In line with the wider literature, far less attention has been paid to depression occurring in the antenatal as opposed to the postnatal period. This is surprising considering that reports published two decades previous documented higher rates of depressive symptoms among young mothers during the antenatal relative to the postnatal period (Troutman and Cutrona 1990). Yet, in their paper, Troutman and Cutrona focused exclusively on their postnatal findings, making little reference to their pregnancy data: a peculiarity common to other studies in this literature (e.g. Rich-Edwards *et al.* 2005). The neglect of the study of antenatal depression among young mothers is further illustrated by the limited number of papers published on this topic. Only seven of the identified studies assessed the mother's mental state during pregnancy (see Table 14.1). Five of these studies were longitudinal, conducting one or two follow-up assessments during the first year postpartum. Overall, the reported prevalence of antenatal depression among young mothers lies between 16% and 42%, with the one diagnostic interview study reporting the lowest rate. Typically however, it is estimated that one in four adolescent mothers suffer from depression during pregnancy.

All of the longitudinal studies report higher rates of depressive symptoms during pregnancy than the post partum, yet due to their focus on PND, the antenatal findings are often not discussed. Indeed, the majority of these studies fail even to report the proportion of participants likely to be suffering from depression during pregnancy. In general, all of the antenatal studies that compared young and older mothers find significantly higher rates of depression in the young mother group. A further two studies compared pregnant teenagers with non-pregnant/parenting teenagers. Both of these studies report significantly more depressive symptoms in the child bearing group (Caputo and Bordin 2007; Troutman and Cutrona 1990). However, in the Troutman and Cutrona study, significant between group differences in the rates of clinically significant depression was not observed (see Table 14.1).

Postnatal depression

Of the 15 studies that assessed the mothers' mental state during the postnatal period (as defined as the first six months postpartum), three were longitudinal with only postnatal assessments, and five were longitudinal with both antenatal and postnatal assessments. Seven of the studies were cross-sectional. The three longitudinal studies that conducted only postnatal assessments evaluated the mother's mental state within the first three months of childbirth, conducting two or three further assessments at 6, 12, or 18 monthly intervals over the following 2 to 3 years (Leadbeater and Linares 1992; Ramos-Marcuse *et al.* 2010; Schmidt *et al.* 2006). Two of these studies documented a peak in depressive symptoms during the first 3 months postpartum, noting a significant decline in symptom severity over the course of subsequent assessments (Leadbeater and Linares 1992; Schmidt *et al.* 2006). The study conducted by Ramos-Marcuse and colleagues (2010) differentiated three groups of participants based on their depressive symptom trajectories. In this study, the low and medium depressive symptom groups displayed a decrease in symptom severity over time, whereas the high symptom group displayed an increase in symptom severity overtime.

The vast majority of studies used self-report questionnaires to assess the mothers' mental state during the postnatal period with only two studies using diagnostic interviews. For the questionnaire studies, prevalence estimates of PND among teenage mothers lie between 22% and 53% (Rich-Edwards *et al.* 2005: Hudson *et al.* 2000). Typically, it is estimated that one in three adolescent mothers are depressed postpartum (see Table 14.1). For the interview studies, 33% and 26% of adolescent mothers have been found to be suffering from clinically significant depression in the first 3 months following childbirth (Beardslee *et al.* 1988; Troutman and Cutrona 1990). Thus, in reference to the broader literature (see O'Hara 1997), adolescent mothers are approximately twice as likely as adult mothers to be depressed postpartum.

Young mothers and perinatal depression: methodological problems

The literature on early parenthood and maternal depression is fraught with methodological limitations. These include sampling problems, measurement inconsistencies, differences in the definition of a young mother, and variability in the construction of the comparison group. In terms of sampling problems, many of the studies included in Table 14.1 recruited their participants from specialized intervention programmes. This recruitment strategy brings the representativeness of the sample into question as it is possible that these young women are at lower risk of depression because of the additional support that they receive. Conversely, it is also possible that women enrolled in specialized programmes are at elevated risk.

Further sampling-related biases that plague this literature concern the fact that the vast majority of studies included in Table 14.1 were conducted in the USA—with many recruiting only ethnic minority samples. Given that the context of early motherhood varies by country, one can question how well these findings generalize to young mothers from other industrialized nations. Furthermore, the presence of high attrition rates and selective attrition among the identified studies also brings into question how representative their findings are. For example, one of the more impressive longitudinal studies included in Table 14.1 (Schmidt *et al.* 2006[2]) suffered a 40% drop out rate over a three year period with greater attrition seen among those women depressed at baseline (Schmidt *et al.* 2006).

Issues of construct validity and measurement inconsistencies also compromise this literature. For example, six different self-report questionnaire measures and one diagnostic interview were used to identify antenatal and/or postnatal depression. Not only do these questionnaires differ in content, but only three of them (the Beck Depression Inventory (BDI), the Edinburgh Postnatal Depression Scale (EPDS), and the General Health Questionnaire (GHQ)) have been validated in pregnant and postpartum populations (Holcomb *et al.* 1996; Kumar and Robson 1984; Murray and Cox 1990). This issue is of particular importance given that the somatic symptoms of depression overlap with the 'symptoms' of pregnancy (e.g. insomnia/hypersomnia, appetite changes, weight gain, and fatigue). Thus, in the questionnaire based studies, somatic symptoms that are often part and parcel of the perinatal experience are recorded as present, regardless of whether they occur in the context of depressed mood. The inevitable inflation of symptom scores that this creates could therefore account for the higher prevalence rates of depression that are found in questionnaire studies. It is only through in-depth interviews that the context and nature of perinatal somatic symptoms can be understood—and, differentiated from those of depression.

Additional methodological inconsistencies can be seen in Table 14.1. In particular, even when different studies have used the same questionnaire scale to assess depression, they often adopt different cut-scores to identify probable cases. The uncertainty and confusion caused by these decisions (e.g. prevalence rates that vary by the threshold used for depression) is avoidable given that each measure has a pre-specified cut-score that has been derived from a series of validity and reliability studies. Furthermore, as shown in Table 14.1, different studies use different ages to define a young mother. Not all studies use age at first birth as the criterion. Instead, some authors use the mother's age at entry into the study to define a young mother. This strategy complicates the interpretation of the findings as women who gave birth as teenagers are then classified as older mothers (see Hand *et al.* 2006). Taken together, the aforementioned methodological limitations not only complicate comparisons between studies, they reduce the applicability of the findings to clinical settings.

Are women in their early 20s also at risk?

As noted previously, there is reason to believe that risks associated with an 'off-time early' entry into parenthood may affect women in their early 20s as well as adolescent mothers. In particular, women in their early 20s may also be at elevated risk for perinatal depression when compared to mothers of normative parenting age. However, in the literature on perinatal mental health problems, adolescent women are often excluded and women in their early 20s are not differentiated from other members of the sample. In contrast, our own studies of the relationship between young maternal age and women's risk for perinatal depression have drawn attention to the fact that women in their early twenties constitute an invisible risk group.

We first examined links between maternal age and perinatal illness in the South London Child Development Study (SLCDS). In this prospective longitudinal study a representative sample of women and their children were recruited from antenatal clinics in two relatively disadvantaged areas of South London and subsequently followed up during infancy, childhood and adolescence (please see Chapter 10 for further details on this sample). The SLCDS was an important part of Professor Kumar's own research programme (Sharp *et al.* 1995; Hay *et al.* 2001). We found that from the pregnancy to adolescence period, almost three in four young mothers—both those who entered parenthood in their teenage and in their early 20s—experienced at least one episode of depression (Waters *et al.* under review). Relative to older mothers, women who entered parenthood during their teenage years and early 20s were particularly vulnerable to depression during pregnancy. During the antenatal months, over a third of the teenage and early 20s mothers were depressed.

In general, prevalence rates for depression are higher than average in the relatively disadvantaged SLCDS sample (see Pawlby *et al.* 2009). However, the demographic characteristics of the South London sample do not account for the fact that young mothers are at elevated risk for perinatal illness. Our current work in a second sample has similarly drawn attention to young mothers' risk for depression during pregnancy. In the Cardiff Child Development Study (CCDS), a nationally representative sample of primiparous women recruited from two catchment areas in South Wales, the overall rate of antenatal depression was almost identical to estimates from the meta-analyses (Gavin *et al.* 2005). In the CCDS sample, young women were also at elevated risk for antenatal depression (Waters 2009). Almost half the women who were 19 years of age or younger and a third of those in their early 20s were diagnosed with depression during pregnancy, compared to only 7% of older women. Put another way, the majority of women suffering from depression in pregnancy in this representative sample were young, a fact that has major implications for clinical services.

Could the elevated rates of perinatal depression among young mothers account for the adverse offspring outcomes?

A small number of studies examining why children born to young mothers are at risk of adverse outcomes have highlighted maternal depression as a key determinant. For example, analyses of three different samples of teenage mothers and their pre-school aged children revealed that the mother's symptoms of anxiety and depression increased their children's risk of adverse outcomes (Berrington *et al.* 2005; Black *et al.* 2002; Sommer *et al.* 2000). However, specific effects of antenatal and postnatal depression were not considered in these studies. Similarly, in as far as these studies of young mothers and their children employed a cross-sectional design, or they relied upon single informants, the causal status of maternal depression is challenged.

In the SLCDS we have examined whether the elevated rates of antenatal and postnatal depression among young mothers (both those who entered parenthood in their teens and early 20s) could account for the greater risk of adverse outcomes among their children. In this prospective longitudinal study from pregnancy to adolescence we found that relative to older mothers, the offspring of both teenage and early 20s mothers showed significant deficits in their cognitive functioning. Nevertheless, only the children born to early 20 mothers were at increased risk of developing a clinically significant emotional disorder. In this study there was evidence that the link between young motherhood and children's emotional disorder was mediated by depression in pregnancy, whereas postnatal depression was found to exert effects on children's cognitive functioning (Waters *et al.* under review). However in these analyses, attention was also drawn to other suboptimal antenatal and postnatal experiences including exposure to smoking during pregnancy and the absence of breast-feeding postpartum. Even after accounting for prior and subsequent sources of risk, the legacy of the antenatal and postnatal insults remained clear for the mothers and children in the South London study.

Summary and conclusions

It is well established that young motherhood is associated with an elevated risk of adverse outcomes for mothers and children. Our review has shown that, relative to older mothers, teenage mothers demonstrate higher rates of depression throughout the perinatal period. What is more, this vulnerability to depression during the antenatal and postnatal months is observed amongst primiparous and multiparous women who began childbearing during their teenage years. Thus, women who entered parenthood during their adolescent years, but who are not necessarily teenagers at the time of a subsequent pregnancy, have been found to be at risk of depression during the antenatal and postnatal months. Our own work has demonstrated that the elevated risk for perinatal mental health problems also characterizes women in their early 20s.

During the months following childbirth, approximately one in three adolescent mothers are reported to be suffering from depression. For the pregnancy period, the limited number of available studies implies that one in four adolescent mothers experience depression, although our own work suggests that the rates may be even higher, particularly in disadvantaged communities. Evidence is also emerging which suggests that the elevated rates of antenatal and postnatal depression among young mothers may partly account for the adverse outcomes often seen among their children. However, our own work has also shown that exposure to depression during the perinatal period is only one of many sources of risk in the context of young motherhood. In the future it will prove important to consider whether younger women present with different profiles of symptoms and risk factors, and whether they require more age-appropriate clinical services that extend beyond the perinatal period.

Notes

1 To ensure that a comprehensive review was conducted studies that assessed the mother's mental state during the perinatal period but did not report prevalence data were included in this review.

2 The studies highlighted here and those selected throughout the discussion of methodological issues are chosen as examples as they represent some of the more prominent papers in terms of publication prestige. They are by no means more flawed than the countless number of other studies not cited.

References

Affonso, D.D., Lovett, S., Paul, S.M., and Sheptak, S. (1990). A standardised interview that differentiates pregnancy and postpartum symptoms from perinatal clinical depression. Birth **17**: 121–30.

American Psychiatric Association (2000). Diagnostic and Statistical Manual of Mental Disorders. 4th Ed, Text revised. Washington, DC, APA.

Anderson, J.W., Johnstone, B.M. and Remley, D.T. (1999). Breast-feeding and cognitive development: A meta-analysis American Journal of Clinical Nutrition **70**: 525–535.

Andreozzi, L., Falanagan, P., Seifer, R., Brunner, S., and Lester, B. (2002). Attachment classifications among 18-month-old children of adolescent mothers. Archives of Paediatrics and Adolescent Medicine **156**: 20–6.

Arnett, J.J. (1992). Reckless behaviour in adolescence: A developmental perspective. Developmental Review **12**: 339–73.

Bachman, J.G., Johnston, L.D., O'Malley, P., and Schulenberg, J. (1996). Transitions in drug use during late adolescence and young adulthood. In Transitions through adolescence: Interpersonal domains and contexts, J.A., Graber, J. Brooks-Gunn, and A.C. Peterson, editors. Mahwah, NJ, Erlbaum, pp. 111–40.

Barnes, A. (2003). Australia's fertility rate: Trends and issues. Department of Family and Community Services Research Fact Sheet, No. 9.

Barnet, B., Joffe, A., Duggan, A.K., Wilson, M., and Repke, J. (1996). Depressive symptoms, stress, and social support in pregnant and post partum adolescents. Archives of Paediatric and Adolescent Medicine **150**: 64–9.

Beardslee, W.R., Zuckerman, B.S., Amaro, H., and McAllister. M. (1988). Depression among adolescent mothers: A pilot study. Developmental and Behavioural Paediatrics **9**: 62–5.

Bennett, H.A., Einarson, A., Taddio, A., Koren, G., and Einarson, T. (2004). Prevalence of depression during pregnancy: systematic review. American College of Obstetrics and Gynaecologists **103**: 698–709.

Berrington, A., Diamond, I., Ingham, R., Stevenson, J., Borgoni, R., Hernandez, I., and Smith, P.W.F. (2005). Consequences of teenage parenthood: Pathways which minimise the long term negative impacts of teenage childbearing. Department of Health. Final report—November 2005. London, Department of Health.

Black, M.M., Papas, M.A., Hussey, J.M., et al. (2002). Behaviour and development of preschool children born to adolescent mothers: Risk and 3-generation households. Journal of Paediatrics **109**: 909–18.

Black, M.M., Papas, M.A., Hussey, J.M., et al. (2002b). Behaviour problems among preschool children born to adolescent mothers: Effects of maternal depression and perceptions of partner relationships. Journal of Clinical Child and Adolescent Psychology **31**: 16–26.

Bonari, L., Pinto, N., Ahn, E., Einarson, A., Steiner, M., and Koren, G. (2004). Perinatal risks of untreated depression during pregnancy. Canadian Journal of Psychiatry **49**: 726–5.

Bosch, X. (1998). Investigating reasons for Spain's falling birth rate. Lancet **352**: 887.

Botting, B., Rosato, M., and Wood, R. (1998). Teenage mothers and the health of their children, Population Trends **93**: 19–28.

Buist, A. (2000). Managing depression in pregnancy. Australian Family Physician **29**: 663–7.

Caldwell, C.H., Anfonucci, T.C., Jackson, J.S., Wolford, M., and Osofsky, J.O. (1997). Perceptions of parental support and depressive symptomatology among African American and White adolescent mothers. Journal of Emotional and Behavioural Disorders **5**: 173–83.

Campbell, S.B., Cohn, J.F., Flanagan, C., Popper, S., and Meyers, T. (1992). Course and correlates of postpartum depression during the transition to parenthood. Development and Psychopathology **4**: 29–47.

Caputo, V.G. and Bordin, I.A. (2007). Mental health problems among pregnant and non-pregnant youth. Rev Saude Publica **41** (4): 1–8.

Coley, R.L. and Chase-Lansdale, P.L. (1998). Adolescent pregnancy and parenthood: Recent evidence and future directions. American Psychologist **53**: 152–166.

Cooper, L.G., Leland, N.L., and Alexander, G. (1995). Effect of maternal age on birth outcomes among young adolescents. Social Biology **42**: 22–35.

Cornelius, M.D., Goldschmidt, L., DeGenna, N., and Day, N.L. (2007). Smoking during teenage pregnancies: effects on behavioural problems in offspring. Nicotine &Tobacco Research **9**: (7), 739–50.

Cummings M.E. and Davies, P. T. (1994). Maternal depression and child development. Journal of Child Psychology and Psychiatry **35**(1): 73–112.

Davis, E.P., Glynn, L.M., Dunkel-Schetter, C., et al. (2005). Corticotropopin-relasing hormone during pregnancy is associated with infant temperament. Developmental Neuroscience **27**: 299–305.

Elder, G.H., Jr. (1997). The life course and human development. In Handbook of child psychology. Vol. 1: Theoretical models of human development, 5th ed., W. Damon., and Lerner, R.M., editors. New York, Cambridge University Press, pp. 939–991.

Elder, G.H., Jr. (1998). The life course as developmental theory. Child Development 69: 1–12.

Elfenbein, D.S. and Felice, M.E. (2003). Adolescent pregnancy. Pediatric Clinical Journal of North America 50: 781–800.

Essex, M.J., Klein, M.H., Miech, R., and Smider, N.A. (2001). Timing of initial exposure to maternal major depression and children's mental health symptoms in kindergarten. British Journal of Psychiatry 179: 151–6.

Evans, J., Heron, J., Francomb, H., Oke, S., and Golding, J. (2001). Cohort study of depressed mood during pregnancy and childbirth. British Medical Journal 323: 257–60.

Fergusson, D.M., and Woodward, L.J. (1999). Maternal age and educational and psychosocial outcomes in early adulthood. Journal of Child Psychology and Psychiatry 43: 479–89.

Field, T., Fox, N. A., Pickens, J., and Nawrocki, T. (1995). Right frontal EEG activation in 3-to 6-month-old infants of depressed mothers. Developmental Psychology 31: 358–63.

Field, T., Diego, M., Dieter, J., et al. (2004). Prenatal depression effects on the foetus and the newborn. Infant Behaviour and Development 27: 216–229.

Figueiredo, B., Pacheco, A., and Costa, R. (2007). Depression during pregnancy and the postpartum in adolescent and adult Portuguese mothers. Archives of Women's Mental Health 10(3): 103–109.

Furstenberg, F.F., Jr. (1992). Teenage childbearing and cultural rationality: A thesis in search of evidence, Family Relations 41: 239–43.

Furstenberg, F.F., Jr., Hughes, M. E., and Brooks-Gunn, J. (1993). The next generation: The children of teenage mothers growing up. In Early parenthood and coming of age in the 1990's, M.K. Rosenheim, and M.F. Testa, editors. New Brunswick, NJ, Rutgers University Press, pp. 119–135.

Galler, J.R. Harrison, R.H., Ramsey, F., Forde, V., and Butler, S.C. (2000). Maternal depressive symptoms affect infant cognitive development in Barbados. Journal of Child Psychology and Psychiatry 41: 747–57.

Gavin, N.I., Gaynes, B.N., Lohr, K.N., Meltzer-Brody, S., Gartlehner, G., and Swinson, T. (2005). Perinatal Depression. A systematic review of prevalence and incidence. American Journal of Obstetrics and Gynaecologists 106: 1071–83.

Goodman, S.H. and Gotlib, I.H. (1999). Risk for psychopathology in the children of depressed mothers: A development model for understanding mechanisms of transmission. Psychological Review 106: 458–90.

Gueorguieva, R.V., Carter, R.L., Ariet, M., Roth, J., Mahan, C.S., and Resnick, M.B. (2001). Effect of teenage pregnancy on educational disabilities in kindergarten. American Journal of Epidemiology 154: 212–20.

Halligan, S.L., Murray, L., Martins, C., and Cooper, P. (2007). Maternal depression and psychiatric outcomes in adolescent offspring: A 13-year longitudinal study. Journal of Affective Disorders 97: 145–54.

Hand, I., Noble, L., North, A., Kim, M., and Yoon, J. (2006). Psychiatric symptoms among postpartum women in an urban hospital setting. American Journal of Perinatology 23: 329–34.

Hay, D.F. (1997). Postpartum depression and cognitive development. In Postpartum depression and child development, L. Murray and P. Cooper, editors. New York, Guilford Press, pp. 85–110.

Hay, D.F. and Kumar, R. (1995). Interpreting the effects of mothers' postnatal depression on children's intelligence: A critique and a reanalysis. Child Psychiatry and Human Development 25: 165–181.

Hay, D.F., Pawlby, S., Sharp, D., et al. (2001). Intellectual problems shown 11-year-old children whose mothers had postnatal depression. Journal of Child Psychology and Psychiatry 42: 871–90.

Hay, D.F., Pawlby, S., Waters, C.S., Perra, O., and Sharp, D. (2010). Mothers' antenatal depression and their children's antisocial outcomes. Child Development **81**: 149–65.

Hay, D.F., Pawlby, S., Waters, C.S., and Sharp, D. (2008). Antepartum and post partum depression: Different effects on different adolescent outcomes. Journal of Child Psychology and Psychiatry **49**: 1079–88.

Hay, D.F., Mundy, L., Roberts, S., *et al.* (2011). Known risk factors for violence predict 12-month-old infants' aggressiveness with peers. Psychological Science **22**: 1205–11.

Hay, D.F., Waters, C.S., Perra, O., *et al.* (in press) Precursors to aggression are evident by six months of age. Developmental Science.

Heron, J., O'Connor, T.G., Evans, J., Golding, J., and Glover, V. (2004). The course of anxiety and depression through pregnancy and the postpartum in a community sample. Journal of Affective Disorders **80**: 65–73.

Hobfoll, S.E., Ritter, C., Lavin, J., Hulsizer, M.R., and Cameron, R.P. (1995). Depression prevalence and incidence among inner-city pregnant and postpartum women. Journal of Consulting and Clinical Psychology **63**: 445–53.

Holcomb, W.L.J., Stone, L.S., Lustman, P.J., Gavard, J.A., and Mostello, D.J. (1996). Screening for depression in pregnancy: Characteristics of the Beck Depression Inventory. Obstetrics and Gynecology **88**(6): 1021–25.

Hudson, D.B., Elak, S. M., and Campbell-Grossman, C. (2000). Depression, self-esteem, loneliness, and social support in adolescent mothers participating in the New Mothers' Network. Adolescence **35**: 443–53.

Huizink, A.C., Robles de Medina, P.R., Mulder, E.J.H., Visser, G.H.A., and Buitelaar, J.K. (2002). Psychological measures of prenatal stress as predictor of infant temperament. Journal of the American Academy of Child and Adolescent Psychiatry **41**: 1078–85.

Huizink, A.C., Robles de Medina, P.G., Mulder, E.J.H., Visser, G.H.A., and Buitelaar, J.K. (2003). Stress during pregnancy is associated with developmental outcome in infancy. Journal of Child Psychology and Psychiatry **44**: 810–18.

Jaffee, S.R., Caspi, A., Moffitt, T.E., Belsky, J., and Silva, P. (2001). Why are children born to adolescent mothers at risk for adverse outcomes in young adulthood? Results from a 20- year longitudinal study. Development and Psychopathology **13**: 377–97.

Kessler, R.C., Berglund, P., Demler, O., Jin, R., Merikangas, K.R., and Walters, E.E. (2005). Lifetime prevalence and age-of-onset distributions of DSM-IV disorders in the National Comorbidity Survey Replication. Archives of General Psychiatry **62**(6): 593–602.

Kiernan, K.E. (1997). Becoming a young parent: A longitudinal study of associated factors. British Journal of Sociology **48**: 406–28.

Kirchengast, S. and Hartmann, B. (2003). Impact of maternal age and maternal somatic characteristics on newborn size. American Journal of Human Biology **15**: 220–8.

Kumar, R. and Robson, K.M. (1984). A prospective study of emotional disorders in childbearing women. British Journal of Psychiatry **144**: 35–47.

Lamb, M. E., Hopps, K., and Elster, A. B. (1987). Strange situation behavior of infants with adolescent mothers. Infant Behavior and Development **10**: 39–48.

Lanzi, R.G., Bert, S.C., and Jacobs, B.K. (2009). Depression among a sample of first-time adolescent and adult mothers. Journal of Child and Adolescent Psychiatric Nursing **22**(4): 194–202.

Leadbeater, B., Bishop, S.J., and Raver, C.C. (1996). Quality of mother-toddler interactions, maternal depressive symptoms, and behaviour problems in preschoolers of adolescent mothers. Developmental Psychology **32**: 280–8.

Leadbeater, B.J.R., and Linares, O. (1992). Depressive symptoms and neglect in Puerto Rican adolescent mothers in the first three years post partum. Development and Psychopathology **4**: 451–68.

Maki, P., Veijula, J., Rasanen, P., *et al.* (2003). Criminality in the offspring of antenatally depressed mothers: A 33-year follow-up of the Northern Finland 1966 Birth Cohort. Journal of Affective Disorders **74**: 273–8.

Manlove, J. (1997). Early motherhood in an intergenerational perspective: The experiences of a British cohort. Journal of Marriage and the Family **59**: 263–79.

Martin, J.A., Kochanek, K.D., Strobino, D.M., Guyer, B., and MacDorman, M.F. (2005). Annual summary of vital statistics—2003. Pediatrics **115**: 619–34.

Maughan, B. and Lindelow, M. (1997). Secular change in psychosocial risks: The case of teenage motherhood. Psychological Medicine **27**: 1129–44.

Miller, C.L., Miceli, P.J., Whitman, T.L., and Borkowski, J.G. (1996). Cognitive readiness to parent and intellectual-emotional development in children of adolescent mothers. Developmental Psychology **32**: 533–541.

Marcus, S.M., Flynn, H.A., Blow, F.C., and Barry, K.L. (2003). Depressive symptoms among pregnant women screened in obstetrics settings. Journal of Women's Health **12**: 373–80.

Mirowsky, J. (2002). Parenthood and health: The pivotal and optimal age at first birth. Social Forces **81**: 315–349.

Moore, K.A. and Snyder, N.O. (1991). Cognitive attainment among firstborn children of adolescent mothers. American Sociological Review **56**: 612–624.

Moffitt, T. E., and the E-Risk Study Team. (2002). Teen-aged mothers in contemporary Britain. Journal of Child Psychology and Psychiatry **43**: 727–42.

Murray, L. (1992). The impact of postnatal depression on infant development. Journal of Child Psychology and Psychiatry **33**: 543–61.

Murray, L., and Cooper, P. (1997). Postpartum depression and child development. New York, NY, Guilford Press.

Murray, D. and Cox. L. (1990). Screening for depression during pregnancy with the Edinburgh Postnatal Depression Scale (EPDS). Journal of Infant and Reproductive Psychology **8**: 99–107.

Murray, L., Kempton, C., Woolgar, M., and Hooper, R. (1993). Depresses mother's speech to their infants and its relation to infant gender and cognitive development. Journal of Child Psychology and Psychiatry **34**: 1083–101.

Murray, L., Sinclair, D., Cooper, P.J., Ducournau, P.,Turner, P., and Stein, A. (1999). The socioemotional development of 5-year old children of postnatally depressed mothers. Journal of Child Psychology and Psychiatry and Allied Disciplines **40**: 1259–71.

Nonacs, R. and Cohen, L.S. (2002). Depression during pregnancy: Diagnosis and treatment options. Journal of Clinical Psychiatry **63**: 24–30.

O'Connor, T.G., Heron, J., Golding, J., Beveridge, M., and Glover, V. (2002). Maternal antenatal anxiety and children's behaviour/emotional problems at 4 years. British Journal of Psychiatry **180**: 502–508.

O'Hara, M., Zekoski, E., Phillips, L., and Wright, E. (1990). Controlled prospective study of postpartum mood disorders: Comparison of childbearing and non-childbearing women. Journal of Abnormal Psychology **99**: 3–15.

O'Hara, M. (1997). The nature of postpartum depressive disorders. In Postpartum depression and child development, L. Murray, and P.J. Cooper, editors (3–34). London, Guilford Press.

O'Keane V. (2006). Mood disorder during pregnancy: Aetiology and management. In Psychiatric disorders and pregnancy V. O'Keane, M. Marsh, and G. Seneviratne, editors. London, Taylor and Francis, pp. 69–105.

Office of National Statistics (2007). Birth statistics. Review of the registrar general on births and patterns of family building in England and Wales, 2005. London, Office of National Statistics.

Office of National Statistics (2010). Social Trends 40, London, The Stationery Office.

Office of National Statistics (2012). Conceptions in England and Wales 2010. Statistical Bulletin. London, Office of National Statistics.

Pardo, R.A., Nazer, J., and Cifuentes, L. (2003). Prevalence of congenital malformations at birth among teenage mothers. Revista Medica De Chile **131**(10): 1165–72.

Pawlby, S., Hay, D.F., Sharp, D.S., Waters, C.S., and O'Keane, V. (2009). Antenatal depression predicts depression in adolescent offspring: prospective longitudinal community-based study. Journal of Affective Disorders **113**: 236–43.

Pevalin, D. (2003). Outcomes in childhood and adulthood by mother's age at birth: Evidence from the 1970 British Cohort Study. Working paper 2003–31, ISER, University of Essex, Colchester.

Pomerleau, A., Scuccimarri, C., and Malcuit, G. (2003). Mother-infant behavioural interactions in teenage and adult mothers during the first six months postpartum: Relations with infant development. Infant Mental Health Journal **24**(5): 495–509.

Prodromidis, M., Abrams, S., Field, T., Scafidi, F., and Rahdert, E. (1994). Psychosocial stressors among depressed adolescent mothers. Adolescence **29**: 331–343.

Quinlivan, J,A., Tan, L,H., Steele, A., and Black, K. (2004). Impact of demographic factors, early family relationships and depressive symtomatology in teenage pregnancy. Australian and New Zealand Journal of Psychiatry **38**: 197–203.

Ramos-Marcuse, F., Oberlander, S.E., Papas, M.A., et al. (2010). Stability of maternal depressive symptoms among urban, low-income, African American adolescent mothers. Journal of Affective Disorders **122**: 68–75.

Rich-Edwards, J.W., Kleinman, K., Abrams, A. et al. (2005). Sociodemographic predictors of antenatal and postpartum depressive symptoms among women in a medical group practice. Journal of Epidemiology and Community Health **60**: 221–227.

Rodgers, M.M., Peoples-Sheps, M.D., and Suchindran, C. (1996). Impact of a social support program on teenage prenatal care use and pregnancy outcomes. Journal of Adolescent Health **19**: 132–140.

Rubertsson, C., Wickberg, B., Gustavsson, P. and Radestad, I. (2005). Depressive symptoms in early pregnancy, two months and one year postpartum: prevalence and psychosocial risk factors in a national Swedish sample. Archives of Women's Mental Health **8**: 97–104.

Secco, M. L., Profit, S., Kennedy, E., Walsh, A., Letourneau, N., and Stewart, M. (2007). Factors affecting postpartum depressive symptoms of adolescent mothers. JOGNN **36**: 47–54.

Sharp, D., Hay, D.F., Pawlby, S., et al. (1995). The impact of postnatal depression on boys' intellectual development. Journal of Child Psychology and Psychiatry and Allied Disciplines **36**: 1315–36.

Shaw, M., Lawlor, D.A., and Najman, J.M. (2006). Teenage children of teenage mothers: Psychological, behavioural and health outcomes from an Australian prospective longitudinal study. Social Science and Medicine **62**: 2526–39.

Schmidt, M.R., Wiemann, C.M., Rickert, V.I., and O'Brian-Smith, E. (2006). Moderate to severe depressive symptoms among adolescent mothers followed four years postpartum. Journal of Adolescent Health **38**: 712–18.

Social Exclusion Unit (1999). Teenage pregnancy. Report to the Prime Minister. London, HMSO.

Sommer, K.S., Whitman, T.L., Borkowski, J.G., et al. (2000). Prenatal maternal predictors of cognitive and emotional delays in children of adolescent mothers. Journal of Adolescence **35**: 87–112.

Spieker, S.J., and Bensley, L. (1994). Roles of living arrangements and grandmother social support in adolescent mothering and infant attachment. Developmental Psychology **30**: 102–11.

Stevens-Simon, C., Nelligan, D., and Kelly, L. (2001). Adolescents at risk for mistreating their children part II: A home and clinic based prevention program. Child Abuse and Neglect **25**: 753–769.

Troutman, B.R. and Cutrona, C. E (1990). Non-psychotic postpartum depression among adolescent mothers. Journal of Abnormal Psychology **99**: 69–78.

Ventura, S., Martin, J.A., Curtain, S.C., Menacker, F., and Hamilton, B.E. (2001). Births: Final data for 1999. National Vital Statistics Reports, **49**: 1–99.

Waters, C.S. (2009). Young motherhood, maternal psychopathology and children's cognitive, behavioural and emotional development. Unpublished Doctoral Thesis. Cardiff, Cardiff University.

Waters, C.S., Hay, D.F., van Goozen, S., and Pawlby, S. (under review). Outcomes for children born to young mothers and their exposure to adverse antenatal and postnatal experiences.

Woodward, L.J., Fergusson, D.M., and Horwood, J. (2006). Gender differences in the transition to early parenthood. Development and Psychopathology **18**: 275–94.

Chapter 15

Childhood and adolescent mental health as developmental predictors of the early caregiving of teenage mothers

Alison E. Hipwell

Introduction

I first met Channi 25 years ago when I applied for a Research Assistant position on the Mother-Baby Unit (MBU) at the Bethlem Royal Hospital. The research project was to improve the process of collecting data on infant functioning and mother–infant interactions among inpatient dyads on the MBU in order to evaluate better the real and potential risks to the infant. Channi had noticed that, soon after an admission, MBU staff often had a hunch about which mothers *could* demonstrate sensitive and responsive caregiving once their florid psychotic episode had improved, and which mothers were likely to have ongoing difficulties. He had developed the Bethlem Mother-Infant Interaction Scale for completion by nurses on the unit to capture and quantify their observations in a more systematic manner. Although my primary responsibility was to test the psychometric properties of the scale, Channi encouraged my nascent interests in the transactional relationships between maternal postpartum psychopathology and infant development. During the next 5 years and beyond, I benefited greatly from his intellectual guidance and mentorship, his exceptional generosity and his visionary thinking. These highly formative experiences have contributed to my sustained interest in early prediction of both maternal caregiving and perinatal psychopathology. In this chapter, I describe results from a prospective study of adolescent mothers that combine both of these elements.

Teenage caregiving

A glance at the literature gives a very strong impression that adolescent mothers and their infants are a highly vulnerable group of dyads. Much has been written about adolescent motherhood as a life transition that is not yet normative, requiring teenagers to cope with the developmental demands of adolescence simultaneously with the new and, not insignificant, challenges of pregnancy and motherhood. Research has shown that adolescence is a period in life that is characterized by mood volatility (Brent and Birmaher 2002;

Nolen-Hoeksema and Girgus 1994) as well as vulnerability for onset and escalation of a wide range of mental health problems, including depression (Lewinsohn et al. 1993), and behaviour problems (Steinberg et al. 2006). Combining this developmental window of risk for psychopathology with the possibility that adolescent mothers may be emotionally and practically unprepared to deal with their infant's capacities and needs, certainly gives cause for concern.

Being born to an adolescent mother often bodes ill for the offspring (Conger et al. 1994). Compared to the offspring of older mothers, infants of adolescent mothers tend to have lower birth weight (Chen et al. 2007; Gilbert et al. 2004), are at greater risk for abuse and neglect (Coley and Chase-Lansdale 1998; Logsdon et al. 2008; Long 2009), and are more likely to show mental health problems (Felice et al. 1999; Fergusson and Woodward 1999), and cognitive and academic deficits later in life (Cornelius et al. 2009; Dahinten et al. 2007). In addition, research has shown that the offspring of adolescent mothers are more susceptible than the children of older mothers to develop aggressive and antisocial behaviour in adolescence, and are more likely to have contact with the criminal justice system as juveniles and/or as adults (Conseur et al. 1997; Shaw et al. 2006).

When comparisons have been made between teenage and adult mothers, studies have typically shown that the caregiving quality of teenage mothers is less optimal. Teenage mothers are reportedly less likely to provide the kinds of supportive and sensitive parenting that fosters social and emotional competence in their infant (Berlin et al. 2002). As a group, teen mothers also tend to display more restrictive, punitive, and impatient behaviours with their infants (Barratt and Roach 1995), make fewer comments about the infant's mental state (Demers et al. 2010), and show a more blunted physiological response to infant cries (Giardino et al. 2008). There is, however, considerable variability in the functioning of teenage mothers; a fact that is often overlooked (East and Felice 1996; Oxford et al. 2006). Thus, for some adolescents early parenting may be normative, expected, and planned, and the experience of becoming a mother may be fulfilling and positively transforming (Barratt et al. 1996; Carey et al. 1998; Lesser et al. 1999). Although research examining putative moderators of teenage caregiving is accumulating, more work in this area is clearly warranted.

Selection effects for teenage pregnancy: implications for caregiving

It is clear that adolescent parenthood is not randomly distributed across the population, and that a complex set of characteristics operate to 'select' which individuals become parents during this developmental period. There is, for example, good evidence that adolescent parenthood is associated with particular demographic and psychosocial circumstances that may impact adolescent parenting more than some capacity or ability inherent to being a teenager (Darroch 2001; Felice et al. 1999; Furstenberg 2003). Thus, compared with their non-childbearing peers, pregnant teenagers are more likely to be urban-living, to be raised in poverty and in a single parent household, and to be of minority race (Al-Sahab et al.

2012; Oxford 2010; Wahn et al. 2005). Such factors are, themselves, associated with more limited financial, social, and educational resources and parenting stress. Consistent with this notion, Hollander (1995) demonstrated that the health problems of infants of teenage mothers reflected the mothers' economic disadvantage, and not an inability of young mothers to care for their children. Adolescent mothers are also more likely to have experienced a poor quality of relationship with their own parents, including exposure to harsh or inconsistent discipline, and low familial support compared with adult mothers (Franklin et al., 2004; Jaffee et al., 2001; Manlove 1997; Talashek et al., 2006). From a social learning perspective, such experiences are likely to make the task of providing sensitive caregiving especially challenging.

The caregiving abilities of adolescent mothers may also be 'selected' by virtue of mental health factors that increase the likelihood of teenage childbearing. For example, conduct disordered girls often develop problems within intimate relationships (Fontaine et al. 2009) and may be three to five times more likely than non-conduct disordered girls to become pregnant as teenagers (Bardone et al. 1998; Bradshaw et al. 2010; Gaudie et al. 2010; Woodward and Fergusson 1999). Thus, in a clinic sample of 83 preadolescent females, Kovacs and colleagues (1994) reported that approximately 55% of girls with conduct disorder (CD) later became pregnant during adolescence compared with only 12% of girls with other psychiatric diagnoses. However, it remains unclear whether there is a specific association between early pregnancy and CD (beyond a link with the CD symptom of early sexual promiscuity), or whether this association reflects aspects of a disadvantaged family background and/or general involvement in risky behaviours (Bardone et al. 1998; Woodward and Fergusson 1999). More recently, data have shown that even after controlling for sociodemographic and family variables, CD symptom severity was a unique predictor of pregnancy by 19 years (Pedersen and Mastekaasa 2011). The results of this study and others (e.g. Miller-Johnson et al. 1999) however, suggest that the strength of the association between CD symptoms and likelihood of teenage pregnancy dissipates with increasing age across the adolescent period.

Evidence that depression in childhood or adolescence heightens risk for early pregnancy is more mixed. It has been postulated that depressed girls may engage in risky sexual behaviour to seek intimacy or reduce social isolation (Kovacs et al. 1994). Although some empirical studies show that psychological distress (DiClemente et al. 2001), low self-esteem (Spencer et al. 2002), and depressive symptoms (Fergusson and Woodward 2002) predict early sexual behaviours and pregnancy, others report no relationship between depressed mood and early onset sexual intercourse (Whitbeck et al. 1993).

Prevalence of postnatal depression among teenage mothers

Despite the fact that the psychosocial stressors of parenting may be especially salient for teenage mothers, the prevalence of postnatal psychopathology for this group of females has yet to be established. Compared with a prevalence rate of about 13% in adult women (O'Hara and Swain 1996), research on adolescent samples has found rates of non-psychotic depression to range widely from 20% to 67%, depending on the measures, the timing, and the impairment definitions used (Colletta 1983; Deal and Holt 1998; Figueiredo et al. 2007; Gaynes et al. 2005; Hudson et al. 2000; Logsdon et al.2005; Schmidt et al. 2006). Troutman and Cutrona (1990) reported on a study that is noteworthy by its use of a structured diagnostic interview to assess major and minor depressive disorder in 128 adolescent mothers at 6 weeks postpartum and a matched control group of 114 non-childbearing adolescents. The results revealed that 6% of the adolescent mothers met diagnostic criteria for major depression and 20% for minor depression, and there were no differences in prevalence from the non-childbearing group. Although this study was one of the first to use a non-childbearing, age- and SES-matched, control group of adolescents, these girls were mostly nominated friends of the childbearing group, and therefore some selection bias may have been introduced. Nevertheless, other investigators have also noted low rates of mental health problems among adolescent mothers (Oxford et al. 2006) indicating that further investigation of the factors differentiating high and low risk is needed.

Homotypic and heterotypic continuities in psychopathology across the perinatal period

Understanding the role of selection effects in the origins, nature and developmental course of postpartum psychopathology among teenage mothers is critical for the development of effective and tailored treatment and prevention programmes. Although a certain degree of continuity in mental health problems over the life course is likely, virtually nothing is known about the risk from symptoms of psychopathology in childhood or early adolescence on postnatal symptomatology in teenagers. It is therefore not known whether symptoms persist or recur in the postnatal period (homotypic continuity), or whether symptoms become expressed in new ways at this time (heterotypic continuity). This information is lacking due to the dearth of longitudinal studies that collect data prior to pregnancy. Prospective studies are essential for this work given that retrospective recall in adulthood of prior episodes of psychopathology and major adverse experiences in childhood and adolescence, are known to be hampered by high rates of false negatives and substantial inaccuracies and biases (Hardt and Rutter 2004; Henry et al. 1994).

In adult samples, there is some support for homotypic continuity in depressive symptomatology. Although there are few large-scale prospective studies documenting mental health prior to conception among adult women, the weight of evidence from retrospective reports suggests that for about one third to one half of recently delivered women, postnatal depression constitutes an exacerbation or recurrence of an earlier episode of depressive illness (e.g. Gotlib et al. 1991; Marcus et al. 2003; Stowe et al. 2005). Other (retrospective) reports have shown that postnatal 'relapse' of depression is associated with an elevated risk for future non-postpartum episodes compared with postnatal depression occurring *de novo* (Cooper and Murray 1995). This information then is critical for targeted prevention efforts.

Little research has examined the impact of childbirth on continuities and discontinuities in conduct problems among teenage girls. Serbin et al. (1998) suggested that rates of antisocial behaviour decrease following delivery simply because the maternal role limits the opportunities to engage in delinquency outside the home. Although this may be the case for certain forms of antisocial behaviour such as property crime, other characteristics such as interpersonal aggression may become exacerbated by the demands of caring for a young infant. The possibility of heterotypic continuity, however, should not be overlooked and pre-pregnancy conduct problems may give rise to other forms of psychopathology in the postnatal period. Thus data from non-childbearing community samples of adolescents shows that CD often precedes or co-occurs with the development of depression (e.g. Hipwell et al. 2011; Moffitt et al. 2001; Wolff and Ollendick 2006), and that negative life events associated with CD often mediate this link (Rowe et al. 2006). Furthermore, the prognosis for adolescents with these conditions, whether occurring concurrently or consecutively, tends to be poor (e.g. Ezpeleta et al. 2006; Marmorstein and Iacono 2001).

Impact of postnatal psychopathology on teenage caregiving

Much research with adult samples has shown that maternal postpartum psychopathology, primarily depression, is associated with negative parenting practices that range from low levels of responsivity and engagement, to high levels of intrusive and controlling behaviours towards the infant (e.g. Field 2010). Studies have also shown that there may be lasting adverse effects on the child's development that are evident long after postnatal symptoms have remitted (e.g. Hay et al. 2003; Stein et al., 1991). However, studies examining the effects of postpartum depression have often intentionally excluded teenage mothers, and little is known about the impact of postpartum disorders over and above 'adolescent-specific' difficulties with the tasks of parenting. Based on the adult literature, however, it is likely that postpartum depression would increase the likelihood of negative parenting practices among teenage mothers. This notion is supported by a small observational study of 21 mother-infant dyads in an adolescent hospital clinic (Cassidy et al. 1996). The mothers were 15 to 20 years old and their infants ranged in age from 3 to 24 months. The severity of the mothers' concurrent depressive symptoms was associated with maternal over-control and infant difficulty. In contrast, the severity of the mother's antisocial history (retrospectively reported) was associated with a lack of maternal responsivity and infant passivity. These results suggested that concurrent depression and antisocial history may have different effects on the quality of mother–infant interactions. These provocative findings clearly demand further investigation and replication.

The current study

Accumulating evidence from cross-sectional and retrospective studies suggests that both 'selection effects' (e.g. disadvantage or disposition that exists prior to adolescent pregnancy), and 'elicitation effects' (e.g. stress from social adversity associated with young motherhood) are likely to have an impact on the quality of caregiving of teenage mothers. The current study presents a unique opportunity to examine some of these relationships within a developmental context. Using data gathered in a subsample of teenage mothers who had been participating in a large-scale prospective study since mid-childhood, the following hypotheses were tested:

1 Teenage mothers, drawn from a representative community sample of adolescents, will be characterized by elevated depression and conduct problems in the postnatal period compared with an age-matched group of non-childbearing peers. Severity of postnatal psychopathology and deficits in the quality of mother-infant interaction will be greater among younger than older adolescents.

2 Trajectories of depression and conduct disorder symptomatology across childhood and adolescence will predict quality of early caregiving and postnatal adjustment after controlling for maternal age at delivery.

The Pittsburgh Girls Study

The Pittsburgh Girls Study (PGS) is an ongoing multiple cohort, longitudinal study examining the development of CD and depression and their comorbid conditions in a community sample of 2,451 inner-city African American and European American girls. The study receives funding from the National Institute of Mental Health (MH056630), National Institute of Drug Abuse (DA012237), the Falk Fund, and FISA. The PGS began in 1998 with a 1-year preparatory phase followed by an enumeration of 103,238 Pittsburgh households in order to locate girls ages 5, 6, 7, and 8 years who, with their parent, could be enrolled into four age cohorts. For the enumeration, a housing database for the City of Pittsburgh was compiled using 911 and post-office databases. Many addresses were entered by hand. The city neighbourhoods were then divided in 23 'disadvantaged' (>25% of families living in poverty) and 66 'non-disadvantaged' neighbourhoods using information on household poverty from the 1990 Census. The goal was to conduct 100% enumeration of the households in the disadvantaged neighbourhoods, and 50% of the remainder over a 1-year period, in order to increase the prevalence of CD in the sample. This process elicited 3,241 5- to 8-year old girls, representing 83.7% of the girls identified by the US Census in 2000. No difference was revealed in the rates of success in identifying girls according to the type of neighbourhood. Of 2,876 girls who were age-eligible and who could also be located subsequently, 2,451 (85%) agreed to participate in the longitudinal study. The final sample consisted of four age cohorts initially aged 5 ($N = 588$), 6 ($N = 630$), 7 ($N = 611$), and 8 ($N = 622$) years (see Hipwell et al. 2002; Keenan et al. 2010 for further details). The 13th annual data collection wave was completed in summer 2013. Thus, in this accelerated longitudinal design completed assessments span the age period from early childhood to early adulthood (age 5 through 20).

Approximately half of the PGS sample is African American (52.5%), 40.7% is European American, and most of the remaining girls are of mixed ethnicity. When weights are applied to correct for the over-sampling of disadvantaged neighbourhoods, the racial distribution is similar to that reported in the 2000 Census for girls aged 5–8. Across the cohorts, 56% to 61% of the parents were cohabiting in wave 1, about 47% of the parents had completed 12 or fewer years of education, and 25% of the sample lived in poverty with a yearly income of less than $15,000. Retention of the original sample has been very high: over the course of the study, the average participation rate has been 91%.

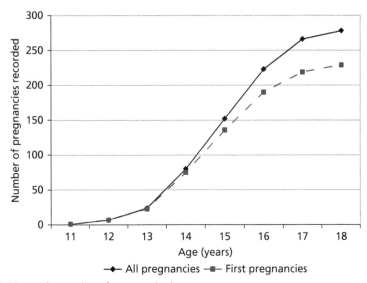

Fig. 15.1 PGS sample: number of pregnancies by age.

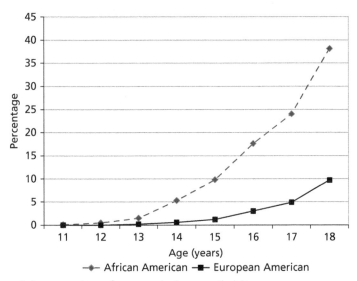

Fig. 15.2 Cumulative percentage of pregnancies by race ethnicity.

Pregnancies, and the outcome of any pregnancies, have been documented as part of the annual PGS face-to-face home interviews. By PGS wave 11, 296 pregnancies among girls aged between 12 and 19 years had been reported by the girl participant and/or her primary caregiver. Twenty-nine girls had had two pregnancies during this time, nine reported three pregnancies, and two girls reported four pregnancies. The cumulative number of PGS pregnancies is shown in Figure 15.1. A larger proportion of the pregnancies were reported among African American than European American girls (14.8% and 3.0% respectively, $\chi2[1] = 92.92$, $p < 0.001$, see Figure 15.2).

Teen Mother sample

At the time of writing, 94 adolescent mothers were identified as being eligible for recruitment into the Teen Mother sub-study. Among these mother–infant pairs, 70 dyads were identified in time for a research visit at around 4 months postpartum (81.9%) and 7 were closer to 1 year postpartum. In order to focus on predictors of early caregiving, this latter group of mothers and infants were excluded from the current analyses. In addition, one adolescent refused participation (.8%), and we were unable to contact or schedule a further 16 potential participants (17%).

The sample of 70 mothers ranged in age from 12 to 19 years, with a mean age of 16 years (SD = 1.4). The majority of the mothers were African American (N = 60, 85%), six (9%) were European American, and four teenagers (6%) self-identified as multiracial. The majority of the young mothers (59%) were raised in household poverty and all were primiparous. Approximately half of the infants were male (58%), and the mean infant age was 4.9 months (SD = 1.7, range = 2.5–9.2).

Procedure and measures

The adolescent mothers and their infants were invited to visit the research laboratory at 4 months postpartum. Consent was obtained from the teen mother's guardian if the adolescent was younger than 18 years, and written consent for the infant's participation was obtained from the teenage mother herself.

Separate face-to-face interviews were administered with the young mother and her guardian and included assessment of psychopathology (e.g. depression, conduct disorder), parenting behaviours, and infant factors. The mother and her infant were also filmed during infant measurement and weighing, a 2-minute period of face-to-face warm-up, followed by toy play (3 minutes), the still face paradigm (Tronick et al. 1978), and a 3-minute recovery period.

Severity of postnatal depression was assessed using the Edinburgh Postnatal Depression Scale (EPDS; Cox et al. 1987). This widely used 10-item measure assesses the severity of depressed mood, anhedonia, guilt, anxiety, and suicidal ideation within the past 7 days. Items are rated on 4-point scales (e.g. 0 = not at all to 3 = most of the time). The scale has been shown to be internally consistent, and has high levels of sensitivity (68–95%) and specificity (79–96%) as compared to a psychiatric diagnosis of major depression, using a cut-off score of 12 (Cox et al. 1987; Murray and Carothers 1990).

Parenting stress was assessed using the 12-item parental distress/role-strain subscale of the Parenting Stress Index (PSI, Abidin et al. 2006). This subscale has good psychometric properties (Abidin et al. 1992) and has been widely used with minority and teenage populations.

Observations of mother–infant interaction: Global ratings of observed infant and maternal behaviour during the warm-up period were made using behaviourally anchored rating scales adapted from the Chicago Baby Project (Keenan 2003). The infant rating scales comprised positive affect, negative affect, and orientation to the mother, each scored on

5-point likert scales (1 = none to 5 = often/a lot). High ratings of positive and negative affect reflected frequent displays of each that were intense, heightened, and prolonged. High ratings of infant orientation to mother were given when the infant made frequent and prolonged eye contact with mother, and appeared attuned and responsive to the mother's bids.

Five dimensions of maternal behaviour (hostility, warmth, involvement, intrusiveness, and maternal attributions of infant agency and intent) were scored on 4-point behaviourally anchored scales (1 = none to 4 = often/a lot). Maternal hostility was defined as the emotional expression of anger, irritation, or impatience toward the child. Examples of maternal warmth and positive affect included expressions conveying pride, pleasure, or empathy for the child, and instances of encouraging or supportive affect. Maternal involvement was indexed by consistent attempts to communicate with the child while also maintaining eye contact. Ratings of maternal intrusiveness included frequent efforts to physically manipulate or restrict the baby, placing face or hands close to the infant's face, or loud or high-pitched talking, vocalizing or laughing. Finally, high levels of maternal attributions were demonstrated by the frequency of comments that attributed skills, intentionality and abilities to the baby, or that indicated the mother's belief that the baby could play an active role in, have an impact on, the environment (e.g. 'Are you talking to me?', 'Do you think that is funny?'). Inter-rater reliability, assessed using Intra-Class Correlation coefficients between raters blind to all other information about the dyads, was greater than .90 for all the rating scales.

Conduct problems and depressive symptomatology were assessed from mid-childhood through adolescence using the Child Symptom Inventory (CSI-4) transitioning into the Adolescent Symptom Inventory (ASI-4; Gadow and Sprafkin1994/1997) from age 13 onwards. The CSI-4/ASI-4 is a DSM-IV-based (American Psychiatric Association 1994) checklist that assesses the severity of 13 clinical symptoms of Conduct Disorder and 11 symptoms of depression using 4-point rating scales (1 = never to 4 = very often). The measure has excellent psychometric properties and has demonstrated good sensitivity and specificity in distinguishing youth with clinical diagnoses from healthy controls (Gadow and Sprafkin1994/1997).

Results

Rates of postnatal psychopathology among teenage mothers

The majority of girls reported no symptoms of either CD or depression at the postpartum visit. Thus, 66.2% of adolescent mothers reported no CD symptoms, and 79.4% reported no depressive symptomatology. However, 7.3% of girls reported two or more symptoms of CD in the postnatal period, a threshold that has been argued as appropriate for DSM-IV criterion for girls (Cote et al. 2001; Zoccolillo et al. 1996). This rate of estimated diagnosis is somewhat higher than CD prevalence in non-childbearing samples of adolescent girls (1.8% to 4.1%; Feehan et al. 1994; Fergusson et al. 1993; Offord et al., 1987). There was a trend for CD severity scores to decrease with age ($r = -0.21$, $p = 0.07$), but the effect did not reach significance.

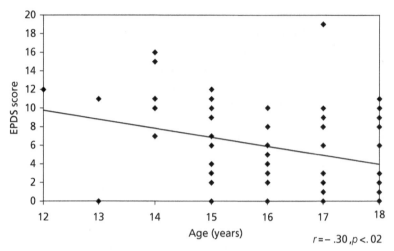

Fig. 15.3 EPDS score is negatively related to maternal age.

This group of adolescent mothers reported few DSM-IV symptoms of depression in the postpartum period: 13.2% reported one symptom, 2.9% reported two and three symptoms, and 1.5% individuals met diagnostic criteria for major depressive disorder. Scores on the EPDS (Cox et al. 1987) were also not especially high, with 8.8% obtaining a score of 12 and higher (indicative of probable depression). Examination of these scores by maternal age revealed a moderate negative association ($r = -0.30$, $p < 0.02$, see Figure 15.3). Thus with increasing age, severity of postnatal depressed mood decreased in this sample. In particular, among the mothers aged 12–15 years ($N = 24$), almost 21% scored in the 'probable depression' range compared with 2% of the 16–19-year-olds ($N = 46$).

Quality of mother–infant interaction by adolescent age

To examine whether quality of mother–infant interaction was similarly distinguished along this age dichotomy, mean scores on the global ratings of infant and maternal warm-up behaviour were compared for the same two age groups: 15 years or younger vs. 16 years or older. The results of ANOVA revealed that the infants of younger mothers showed lower levels of positive affect during the 2-minute warm-up period (mean = 2.29, SD = 1.30 for 12–15-year-olds, and mean = 2.91, SD = 1.18 for 16–18-year-olds, $F[1,68] = 4.2$, $p < 0.05$). The younger group of mothers showed higher levels of intrusive behaviour compared with the older group (mean = 2.13, SD = 1.08, and mean = 1.63, SD = 0.92 respectively, $F[1,68] = 4.9$, $p < 0.05$). These younger mothers were also less likely to attribute intentionality or agency to their baby (mean = 2.00, SD = 0.83 for 12–15-year-olds, and mean = 2.53, SD = 1.00 for 16–18-year-olds, $F[1,68] = 3.98$, $p < 0.05$). No group differences were revealed on the remaining dimensions of infant negative affect, orientation to mother, maternal hostility, warmth or involvement.

The eight dimensions of mother–infant interaction were then reduced using principal components analysis. Following varimax rotation, the results revealed three components with eigenvalues greater than 1.0. The factor loadings of all items were greater than 0.60. The first component comprised infant positive affect, maternal warmth, and maternal involvement, was labelled 'Positive involvement' and explained 33.4% of the variance. The second component ('Negative-dismissing') consisted of infant negative affect, maternal hostility, and maternal attributions (reversed scale) and described an additional 16.9% of the variance in scores. Finally, a component labelled 'Intrusive-withdrawn' accounted for 13.2% variance, and comprised low levels of infant orientation to the mother and high maternal intrusiveness.

A series of hierarchical linear regression analyses was then conducted to examine the predictive utility of maternal age, the severity of EPDS scores and the interaction between age and EPDS severity on the quality of mother-infant interaction after controlling for sociodemographic variables (poverty, minority race, and living in a single parent household) and parenting stress. In the first model with Positive involvement as the dependent variable, the results showed significant effects of both maternal age and postnatal depression severity. Thus, younger adolescent mothers ($\beta 1 = -0.27$, $t = 1.99$, $p < 0.05$), plus adolescent mothers reporting depressed mood in the postnatal period ($\beta = 0.27$, $t = 2.01$, $p < 0.05$) showed less positive involvement after parenting stress and sociodemographic covariates were taken into account. The interaction between maternal age and EPDS score, however, did not add anything further to the model. Neither maternal age nor depressed mood, or the interaction between them, predicted the Negative-dismissive and Intrusive-withdrawn components after controlling for sociodemographic covariates and parenting stress.

Depression and CD across childhood and adolescence as developmental predictors of mother–infant interactions

Latent class and growth mixture modelling analyses were conducted to examine developmental trajectories of depression and CD severity from age 5–14 years to quality of observed maternal caregiving. Trajectories of data from the entire PGS sample were modelled using Mplus 5.2 (Muthen and Muthen 2008). This analytic approach allows estimation of trajectory shapes as random rather than fixed effects, thus modelling individual variation in trajectory shape within each latent class. For each of these models, a single-class latent growth curve model was specified first and then a series of models were tested with reference to the Bayes Information Criterion (Schwartz 1978), the likelihood ratio test statistic, the bootstrap likelihood ratio test, and the entropy measure (e.g. Ramaswamy et al. 1993). For depression severity, a four group quadratic growth solution best fitted the data between ages 5 and 14 years. The trajectories groups comprised 'high' (4%), 'low' (68.1%), 'increasing' (15.4%), and 'decreasing' (12.6%). For conduct problems, a three group solution (low = 92.2%, increasing = 4.1% and decreasing = 3.7%) best fitted the data.

Trajectory class membership was then determined for the 70 teenage mothers included in the current sample. Of the depression trajectories, 5 girls were classified in the 'high' group (7.1%), 35 in the 'low' group (50%), 19 in the 'increasing' (27.1%), and 11 in the 'decreasing' (15.7%) groups. Due to their small number, the five girls in the 'high' trajectory group were combined with the 'increasing' group for the following analyses. Of the

CD severity trajectories, 60 girls (85.7%) were classified within the low CD group, and 10 (14.3%) showed increasing levels of conduct problems across childhood.

The previous hierarchical regression models were re-run to examine whether the developmental course of depression and CD across childhood and early adolescence added further prediction to the models. In the first set of these analyses, the three depression trajectory groups were entered, and in the second set, the low and increasing CD groups were entered as additional predictors.

In the case of positive involvement, there was a trend for the depression trajectory groups to explain additional variance after accounting for sociodemographic variables, maternal age, parenting stress, and postnatal mood ($\beta = -0.27$, $t = 1.81$, $p < 0.10$). In this model, low EPDS severity score remained a significant predictor ($\beta = -0.34$, $t = 2.19$, $p < 0.05$), but the effect of older maternal age became negligible. In contrast, the two CD trajectory groups did not significantly predict Positive involvement scores. In this model, severity of EPDS score remained a significant predictor ($\beta = -0.28$, $t = 1.91$, $p < 0.05$), but maternal age again became non-significant. Thus, although the trajectories of psychopathology across childhood and adolescence explained only a marginal amount of variance in Positive involvement, consideration of developmental change in psychopathology accounted for the previously obtained effects of maternal age. The results however also revealed that depressed mood in the postnatal period remained an important risk factor for reduced levels of positive involvement in the current sample.

The prior results of the regression analyses for the Negative-dismissing component were unchanged with the inclusion of the depression and CD trajectory groups. However, in the models predicting the Intrusive-withdrawn factor, the results revealed a unique significant effect of CD trajectory group ($\beta = 0.22$, $t = 1.62$, $p < 0.05$), despite the small sample size. Thus an increasing trajectory of CD severity between ages 5 and 14 years predicted higher levels of intrusive behaviour by the mother and reduced infant orientation to the mother during the warm-up interaction. None of the other variables, including EPDS score, were significantly associated with this aspect of the mother-infant interaction. These results are congruent with, and extend the findings obtained by Cassidy and colleagues (1996), which suggested that an antisocial history and concurrent depression may have differential effects on caregiving quality. The current results, however, suggest a trend for the course of depression across childhood and adolescence to adversely affect dyadic positive involvement over and above the effects of postnatal depressed mood. In contrast, increasing levels of CD prior to childbearing are associated with higher levels of intrusiveness by the mother and reduced maternal orientation by the infant, behaviours which were unaffected by postnatal depressed mood in the current sample.

Conclusions

The preliminary results presented here indicate that, *as a group*, teenage mothers are not at especially high risk for postnatal depression. However, age appears to be a critical factor and more than one in five of the youngest mothers in this group fell into the 'probably' depressed range of the EPDS. Very young adolescent mothers may be at increased risk because their circumstance is much less normative relative to their peers, but individual, family, school, and neighbourhood factors are likely to also play a role. The results of the current study further suggested that younger maternal age and low mood in the postnatal period are specific risk factors for reduced levels of positive involvement between the mother and her infant, but do not increase the likelihood of negative or intrusive engagement. This finding has implications for the design of interventions, and suggests that scant clinical resources may be best used to improve positive aspects of parenting, before focusing on ameliorating negative behaviours. Several effective parent-child interventions in other populations of high-risk dyads (e.g. Eyberg 1979; Webster-Stratton *et al.* 2001) take such an approach. In contrast, girls who show increasing levels of CD symptomatology during childhood and adolescence may need tailored interventions for reducing intrusive or hostile behaviours with their infant.

However, much further work is needed to understand the relative import of selection and elicitation effects of psychopathology on teenage caregiving. Cross-sectional and retrospective studies conducted to date suggest that these effects are likely to be highly relevant for postnatal functioning but prospective studies have been rare. The teen mother sub-study of the Pittsburgh Girls Study provides a unique opportunity to test these hypotheses with a broad range of mental health problems assessed over an extended developmental period. As the subsample increases in size, it will become possible to investigate whether the perinatal period is a time of risk (or in some cases, protection) for childbearing vs. demographically matched non-childbearing teenagers within the context of both prior and subsequent mental health. The design will also enable homotypic and heterotypic continuities in psychopathology to be examined, and developmentally specific risk and protective factors and moderators of postnatal adjustment to be identified, in order for the evident heterogeneity within this population to be better understood.

Efforts to identify the developmental and contextual factors that influence the caregiving of teenage mothers clearly face significant methodological challenges. Tackling these challenges, however, has the potential to fill critical gaps in knowledge with far-reaching benefits for the teenager, her baby and beyond, and are therefore well-worth pursuing.

References

Abidin, R., Flens, J.R., and Austin, W.G. (2006). The Parenting Stress Index Forensic uses of clinical assessment instruments Mahwah, NJ: Lawrence Erlbaum Associates Publishers, pp. 297–328.

Abidin, R. R., Jenkins, C. L., and McGaughey, M. C. (1992). The relationship of early family variables to children's subsequent behavioral adjustment. Journal of Clinical Child Psychology, 21(1), 60–69.

Al-Sahab, B., Heifetz, M., Tamim, H., Bohr, Y., and Connolly, J. (2012). Prevalence and characteristics of teen motherhood in Canada. Maternal and Child Health Journal 16(1): 228–34.

American Psychiatric Association (1994). Diagnostic and Statistical Manual of Mental Disorders (4th ed.). Washington, DC, American Psychiatric Association.

Bardone, A.M., Moffitt, T.E., Caspi, A., *et al.* (1998). Adult physical health outcomes of adolescent girls with conduct disorder, depression, and anxiety. Journal of the American Academy of Child and Adolescent Psychiatry 37(6): 594–601.

Barratt, M., and Roach, M. (1995). Early Interactive processes: Parenting by adolescent and adult single mothers. Infant Behavior and Development **18**(1): 97–109.

Barratt, M., Roach, M., Morgan, K., and Colbert, K. (1996). Adjustment to motherhood by single adolescents. Family Relations **45**: 209–15.

Berlin, L. J., Brady-Smith, C., and Brooks-Gunn, J. (2002). Links between childbearing age and observed maternal behaviors with 14-month-olds in the Early Head Start Research and Evaluation Project. Infant Mental Health Journal **23**(1–2): 104–29.

Bradshaw, C.P., Schaeffer, C.M., Petras, H., and Ialongo, N. (2010). Predicting negative life outcomes from early aggressive-disruptive behavior trajectories: gender differences in maladaptation across life domains. Journal of Youth and Adolescence **39**(8): 953–66.

Brent, D., and Birmaher, B. (2002). Adolescent depression. New England Journal of Medicine **347**(9): 667–671.

Carey, G., Ratliff, D., and Lyle, R.R. (1998). Resilient adolescent mothers: Ethnographaic interviews. Families, Systems, and Health **16**(4): 347–364.

Cassidy, B., Zoccolillo, M., and Hughes, S. (1996). Psychopathology in adolescent mothers and its effects on mother-infant interactions: a pilot study. Canadian Journal of Psychiatry **41**(6): 379–84.

Chen, X.-K., Wen, S.W., Fleming, N., Demissie, K., Rhoads, G.G., and Walker, M. (2007). Teenage pregnancy and adverse birth outcomes: a large population based retrospective cohort study. International Journal of Epidemiology **36**(2): 368–73.

Coley, R.L., and Chase-Lansdale, P.L. (1998). Adolescent pregnancy and parenthood. Recent evidence and future directions. American Psychologist **53**(2): 152–66.

Colletta, N. D. (1983). At risk for depression: a study of young mothers. [Research Support, Non-U.S. Gov't]. Journal of Genetic Psychology **142**(2d Half): 301–10.

Conger, R.D., Ge, X., Elder, G.H., Jr., Lorenz, F.O., and Simons, R.L. (1994). Economic stress, coercive family process, and developmental problems of adolescents. Child Development **65**(2 Spec No): 541–61.

Conseur, A., Rivara, F.P., Barnoski, R., and Emanuel, I. (1997). Maternal and perinatal risk factors for later delinquency. Pediatrics **99**(6): 785–90.

Cooper, P.J., and Murray, L. (1995). Course and recurrence of postnatal depression: Evidence for the specificity of the diagnostic concept. British Journal of Psychiatry **166**(2): 191–95.

Cornelius, M.D., Goldschmidt, L., Willford, J.A., et al. (2009). Body size and intelligence in 6-year-olds: are offspring of teenage mothers at risk? Maternal and Child Health Journal **13**(6): 847–56.

Cote, S., Zoccolillo, M., Tremblay, R., Nagin, D. S., and Vitaro, F. (2001). Predicting girls' conduct disorder in adolescence from childhood trajectories of disruptive behaviors. Journal of the American Academy of Child and Adolescent Psychiatry **40**: 678–84.

Cox, J., Holden, J., and Sagovsky, R. (1987). Detection of postnatal depression: Development of the 10-item Edinburgh Postnatal Depression Scale. British Journal of Psychiatry **150**: 782–86.

Dahinten, V., Shapka, J. D., and Willms, J. (2007). Adolescent children of adolescent mothers: The impact of family functioning on trajectories of development. Journal of Youth and Adolescence **36**(2): 195–212.

Darroch, J.E. (2001). Adolescent pregnancy trends and demographics. Current Women's Health Reports, **1**(2), 102–110.

Deal, L.W., and Holt, V.L. (1998). Young maternal age and depressive symptoms: results from the 1988 National Maternal and Infant Health Survey. American Journal of Public Health **88**(2): 266–70.

Demers, I., Bernier, A., Tarabulsy, G.M., and Provost, M.A. (2010). Mind-mindedness in adult and adolescent mothers: Relations to maternal sensitivity and infant attachment. International Journal of Behavioral Development **34**(6): 529–37.

DiClemente, R., Wingood, G., Crosby, R., *et al.* (2001). A prospective study of psychological distress and sexual risk behavior among black adolescent females. Pediatrics **108**(5): E85.

East, P.L., and Felice, M.E. (1996). Adolescent pregnancy and parenting: Findings from a racially diverse sample. Mahwah, NJ, Lawrence Erlbaum Associates Publishers

Eyberg, S. (1979). A parent–child interaction model for the treatment of psychological disorders in young children. Paper presented at the Western Psychological Association, San Diego.

Ezpeleta, L., Domenech, J., and Angold, A. (2006). A comparison of pure and comorbid CD/ODD and depression. Journal of Child Psychology and Psychiatry **47**(7): 704–12.

Feehan, M., McGee, R., Raja, S.N., and Williams, S.M. (1994). DSM-III-R disorders in New Zealand 18-year-olds. Australian and New Zealand Journal of Psychiatry **28**(1): 87–99.

Felice, M.E., Feinstein, R.A., Fisher, M.M., *et al.* (1999). Adolescent pregnancy—current trends and issues: 1998 American Academy of Pediatrics Committee on Adolescence, 1998–1999. Pediatrics **103**(2): 516–20.

Fergusson, D.M., and Woodward, L.J. (1999). Maternal age and educational and psychosocial outcomes in early adulthood. Journal of Child Psychology and Psychiatry and Allied Disciplines **40**(3): 479–89.

Fergusson, D., and Woodward, L. (2002). Mental health, educational, and social role outcomes of adolescents with depression. Archives of General Psychiatry **59**(3): 225–31.

Fergusson, D.M., Horwood, L., and Lynskey, M.T. (1993). Prevalence and comorbidity of DSM-III-R diagnoses in a birth cohort of 15 year olds. Journal of the American Academy of Child and Adolescent Psychiatry **32**(6): 1127–34.

Field, T. (2010). Postpartum depression effects on early interactions, parenting, and safety practices: A review. Infant Behavior and Development **33**(1): 1–6.

Figueiredo, B., Pacheco, A., and Costa, R. (2007). Depression during pregnancy and the postpartum period in adolescent and adult Portuguese mothers. Archives of Womens Mental Health **10**(3): 103–9.

Fontaine, N., Carbonneau, R., Vitaro, F., Barker, E.D., and Tremblay, R.E. (2009). Research review: a critical review of studies on the developmental trajectories of antisocial behavior in females. Journal of Child Psychology and Psychiatry and Allied Disciplines **50**(4): 363–85.

Franklin, C., Corcoran, J., and Harris, M. (2004). Risk and protective factors for adolescent pregnancy. In Risk and resilience in childhood: an ecological perspective, 2nd ed., M.W. Fraser, editor. Washington, DC, NASW Press, pp. 281–313.

Furstenberg, F.F., Jr. (2003). Teenage childbearing as a public issue and a private concern. Annual Review of Sociology **29**: 23–39.

Gadow, K., and Sprafkin, J. (1994/1997). Child/adolescent symptom inventories manual. Stonybrook, NY, Checkmate Plus.

Gaudie, J., Mitrou, F., Lawrence, D., Stanley, F.J., Silburn, S.R., and Zubrick, S.R. (2010). Antecedents of teenage pregnancy from a 14-year follow-up study using data linkage. BMC Public Health **10**: 63.

Gaynes, B.N., Gavin, N., Meltzer-Brody, S., *et al.* (2005). Perinatal depression: prevalence, screening accuracy, and screening outcomes. AHRQ Evidence Report Summaries, **119**, 1–8.

Giardino, J., Gonzalez, A., Steiner, M., and Fleming, A.S. (2008). Effects of motherhood on physiological and subjective responses to infant cries in teenage mothers: a comparison with non-mothers and adult mothers. Hormones and Behavior **53**(1): 149–58.

Gilbert, W., Jandial, D., Field, N., Bigelow, P., and Danielsen, B. (2004). Birth outcomes in teenage pregnancies. Journal of Maternal-Fetal and Neonatal Medicine **16**(5): 265–70.

Gotlib, I. H., Whiffen, V.E., Wallace, P.M., and Mount, J.H. (1991). Prospective investigation of postpartum depression: Factors involved in onset and recovery. Journal of Abnormal Psychology **100**(2): 122–32.

Hardt, J., and Rutter, M. (2004). Validity of adult retrospective reports of adverse childhood experiences: review of the evidence. Journal of Child Psychology and Psychiatry and Allied Disciplines **45**(2): 260–73.

Hay, D.F., Pawlby, S., Angold, A., Harold, G.T., and Sharp, D. (2003). Pathways to violence in the children of mothers who were depressed postpartum. Developmental Psychology **39**(6): 1083–94.

Henry, B., Moffitt, T.E., Caspi, A., Langley, J., and Silva, P.A. (1994). On the 'remembrance of things past': A longitudinal evaluation of the retrospective method. Psychological Assessment **6**(2): 92–101.

Hipwell, A.E., Loeber, R., Stouthamer-Loeber, M., *et al.* (2002). Characteristics of girls with early onset disruptive and antisocial behaviour. Criminal Behaviour and Mental Health **12**(1): 99–118.

Hipwell, A.E., Stepp, S., Feng, X., *et al.* (2011). Impact of oppositional defiant disorder dimensions on the temporal ordering of conduct problems and depression across childhood and adolescence in girls. Journal of Child Psychology and Psychiatry **52**(10): 1099–08.

Hollander, D. (1995). Mother's socioeconomic background may play greater role in childhood development than maternal age. Family Planning Perspectives **27**: 129–30.

Hudson, D.B., Elek, S.M., and Campbell-Grossman, C. (2000). Depression, self-esteem, loneliness, and social support among adolescent mothers participating in the new parents project. Adolescence **35**(139): 445–53.

Jaffee, S., Caspi, A., Moffitt, T.E., Belsky, J., and Silva, P. (2001). Why are children born to teen mothers at risk for adverse outcomes in young adulthood? Results from a 20-year longitudinal study. Development and Psychopathology **13**(2): 377–97.

Keenan, K. (2003). Chicago Baby Project: Global rating of child response, child distress, maternal response and maternal soothing. Unpublished manual, University of Chicago.

Keenan, K., Hipwell, A., Chung, T., *et al.* (2010). The Pittsburgh girls study: Overview and initial findings. Journal of Clinical Child and Adolescent Psychology **39**(4): 506–21.

Kovacs, M., Krol, R.S., and Voti, L. (1994). Early onset psychopathology and the risk for teenage pregnancy among clinically referred girls. Journal of the American Academy of Child and Adolescent Psychiatry **33**(1): 106–13.

Lesser, J., Koniak-Griffin, D., and Anderson, N. (1999). Depressed adolescent mothers' preceptions of their own maternal role. Issues in Mental Health Nursing **20**: 131–49.

Lewinsohn, P., Hops, H., Roberts, R., Seeley, J., and Andrews, J. (1993). Adolescent psychopathology: I. Prevalence and incidence of depression and other DSM-III-R disorders in high school students. Journal of Abnormal Psychology **102**(1): 133–44.

Logsdon, M., Birkimer, J., Simpson, T., and Looney, S. (2005). Postpartum depression and social support in adolescents. Journal of Obstetric, Gynecologic, and Neonatal Nursing **34**(1): 46–54.

Logsdon, M., Ziegler, C., Hertweck, P., and Pinto-Foltz, M. (2008). Testing a bioecological model to examine social support in postpartum adolescents. Journal of Nursing Scholarship **40**(2): 116–23.

Long, M.S. (2009). Disorganized attachment relationships in infants of adolescent mothers factors that may augment positive outcomes. Adolescence **44**(175): 621–33.

Manlove, J. (1997). Early motherhood in an intergenerational perspective: The experiences of a British cohort. Journal of Marriage and Family **59**(2): 263–79.

Marcus, S.M., Flynn, H.A., Blow, F.C., and Barry, K.L. (2003). Depressive symptoms among pregnant women screened in obstetrics settings. Journal of Women's Health **12**(4): 373–80.

Marmorstein, N.R., and Iacono, W.G. (2001). An investigation of female adolescent twins with both major depression and conduct disorder. Journal of the American Academy of Child and Adolescent Psychiatry **40**(3): 299–306.

Miller-Johnson, S., Winn, D.M., Coie, J., *et al.* (1999). Motherhood during the teen years: a developmental perspective on risk factors for childbearing. Development and Psychopathology **11**(1): 85–100.

Moffitt, T.E., Caspi, A., Rutter, M., and Silva, P.A. (2001). Sex differences in antisocial behaviour: Conduct disorder, delinquency, and violence in the Dunedin Longitudinal Study. New York, NY, Cambridge University Press.

Murray, L., and Carothers, A. (1990). The validation of the Edinburgh Post-natal Depression Scale on a community sample. The British Journal of Psychiatry **157**: 288–90.

Muthen, L., and Muthen, R. (2008). Mplus: The comprehensive modeling program for applied researchers, (version 5.2). Los Angeles, CA, Muthen and Muthen.

Nolen-Hoeksema, S., and Girgus, J. (1994). The emergence of gender differences in depression during adolescence. Psychological Bulletin **115**(3): 424–43.

O'Hara, M.W., and Swain, A.M. (1996). Rates and risks of postpartum depression–a meta-analysis. International Review of Psychiatry **8**(1): 37–54.

Offord, D.R., Boyle, M. H., Szatmari, P., et al. (1987). Ontario Child Health Study: II. Six-month prevalence of disorder and rates of service utilization. Archives of General Psychiatry **44**(9): 832–6.

Oxford, M. (2010). Predicting markers of adulthood among adolescent mothers. Social Work Research **34**(1): 33.

Oxford, M., Gilchrist, L., Gillmore, M., and Lohr, M. (2006). Predicting variation in the life course of adolescent mothers as they enter adulthood. Journal of Adolescent Health **39**(1): 20–6.

Pedersen, W., and Mastekaasa, A. (2011). Conduct disorder symptoms and subsequent pregnancy, child-birth and abortion: A population-based longitudinal study of adolescents. Journal of Adolescence **34**(5): 1025–33.

Ramaswamy, V., DeSabro, W., Reibstein, D., and Robinson, W. (1993). An empirical pooling approach for estimating marketing mix elasticities with PIMS data. Marketing Sciences **12**: 103–24.

Rowe, R., Maughan, B., and Eley, T. (2006). Links between antisocial behavior and depressed mood: The role of life events and attributional style. Journal of Abnormal Child Psychology **34**(3): 293–302.

Schmidt, R., Wiemann, C., Rickert, V., and Smith, E. (2006). Moderate to severe depressive symptoms among adolescent mothers followed four years postpartum. Journal of Adolescent Health **38**(6): 712–18.

Schwartz, G. (1978). Estimating the dimension of a model. Annals of Statistics **6**: 461–4.

Serbin, L.A., Cooperman, J.M., Peters, P.L., et al. (1998). Intergenerational transfer of psychosocial risk in women with childhood histories of aggression, withdrawal, or aggression and withdrawal. Developmental Psychology **34**(6): 1246–62.

Shaw, M., Lawlor, D.A., and Najman, J.M. (2006). Teenage children of teenage mothers: Psychological, behavioural and health outcomes from an Australian prospective longitudinal study. Social Science and Medicine **62**(10): 2526–39.

Spencer, J.M., Zimet, G.D., Aalsma, M.C., and Orr, D.P. (2002). Self-esteem as a predictor of initiation of coitus in early adolescents. Pediatrics **109**(4): 581–4.

Stein, A., Gath, D., Bucher, J., Bond, Al., Day, A., and Cooper, P. (1991). The relationship between post-natal depression and mother-child interaction. British Journal of Psychiatry **158**: 46–52.

Steinberg, L., Dahl, R., Keating, D., Kupfer, D., Masten, A., and Pine, D. (2006). The study of developmental psychopathology in adolescence: Integrating affective neuroscience with the study of context. In Developmental psychopathology, Vol 2: Developmental neuroscience, 2nd ed., D. Cicchetti and D. Cohen, editors. Hoboken, John Wiley and Sons Inc., pp. 710–41.

Stowe, Z.N., Hostetter, A.L., and Newport, D.J. (2005). The onset of postpartum depression: Implications for clinical screening in obstetrical and primary care. Americal Journal of Obstetrics and Gynecology **192**: 522–6.

Talashek, M.L., Alba, M.L., and Patel, A. (2006). Untangling the health disparities of teen pregnancy. Journal for Specialists in Pediatric Nursing **11**(1): 14–27.

Tronick, E., Als, H., Adamson, L., Wise, S., and Brazelton, T.B. (1978). The infant's response to entrapment between contradictory messages in face-to-face interaction. Journal of the American Academy of Child Psychiatry 17(1): 1–13.

Troutman, B., and Cutrona, C. (1990). Nonpsychotic postpartum depression among adolescent mothers. Journal of Abnormal Psychology 99(1): 69–78.

Wahn, E.H., Nissen, E., and Ahlberg, B.M. (2005). Becoming and being a teenage mother: how teenage girls in South Western Sweden view their situation. Health Care for Women International 26(7): 591–603.

Webster-Stratton, C., Reid, M., and Hammond, M. (2001). Preventing conduct problems, promoting social competence: A parent and teacher training partnership in Head Start. Journal of Clinical Child Psychology 30(3): 283–302.

Whitbeck, L., Conger, R., Simons, R., and Kao, M.-Y. (1993). Minor deviant behaviors and adolescent sexual activity. Youth and Society 25(1): 24–37.

Wolff, J. C., and Ollendick, T. H. (2006). The comorbidity of conduct problems and depression in childhood and adolescence. [Review]. Clinical Child and Family Psychology Review 9(3–4): 201–20.

Woodward, L. J., and Fergusson, D.M. (1999). Early conduct problems and later risk of teenage pregnancy in girls. Development and Psychopathology 11(1): 127–41.

Zoccolillo, M., Tremblay, R., and Vitaro, F. (1996). DSM-III-R and DSM-III criteria for conduct disorder in preadolescent girls: Specific but insensitive. Journal of the American Academy of Child and Adolescent Psychiatry 30: 973–81.

Section 4

Biological aspects of perinatal mental disorders

Section 4

Biological aspects
of perinatal mental
disorders

Chapter 16

The intergenerational transmission of stress: psychosocial and biological mechanisms

Carmine M. Pariante

A tribute to Channi

I met Channi for the first time when I was a senior house officer (trainee) in psychiatry at the Maudsley Hospital, and I worked under his supervision for 6 months, in 1998. At that time, Channi was the only Consultant Perinatal Psychiatrist at the Maudsley, covering the Liaison Services at King's College Hospital, the outreach work, and the Mother and Baby Unit. And, of course, he was leading the academic section. It is perhaps the best tribute to his memory that it takes now three consultants and two academics to do the work that he was then doing all by himself!

I was already interested in neuroendocrinology, and Channi was fascinated by the possibility that hormones might have a role in the mental health problems of the perinatal period. At that time, the notion that hormonal changes in pregnancy could have long-lasting effects on the offspring was still at its infancy, and I remember fondly the many discussions on this topic with Channi, sitting at his famous old desk.

Channi was a pioneer in this field: he was the first to emphasize the dramatic impact of depression in pregnancy on the wellbeing of mothers and children. I am honoured to be able to continue this line of research today.

Introduction

Importance

The intergenerational transmission of stress has powerful clinical and social consequences, consolidating social adversity and psychopathology in future generations. The 2007 Policy Briefing by the World Health Organization Regional Office for Europe, 'Preventing child maltreatment in Europe: a public health approach' (WHO 2007), recognizes that 'there is an association between maltreatment in childhood and the risk of later . . . becoming a perpetrator of violence or other antisocial behaviour as a teenager or adult'. The report also highlights that the costs are both overt (for example, medical care for victims, treatment of offenders, and legal costs for social care) and less obvious (for example, criminal justice and prosecution costs, specialist education, and mental health provision). In Europe, only the United Kingdom has calculated the total economic burden, estimated to be £735 million in 1996 (WHO 2007). There is no doubt that an enormous amount of work and resources are going into prevention strategies and public health approaches; however, it is surprising that very little research has been conducted in humans to try to understand why childhood maltreatment is passed from one generation to the next, and what are the biological and molecular mechanisms underlying this intergenerational effect. With the recent document on the 'Grand Challenges in Global Mental Health' (Collins *et al.* 2011) underscoring the need for research that uses a life-course approach, and indicating the identification of 'modifiable social and biological risk factors across the life course' as one of the grand challenges to be addressed urgently, this issue is also extremely timely.

Aim of this chapter

This chapter will review the clinical evidence in relationship with the intergenerational transmission of exposure to stress, and in particular of exposure to childhood maltreatment. We will focus in particular on the mechanisms by which exposure to stress and maltreatment in the childhood of women translate into exposure to stress and maltreatment in their offspring, highlighting pregnancy and the in utero environment as the crucial timing and biological setting where these mechanisms operate. In summary, this chapter will propose that experiences of childhood maltreatment in mothers induce persistent behavioural and biological changes in the regulation of maternal stress response, which in turn alter the biology of the in utero environment during their pregnancies, especially in more vulnerable mothers who also experience stress and depression during pregnancy. This abnormal biology of the in utero environment induces further changes in both mothers and offspring, which in turn contribute to the transmission of the stress exposure: in mothers, by altering the quality of the interaction with their offspring and predisposing to less vigilance and protective behaviour; and, in the offspring, by programming an altered stress response and a disturbed behavioural trajectory. Crucially, the evidence points to the pregnancy period as a uniquely sensitive period for preventative intervention aimed at breaking the cycle of transmission.

The intergenerational transmission of exposure to violence

After years of accumulating anecdotal evidence, recently some studies have provided controlled evidence that women who experience childhood exposure to stress tend to have children who also experience exposure to stress. For example, in an American sample of almost 500 mother–child dyads, a history of maternal physical and sexual abuse was found to predict offspring maltreatment in the first two years of life, as measured by county court records of allegations and substantiations (Appleyard *et al.* 2011; Berlin *et al.* 2011). In a study conducted in the large UK cohort study, the Avon Longitudinal Study of Parents and Children, out of 14,256 children participating in the study, 293 were investigated by social services for suspected maltreatment and 115 were placed on local child protection registers; and a history of childhood abuse in parents was a risk factor for the children being investigated for maltreatment or being placed on the child protection register (Sidebotham and Heron 2006). It is of note also our recent work conducted in the South London Child Development Study (from data collected up to offspring age 16) also reveals an association between maternal childhood maltreatment and offspring childhood maltreatment in the period from birth to eleven years ($r = 0.28$, $p < 0.001$; Plant *et al.* 2013). The mechanisms underlying this transmission are, however, unknown.

Risk factors and mechanisms for the intergenerational transmission of stress

Classical risk factors for transmission of stress exposure include mothers' mental health problems, social isolation, unemployment and single parenthood (Berlin *et al.* 2011; Sidebotham and Heron 2006). Appleyard *et al.* (2011) identify a clear pathway from maternal sexual and physical abuse, to maternal substance use problems, to childhood victimization. Indeed, the association between psychopathology in parents and offspring exposure to maltreatment is well recognized (see also the following sections). Interestingly, Berlin *et al.* (2011) identify that maternal cognitive process related to social information (hostile attributions and aggressive response biases) are also involved in the pathway between maternal exposure to maltreatment and offspring maltreatment, thus identifying a potential mechanism. Indeed, children of mothers who have (during offspring childhood) comorbid depression and antisocial disorders are at an elevated risk of experiencing multiple caregiving abuses, including physical maltreatment, high levels of maternal hostility, and exposure to domestic violence (Kim-Cohen *et al.* 2006). Moreover, within twin pairs, the twin receiving more maternal negativity and less warmth have more antisocial behavior problems, suggesting that maternal emotional attitudes toward children may play a causal role in the development of antisocial behaviour (Caspi *et al.* 2004) (see 'Pathway A, Mother-driven').

Evidence pointing to yet another, non mutually-exclusive mechanism, is that a maternal history of exposure to stress in childhood is associated with the children developing behavioral problems, which in turn may predispose them to be exposed to violence (see also 'Pathway B: Child-driven'). For example, in a large British sample of over four thousand mother–child dyads, children of mothers who experienced childhood abuse were at an elevated risk for emotional and behavioural adjustment problems at four and seven years (Roberts *et al.* 2004; Collishaw *et al.* 2007). More recently, in a Spanish study, maternal childhood abuse was found to predict symptoms of disruptive behaviour disorders in offspring during adolescence (Miranda *et al.* 2011). Moreover, there is evidence that children's behaviour may elicit harsh discipline and abnormal parenting practices (Ge *et al.* 1996). Of note, Jaffee *et al.* (2004) have found that environmental factors account for most of the variation in corporal punishment and physical maltreatment in the E-Risk cohort: moreover, and reassuringly, a 'child-driven' effect was only present for corporal punishment, not for physical maltreatment.

The role of the antenatal period

Women who have experienced childhood maltreatment tend to be depressed during pregnancy

Epidemiological and clinical studies have already described an association between experiences of childhood maltreatment and depressive symptomatology in pregnancy ('antenatal depression'), but all have examined predominantly 'at risk' mothers (Romano *et al.* 2006; Chung *et al.* 2008; Rich-Edwards *et al.* 2011), such as pregnant adolescents or low-income women. In our recent work in the South London Child Development Study, we show an association between maternal childhood maltreatment and maternal antenatal depression in an epidemiological sample, as indicated by an incredibly high odds ratio (OR) of 10 (Plant *et al.* 2012). Our study indeed shows that (maternal) history of exposure to maltreatment and stress in childhood is the single most powerful risk factor for the development of depression in pregnancy, even after adjusting for psychopathology at any time during the mother's lifetime. This also indicates that pregnancy is an incredibly delicate period for women who have had a difficult and stressful childhood, and thus perhaps the best time to intervene therapeutically.

Women depressed during pregnancy have an increased risk of their children being victims of maltreatment

The association between *lifetime* psychopathology in mothers and increased risk of childhood maltreatment in offspring has been well described. Specifically, certain parental personality attributes have been associated with offspring maltreatment, such as low self-esteem, negative affectivity (depression and anxiety), and antisocial behaviours (Oliver 1985). More importantly, in our recent paper (Pawlby *et al.* 2011) we have clearly demonstrated, using data from the South London Child Development Study, that *antenatal depression* is associated with increased risk of the offspring being subjected to childhood maltreatment (see Table 16.1). Specifically, we have found that, compared with children who had not been exposed to depression 'in utero', children who were exposed were approximately four times more likely to have experienced childhood maltreatment by the age

Table 16.1 Exposure to maternal depression in utero and experience of childhood maltreatment

	Childhood maltreatment	
	No % (*n*)	Yes % (*n*)
Exposure to depression in utero		
	84.2 (80)	15.8 (15)
	60.0 (15)	40.0 (10)

χ^2 (1) = 7.03, p = 0.008.
Modified from Pawlby, S., Hay, D., Sharp, D., Waters, C.S., and Pariante, C.M. (2011). Antenatal depression and offspring psychopathology: the influence of childhood maltreatment. The British Journal of Psychiatry, **199**(2): 106–12.

of 11 years. Of note, our data point to a specific effect of antenatal, rather than postnatal, depression, in increasing the risk of childhood maltreatment (Pawlby *et al.* 2011). Taken together with the evidence already summarized, it is plausible that persistent behavioural and biological abnormalities in women, induced by their experience of childhood exposure to violence, increase the risk for maternal depression in pregnancy, which in turn confers risk for offspring maltreatment, and provides a vehicle for the intergenerational transmission of childhood maltreatment. However, the pathways by which this vehicle operates are yet unknown. Indeed, it is important to emphasis that our study *does not* indicate that women who are depressed during pregnancy go on to be violent to their children, as the excess of maltreatment (which, in our study, also included harsh discipline) was originated not by the mothers alone but also by other members of the family or of the social environment. Nevertheless, it is possible to speculate that lack of vigilance from the mothers might have played a role.

Potential pathways by which antenatal depression increases the risks of offspring maltreatment

As mentioned previously, two, non-mutually exclusive pathways can be proposed:

◆ *Pathway A, mother-driven:* the behavioural and biological abnormalities induced by antenatal depression disrupt future maternal care, which then account for the increased risk of exposure to violence.

◆ *Pathway B, child-driven:* the behavioural and biological abnormalities induced by antenatal depression programme the child onto a trajectory for behavioural problems, which then account for the increased risk of exposure to violence.

Biological and behavioural mechanisms

Childhood exposure to violence induces persistent behavioural and biologic abnormalities

Both these pathways start with maternal childhood exposure to violence, and with the persistent molecular abnormalities that are induced by these experiences. Hence, we will briefly review these molecular abnormalities, before discussing the two pathways more in details. There is clear evidence that childhood maltreatment predisposes to a persistent activation of the two main biological systems involved in the stress response, the hypothalamic–pituitary–adrenal (HPA) axis and the inflammatory system. Both these systems are also hyperactive in depression, and indeed this hyperactivity is considered part of the pathogenesis of depression (Heim *et al.* 2008; Pariante and Lightman 2008; Danese *et al.* 2007; Binder 2009). We, and others, have extensively contributed to the understanding of the mechanism underlying HPA axis and inflammation hyperactivity in adults who have experienced childhood trauma, and have proposed an explanatory model centred on the glucocorticoid receptor (GR), that is, one of the most important receptors and transcription factors governing the stress response (Heim *et al.* 2008; Pariante and

Lightman 2008; Danese *et al.* 2007; Binder 2009). Glucocorticoid hormones, like cortisol in humans and corticosterone in rodents, are the final output of the HPA axis, and the main hormones involved in the stress response. By binding to the GR (and to the mineralocorticoid receptor, MR), cortisol effects its cellular actions, including the negative feedback regulation of the HPA axis (by which stress-induced activation of the HPA axis is followed by a rapid return to normal functioning), and the restraint of the inflammatory response (which maintains a physiological control on excessive immune processes). Childhood maltreatment has been shown to induce glucocorticoid resistance, that is, a reduction of GR function, which in turn leads to both the HPA axis hyperactivity and the increased inflammation, because of the lack of, respectively, the GR-mediated negative feedback on the HPA axis and the GR-mediated restraint of inflammation (Heim *et al.* 2008; Pariante and Lightman 2008; Danese *et al.* 2007; Binder 2009). Based on this evidence, it is plausible to speculate that women who have suffered childhood exposure to violence develop glucocorticoid resistance, which in turn predisposes them to develop depression later in adult life, and especially during pregnancy, a period naturally associated with glucocorticoid resistance (see below).

Stress and depression during pregnancy affect the HPA axis of both the mother and the child

There is evidence that normal pregnancy is associated with abnormalities in the function of the HPA axis, the main hormonal stress response system. Specifically, pregnancy is also associated with 'glucocorticoid resistance', as indicated by studies showing impaired GR-mediated negative feedback regulation of the HPA axis by dexamethasone (Smith and Thomson 1991), and reduced GR function in peripheral blood mononuclear cells (PBMCs) (Katz *et al.* 2011). Consistent with the presence of glucocorticoid resistance, both the HPA axis and the inflammatory system are hyperactive during normal pregnancy, and both regulate human parturition. More importantly within this context, there is also some evidence that GR resistance is more marked in women who experience depressive symptoms or stress during pregnancy, as shown by both a further reduction of GR function in PBMC binding (Katz *et al* 2011), as well as an even higher activity of the HPA axis and the inflammatory system (Field *et al.* 2009; O'Keane *et al.* 2011; Coussons-Read *et al.* 2005, 2007; Christian *et al.* 2009; Blackmore *et al.* 2011). Finally, animal and clinical studies have shown that stress during pregnancy leads to increased stress response in the offspring. Many authors have critically reviewed this literature (Weinstock 2005; Glover *et al.* 2010), and overall found that stress in pregnancy tends to increase both basal- and stress-induced HPA axis activity in the offspring, and that there is concordance between maternal cortisol levels and children's cortisol levels. Indeed, one study has found that a lifetime history of maternal depression was enough to predict higher baseline cortisol in the infant (Brennan *et al.* 2008). Finally, it is of note that animal studies have shown that increased inflammation during gestation, via injection of lipopolysaccharide (LPS), also induces a persistent hyperactivity of the HPA axis in the offspring, as well as reduced maternal care and changes in offspring behaviour (see later) (Graciarena *et al.* 2010; Kentner and Pittman 2010). It is therefore plausible that maternal experiences of childhood mal-treatment (and the putative associated changes in the HPA axis and inflammation during pregnancy, especially in women who are also depressed, influence brain mechanisms rel-evant for stress regulation in offspring, and modify their HPA axis activity.

Stress and depression during pregnancy compromise maternal care (Pathway A)

Animal models have been used extensively to understand how stress during gestation alters maternal behaviour. In the best such characterized model, the rat 'licking and grooming' behaviour, pregnant rats receiving a restraint stress in the last 7 days of preg-nancy show, at day 6 postnatal, reduced maternal care behaviour, increased HPA axis activity, and reduced brain expression of the receptor for oxytocin, a neurotransmitter regulating maternal care and social behaviour (Champagne and Meaney 2006). These biological findings are likely related, since administration of the synthetic HPA axis hor-mone, dexamethasone, has also been shown to decrease oxytocin secretion, brain oxy-tocin receptor, and maternal care behaviour (Patchev *et al.* 1993). Interestingly, there is evidence that higher maternal oxytocin levels in pregnancy are associated with maternal bonding behaviour (Feldman *et al.* 2007) and are protective against the occurrence of postnatal depression (Skrundz *et al.* 2011). Taken together with the evidence discussed above, these data support the notion that mothers with a history of exposure to stress in childhood, especially if also depressed, have increased HPA axis activity during preg-nancy, which in turn may alter the oxytocin system and ultimately contribute to im-paired maternal care.

Stress and depression during pregnancy affect offspring behaviour (Pathway B)

Clinical studies have shown that antenatal anxiety and depressive symptoms predict de-layed motor development in infancy, and childhood emotional and behavioural prob-lems, such as attention deficit hyperactivity disorder and disruptive behaviour disorder (Glover *et al.* 2010; Glover and Connor 2002). Moreover, studies examining later off-spring outcomes have found an association between exposure to antenatal depression/anxiety and offspring depression, antisocial behaviour and violence during adolescence (Hay *et al.* 2010; Pawlby *et al.* 2009). These studies have also demonstrated that the as-sociation between exposure to maternal psychopathology in utero and offspring psycho-pathology is independent from the effects of the postnatal environment, thus suggesting a 'fetal programming hypothesis' (Hay *et al.* 2010; Pawlby *et al.* 2009). This advocates that the maternal biological environment in utero induced persistent fetal brain changes (see later). Taken together with the previously-discussed studies, it is possible to speculate that offspring of mothers with experiences of childhood maltreatment, especially if mothers have also been depressed during pregnancy, will show abnormal offspring behavioural development, which finally will predispose to elicit exposure to maltreatment and other stressors.

Implications for the treatment of depression during pregnancy

Around one in eight pregnant women experience a major depressive disorder (MDD) during pregnancy, and one in five experience some depressive symptoms (Grote *et al.* 2010). Therefore, even if depression in pregnancy is linked to a very small increase in the risk of disrupting maternal care, the sheer prevalence of this phenomenon makes it clinically relevant for the intergenerational transmission of exposure to stress. Moreover, depression in pregnancy is associated exactly to the same sociodemographic risk factors that affect intergenerational transmission of exposure to stress, such being a single mother and having a socioeconomically deprived background. Both antidepressants and brief psychotherapies are effective in pregnancy, and some antidepressants are advised as preferable (NICE 2007). Clearly, the positive impact of a larger number of women taking antidepressants during pregnancy has to be considered against the background of small, but significantly increased, risks for the neonates, including for cardiac malformation (Reis and Kallen 2010), pulmonary hypertension (Reis and Kallen 2010) and, in very recent studies, for autism (Croen *et al.* 2011)—a 'health-scare' story that has had much publicity (see for example, CNN 2011). Therefore, any recommendation will have enormous consequences for both future mothers and the health community.

Conclusions

This chapter proposes that the pregnancy and the in utero environment as the crucial *timing* and *biological setting* where the intergenerational transmission of childhood exposure to stress and maltreatment occurs. While there has been extensive research on both the persistent biological effects of exposure to violence and the role of the in utero environment on offspring outcome, there is a lack of research putting these two areas together, and using a fully integrated approach, including clinical and psychosocial assessments, blood and saliva biomarkers, gene expression and epigenetics. Of course, while studying 'risk' mechanisms, this research will also be able to identify protective factors that prevent the intergenerational transmission, and ultimately generate novel therapeutic pathways that will break the intergenerational transmission.

References

Appleyard, K., Berlin, L.J., Rosanbalm, K.D., and Dodge, K.A. (2011). Preventing early child maltreatment: implications from a longitudinal study of maternal abuse history, substance use problems, and offspring victimization. Prevention science: the official journal of the Society for Prevention Research 12(2): 139–49.

Berlin, L.J., Appleyard, K., and Dodge, K.A. (2011). Intergenerational continuity in child maltreatment: mediating mechanisms and implications for prevention. Child Development 82(1): 162–76.

Binder, E.B. (2009) The role of FKBP5, a co-chaperone of the glucocorticoid receptor in the pathogenesis and therapy of affective and anxiety disorders. Psychoneuroendocrinology 34(Suppl 1): S186–95.

Blackmore, E.R., Moynihan, J.A., Rubinow, D.R., *et al.* (2011). Psychiatric symptoms and proinflammatory cytokines in pregnancy. Psychosomatic Medicine 73(8): 656–63.

Brennan, P.A., Pargas, R., Walker, E.F., *et al.* (2008). Maternal depression and infant cortisol: influences of timing, comorbidity and treatment. Journal of Child Psychology and Psychiatry, and Allied Disciplines 49(10): 1099–107.

Caspi, A., Moffitt, T.E., Morgan, J., *et al.* (2004). Maternal expressed emotion predicts children's antisocial behavior problems: using monozygotic-twin differences to identify environmental effects on behavioral development. Developmental Psychology **40**(2): 149–61.

Champagne, F.A. and Meaney, M.J. (2006). Stress during gestation alters postpartum maternal care and the development of the offspring in a rodent model. Biological psychiatry **59**(12): 1227–35.

Christian, L.M., Franco, A., Glaser, R., and Iams, J.D. (2009). Depressive symptoms are associated with elevated serum proinflammatory cytokines among pregnant women. Brain, Behavior, and Immunity **23**(6): 750–4.

Chung, E.K., Mathew, L., Elo, I.T., Coyne, J.C., and Culhane, J.F. (2008). Depressive symptoms in disadvantaged women receiving prenatal care: the influence of adverse and positive childhood experiences. Ambulatory Pediatrics: the Official Journal of the Ambulatory Pediatric Association **8**(2): 109–16.

CNN (2011). Antidepressant use in pregnancy may raise autism risk. July 6 2011.

Collins, P.Y., Patel, V., Joestl, S.S., *et al.* (2011). Grand challenges in global mental health. Nature **475**(7354): 27–30.

Collishaw, S., Dunn, J., O'Connor, T.G., and Golding, J. (2007). Avon Longitudinal Study of Parents and Children Study Team Maternal childhood abuse and offspring adjustment over time. Developmental Psychopathology **19**(2): 367–83.

Coussons-Read, M.E., Okun, M.L., Schmitt, M.P., and Giese, S. (2005). Prenatal stress alters cytokine levels in a manner that may endanger human pregnancy. Psychosomatic Medicine **67**(4): 625–31.

Coussons-Read, M.E., Okun, M.L., and Nettles, C.D. (2007). Psychosocial stress increases inflammatory markers and alters cytokine production across pregnancy. Brain, Behavior, and Immunity **21**(3): 343–50.

Croen, L.A., Grether, J.K., Yoshida, C.K., Odouli, R., and Hendrick, V. (2011). Antidepressant use during pregnancy and childhood autism spectrum disorders. Archives of General Psychiatry **68**(11): 1104–12.

Danese, A., Pariante, C.M., Caspi, A., Taylor, A., and Poulton, R. (2007). Childhood maltreatment predicts adult inflammation in a life-course study. Proceedings of the National.Academy of Sciences of the U S A **104**(4): 1319–24.

Feldman, R., Weller, A., Zagoory-Sharon, O., and Levine, A. (2007). Evidence for a neuroendocrinological foundation of human affiliation: plasma oxytocin levels across pregnancy and the postpartum period predict mother-infant bonding. Psychological Science **18**(11): 965–70.

Field, T., Diego, M., Hernandez-Reif, M., *et al.* (2009). Depressed pregnant black women have a greater incidence of prematurity and low birthweight outcomes. Infant Behavior and Devlopment **32**(1): 10–16.

Ge, X.C., Rand, D., Cadoret, R.J., *et al.* (1996). The developmental interface between nature and nurture: A mutual influence model of child antisocial behavior and parent behaviors. Developmental Psychology **32**(4): 574–89.

Glover, V., O'Connor, T.G., O'Donnell, K. (2010). Prenatal stress and the programming of the HPA axis. Neuroscience and Biobehavioral Reviews **35**(1): 17–22.

Glover, V. and O'Connor, T.G. (2002). Effects of antenatal stress and anxiety: Implications for development and psychiatry. British Journal of Psychiatry **180**: 389–91.

Graciarena, M., Depino, A.M., and Pitossi, F.J. (2010). Prenatal inflammation impairs adult neurogenesis and memory related behavior through persistent hippocampal TGFbeta1 downregulation. Brain, Behavior, and Immunity **24**(8): 1301–9.

Grote, N.K., Bridge, J.A., Gavin, A.R., *et al.* (2010). A meta-analysis of depression during pregnancy and the risk of preterm birth, low birth weight, and intrauterine growth restriction. Archives of General Psychiatry **67**(10): 1012–24.

Hay, D.F., Pawlby, S., Waters, C.S., Perra, O., and Sharp, D. (2010). Mothers' antenatal depression and their children's antisocial outcomes. Child Development **81**(1): 149–65.

Heim, C., Newport, D.J., Mletzko, T., Miller, A.H., and Nemeroff, C.B. (2008). The link between childhood trauma and depression: insights from HPA axis studies in humans. Psychoneuroendocrinology **33**(6): 693–710.

Jaffee, S.R., Caspi, A., Moffitt, T.E., *et al.* (2004). The limits of child effects: evidence for genetically mediated child effects on corporal punishment but not on physical maltreatment. Developmental Psychology **40**(6): 1047–58.

Katz, E.R., Stowe, Z.N., Newport, D.J., *et al.* (2011). Regulation of mRNA expression encoding chaperone and co-chaperone proteins of the glucocorticoid receptor in peripheral blood: association with depressive symptoms during pregnancy. Psychological Medicine: **42**(5): 943–56.

Kentner, A.C. and Pittman, Q.J. (2010). Minireview: early-life programming by inflammation of the neuroendocrine system. Endocrinology **151**(10): 4602–6.

Kim-Cohen, J., Caspi, A., Rutter, M., Tomas, M.P., and Moffitt, T.E. (2006). The caregiving environments provided to children by depressed mothers with or without an antisocial history. American Journal of Psychiatry **163**(6): 1009–18.

Miranda, J.K., de la Osa, N., Granero, R., and Ezpeleta, L. (2011). Maternal experiences of childhood abuse and intimate partner violence: Psychopathology and functional impairment in clinical children and adolescents. Child Abuse and Neglect **35**(9): 700–11. doi: 10.1016/j.chiabu.2011.05.008. Epub 2011 Sep 7.

NICE (2007). Antenatal and postnatal mental health. Oxford, Alden Press.

O'Keane, V., Lightman, S., Marsh, M., *et al.* (2011). Increased pituitary-adrenal activation and shortened gestation in a sample of depressed pregnant women: A pilot study. Journal of Affective Disorders **130**(1–2): 300–5.

Oliver, J.E. (1985). Successive generations of child maltreatment: social and medical disorders in the parents. The British Journal of Psychiatry: the Journal of Mental Science **147**: 484–90.

Pariante, C.M. and Lightman, S.L. (2008). The HPA axis in major depression: classical theories and new developments. Trends in Neurosciences **31**(9): 464–68.

Patchev, V.K., Schlosser, S.F., Hassan, A.H., and Almeida, O.F. (1993). Oxytocin binding sites in rat limbic and hypothalamic structures: site-specific modulation by adrenal and gonadal steroids. Neuroscience **57**(3): 537–43.

Pawlby, S., Hay, D.F., Sharp, D., Waters, C.S., and O'Keane, V. (2009). Antenatal depression predicts depression in adolescent offspring: prospective longitudinal community-based study. Journal of affective disorders **113**(3): 236–43.

Pawlby, S., Hay, D., Sharp, D., Waters, C.S., and Pariante, C.M. (2011). Antenatal depression and offspring psychopathology: the influence of childhood maltreatment. The British Journal of Psychiatry: the Journal of Mental Science **199**(2): 106–12.

Plant, D.T., Barker, E.D., Waters, C.S., Pawlby, S., and Pariante, C.M. (2013). Intergenerational transmission of maltreatment and psychopathology: the role of antenatal depression. Psychological Medicine **43**(3): 519–28. doi: 10.1017/S0033291712001298. Epub 2012 Jun 14.

Reis, M. and Kallen, B. (2010). Delivery outcome after maternal use of antidepressant drugs in pregnancy: an update using Swedish data. Psychological Medicine **40**(10): 1723–33.

Rich-Edwards, J.W., James-Todd, T., Mohllajee, A., *et al.* (2011). Lifetime maternal experiences of abuse and risk of pre-natal depression in two demographically distinct populations in Boston. International Journal of Epidemiology **40**(2): 375–84.

Roberts, R., O'Connor, T., Dunn, J., Golding, J. and the ALSPAC Study Team (2004). The effects of child sexual abuse in later family life; mental health, parenting and adjustment of offspring. Child Abuse and Neglect **28**(5): 525–45.

Romano, E., Zoccolillo, M., and Paquette, D. (2006). Histories of child maltreatment and psychiatric disorder in pregnant adolescents. Journal of the American Academy of Child and Adolescent Psychiatry **45**(3): 329–36.

Sidebotham, P. and Heron, J. (2006). Child maltreatment in the 'children of the nineties': a cohort study of risk factors. Child Abuse & Neglect **30**(5): 497–522.

Skrundz, M., Bolten, M., Nast, I., Hellhammer, D.H., and Meinlschmidt, G. (2011). Plasma oxytocin concentration during pregnancy is associated with development of postpartum depression. Neuropsychopharmacology: official publication of the American College of Neuropsychopharmacology **36**(9): 1886–93.

Smith, R. and Thomson, M. (1991). Neuroendocrinology of the hypothalamo-pituitary-adrenal axis in pregnancy and the puerperium. Bailliere's clinical endocrinology and metabolism. **5**(1): 167–86.

Weinstock, M. (2005). The potential influence of maternal stress hormones on development and mental health of the offspring. Brain, Behavior, and Immunity **19**(4): 296–308.

WHO (2007). Policy Briefing. Preventing child maltreatment in Europe: a public health approach World Health Organization Regional Office for Europe. Copenhagen, Denmark.

Chapter 17

Associations between prenatal stress, anxiety and depression and child behavioural and cognitive development. Is it causal?

Vivette Glover, Kieran O'Donnell,
and Thomas G. O'Connor

Personal note

I (V.G.) first got to know Channi at the inaugural Indian Biological Psychiatry meeting In Bombay over 20 years ago. I was working on monoamine oxidase at the time. It was my first trip to India and his first to Bombay for several decades. We spent much time talking together, and by the end of it, as well as visiting temples, the Gateway of India, and the Elephanta Caves. Channi had persuaded me to carry out research on maternal mood in the perinatal period, the effects on the child, and the underlying biological mechanisms. This I have been doing ever since. Thus for me, like many others, Channi changed the direction of my career. His infectious enthusiasm, and very wide range of interests, have directed and inspired world research in perinatal psychiatry.

Introduction

There is now considerable evidence from both human and animal studies that the children of stressed, anxious, or depressed mothers are more likely to experience a range of neurodevelopmental problems than the children of unstressed mothers. (Glover 2011; O'Donnell et al. 2009; Talge et al. 2007; Van den Bergh et al. 2007,). With animal studies it is much easier to establish that these associations are causal. Newborn rat pups of prenatally stressed mothers can be cross-fostered to non-stressed mothers on the first day after birth, with control pups of unstressed mothers cross-fostered also. This can establish that any differences in outcome are caused by stress in the prenatal period. Many such studies have shown that there are definite fetal programming effects of prenatal stress on behaviour, cognitive development, the hypothalamuspituitaryadrenal (HPA) axis, and brain structure and function of the offspring (e.g. Henry et al. 1994; Weinstock 2001, 2008; Afadlal et al. 2010). The nature of the effects can be affected by the timing of the exposure in gestation, the type of the stress, the strain of the animal, the age at which the offspring was tested, and the sex of the offspring (Weinstock 2008), The effects of prenatal stress on the offspring can often be mimicked by giving the stress hormone corticosterone, or a synthetic glucocorticoid, to the pregnant animal (Matthews 2000; Afadlal *et al.* 2009).

Some of the effects of prenatal stress can also be moderated by the quality of the postnatal maternal care (Maccari *et al.* 1995; Del Cerro *et al.* 2010). Del Cerro and colleagues have shown that pregnant rats, stressed during the last week of gestation, also show less nurturing mothering behaviour themselves, relative to pregnant rats who were not stressed. In an elegant cross-fostering design, which included studying stressed offspring reared by non-stressed dams and non-stressed offspring reared by stressed dams, these authors showed that maternal care by a non-stressed mother could counteract the effects of the prenatal stress on the later mothering behaviour of the female offspring, although not the hormonal and neurological morphological alterations. They conclude that both prenatal stress and early mothering are important for the later behaviour and functioning of the female offspring, although the contribution of each differs with outcome.

In monkeys, some studies have nursery reared prenatally stressed and control infants together to control for postnatal or rearing effects. The offspring of prenatally stressed mother monkeys have been shown to have both increased anxiety and reduced attention span (Schneider *et al.* 2002), as well as changes in brain structure, including reduced hippocampal volume (Coe *et al.* 2003) and altered size of the corpus callosum (Coe *et al.* 2002) relative to the offspring of nonstressed mothers.

Research in humans

Although this type of research has been conducted in animals since the 1950s, it is relatively recently that similar research has been carried out in humans. The prospective human studies mostly date from the last 10 years. Almost all these studies have shown an association between maternal prenatal stress, anxiety, or depression and altered child behavioural, or cognitive outcome or function of the HPA axis (Glover *et al.* 2010). The animal findings concerning timing of exposures and different effects depending on the sex of the child have not yet been extended convincingly to humans, and more research is needed in this area. Some studies have examined large population cohorts such as the Avon Longitudinal Study of Parents and Children (ALSPAC) cohort in Bristol, UK, (e.g. O'Connor *et al.* 2002; Glover *et al.* 2004), and of necessity used maternal report. Others have been small observational studies, such as those of Van den Bergh and her colleagues (e.g. Van Den Bergh and Marcoen 2004), and that of Bergman and colleagues (e.g. Bergman *et al.* 2007).

A notable finding is the wide range of outcomes which have been found to be altered. Different studies have examined offspring at anytime from birth until adulthood. At birth, an increase in congenital malformations has been found to be associated with very severe stress in the first trimester, such as the death of an older child (Hansen *et al.* 2000). Many studies have shown that less severe stress is associated with somewhat lower birthweight and reduced gestational age (e.g. Rice *et al.* 2010; Wadhwa *et al.* 1993). Some investigators have looked at the newborns of mothers who report stress during pregnancy and found a poorer performance on the Neonatal Behavioral Assessment Scale relative to newborns of mothers who do not report stress during pregnancy (Diego *et al.* 2004) showing that adverse behavioural outcomes are observable from the very beginning. Studies of infants and toddlers have shown more difficult temperament (e.g Austin *et al.* 2005; Buitelaar *et al.* 2003) sleep problems (O'Connor *et al.* 2007), and lower cognitive performance and increased fearfulness (Bergman *et al.* 2007) associated with higher maternal stress during pregnancy.

Other studies have examined the association between prenatal stress and neurodevelopmental outcomes in children, age 3 to 16 years, rather than babies, infants or adults. Many independent groups have shown that prenatal stress is associated with increased child emotional problems, especially anxiety and depression, and symptoms of attention deficit hyperactivity disorder (ADHD) and conduct disorder (e.g. O'Connor *et al.* 2002, and 2003; Van Den Bergh and Marcoen 2004; Rodriguez and Bohlin, 2005; Huizink *et al.* 2007; Rice *et al.* 2010). Other studies have shown a reduction in cognitive performance (e.g. Laplante *et al.* 2008; Mennes *et al.* 2006) associated with prenatal stress.

Some studies have found an association between prenatal stress and increased risk of autism (Beversdorf *et al.* 2005; Kinney *et al.* 2008), although a large population study has failed to confirm this (Li *et al.* 2009). Two studies have found an increased risk of schizophrenia in adults born to mothers who experienced stress during pregnancy. Both showed effects with severe stress, the death of a relative (Khashan *et al.* 2008) or exposure to the invasion of the Netherlands in 1940 (van Os and Selten, 1998), and both showed that the sensitive period of exposure was during the first trimester. Prenatal stress has also been associated with specific regional reductions in brain grey matter density (Buss *et al.* 2010). Such altered grey matter may be associated with neurodevelopmental and psychiatric disorders as well as cognitive and intellectual impairment.

Several studies have shown that prenatal stress is associated with an altered diurnal pattern or altered function of the HPA axis, although the pattern of alteration is quite complex (Glover *et al.* 2010). A recent study has shown prenatal stress is associated with reduced telomere length (Entringer *et al.* 2011). This is an intriguing finding, as well as of concern, as reduced telomere length is associated with a reduced life span.

There is little consistency in the literature as to the most sensitive time in gestation for the influence of prenatal stress. It is likely that there are different times of sensitivity dependant on the outcome studied, and the stage of development of the relevant brain or other structures. The two studies of schizophrenia found the most sensitive period was in the first trimester (van Os andSelten, 1998; Khashan *et al.* 2008). This is when neuronal cells are migrating to their eventual site in brain, a process previously suggested to be disrupted in schizophrenia. Other studies have found the greatest associations between emotional or behavioural outcomes stress in later pregnancy (O'Connor *et al.* 2003; Rice *et al.*, 2010) although neither study suggests that late pregnancy is a significantly more sensitive period.

Many types of prenatal stress have been found to be associated with altered outcomes for the child. They vary from maternal anxiety (O'Connor *et al.* 2002; Austin *et al.* 2005; Mennes *et al.* 2006; Obel *et al.* 2003) and depression (O'Connor *et al.* 2002; Obel *et al.* 2003; Pawlby *et al.* 2011), pregnancy specific anxiety (Huizink *et al.* 2003), daily hassles (Huizink *et al.* 2003), bereavement (Khashan *et al.* 2008), life events, including a bad relationship with the partner (Bergman *et al.* 2007), to acute disasters such as exposure to a Canadian ice storm (Laplante *et al.* 2008), 9/11 (Yehuda *et al.* 2005), Chernobyl (Huizink *et al.* 2008), a Louisiana hurricane (Kinney *et al.* 2008), or war (van Os andSelten 1998). It is clear that it is not just a diagnosable mental illness or very extreme or 'toxic stress' that can alter outcome. Exposures which can have an effect vary from the very severe, such as the death of an older child to quite mild stresses, such as daily hassles. Stress is a generic term, which includes this wide range of different types of exposure. What these findings imply is that an effect of prenatal anxiety (or stress or depression) is not limited to those mothers with clinical impairment; indeed, almost all studies on the impact of prenatal anxiety have assessed non-clinical samples.

One study has shown an improvement in cognitive ability and motor development with mild prenatal stress (DiPietro *et al.* 2006). Laplante and colleagues (2008) showed a curvilinear relationship with prenatal stress and cognitive functioning. DiPietro *et al.* (2006) have suggested that there might be an inverted U-shaped doseresponse curve, with mild to moderate stress improving outcome in healthy populations. This is an interesting idea and deserves further investigation. In the studies with the ALSPAC cohort we found a linear dose response between prenatal maternal anxiety and emotional/behavioural outcomes for the child (O'Connor *et al.* 2002). It is possible that prenatal stress has different patterns and direction of effect on different outcomes. One issue of interest is whether some forms of stress have a greater effect than others, but little is yet known about this. Of course, anxiety and depression are quite strongly co-morbid and it is hard to disentangle the effects of the two. However, is possible that they can both affect outcome but in somewhat different ways. Barker *et al.* (2011) found that in both the prenatal and postnatal periods, maternal depression had a wider impact on different types of child maladjustment than maternal anxiety, which appeared more specific to internalizing difficulties in the child.

Is this association causal?

Many human studies, as discussed previously, have shown that there is an association between maternal stress during pregnancy and an altered outcome for the child. The evidence for this is very strong and has been shown in many independent prospective studies from around the world. What is harder to establish is that the association is causal. If a mother is stressed while she is pregnant she may well be stressed postnatally, and this could affect her parenting. There can be other associated, confounding factors, such as smoking or alcohol consumption, which may affect both behaviour and birthweight. There also could be genetic continuity. The mother may have certain genetic risk factors which make her more likely to become anxious or depressed and she may pass these on to her child, which in turn makes them more prone to emotional or behavioural problems.

The prenatal anxiety effect on child outcomes may be indirect, as several studies have shown that maternal stress during pregnancy is associated with altered outcomes at birth that may also predict behavioural and cognitive outcomes, especially reduced birthweight (e.g, Wadhwa *et al*. 1993; Rice *et al*. 2010). Many, but not all, studies reported in the literature account for confounds including birthweight, and continue to find a significant prenatal effect. Other studies have shown reduced scores on the Brazelton assessment (Field *et al*. 2002) and a more difficult temperament (Huizink *et al*. 2002) soon after birth. This is some evidence for prenatal, independent of postnatal, effects.

An interesting recent study by Rice and co-workers compared, in children born after *in vitro* fertilization, the association between prenatal stress (based on a retrospective report of a limited measure) and child outcome in those who were genetically related to the mother with those who were not (Rice *et al*. 2010). They showed that there was an association between maternal stress in pregnancy and child symptoms of ADHD and conduct disorder, and that the association with conduct disorder was apparent in the unrelated mothers. This gives strong support to the idea that the association between prenatal stress and child conduct disorder is independent of genetic factors. However, the fact that the increase in symptoms of ADHD was apparent only in those with related mothers does not conclusively rule out a prenatal environmental component. There may be a gene environment interaction. Prenatal stress may only have the effect of increasing symptoms of ADHD in the genetically vulnerable mother and child pairs. More research is needed to disentangle the role of genetic factors for all outcomes.

Another indication that the effects of prenatal stress are not just due to genetic continuity are the group of studies that have shown children of mothers exposed to acute disasters These have included a Canadian ice storm (Laplante *et al*. 2008), 9/11 (Yehuda *et al*. 2005), and Chernobyl (Huizink *et al*. 2008). With these 'natural or man made experiments', as for example in the ice storm study, the level of stress was objectively assessed, and the exposure has a specific onset. This reduces the confounding effects of pre-existing emotional problems and genetic continuity, and also postnatal emotional and parenting effects.

ALSPAC study

We have recently carried out further studies with the ALSPAC population cohort, using Strengths and Difficulties (SDQ) data from the children up to age 13 years (ODonnell *et al*. in press), trying to allow for a large range of potential confounding factors. These included postnatal maternal mood, and paternal pre and postnatal maternal mood, as well as an index of parenting. We still found that if a mother was in the top 15% for anxiety or depression prenatally, her child was at twice the risk for having a probable mental disorder at age 13 years (raised from about 6% to 12%). This is the first time that paternal pre- and postnatal mood has been included in such analyses. Including it made little difference to the overall findings, suggesting that genetics were not a major determinant of outcome.

We also compared the growth curves for three subscales of the SDQ (emotional problems, ADHD, and conduct disorder) divided by sex, and compared the pattern for children

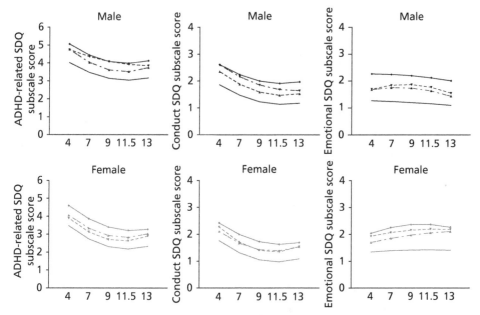

Fig. 17.1 Maternal anxiety and child Strengths and Difficulties scores (SDQ) across childhood.

Growth curve analysis describes SDQ subscores in four groups of children formed on the presence or absence of high maternal anxiety in the prenatal period (32 weeks gestation and at 33 months postpartum, for symptoms of ADHD, conduct disorder, and emotional problems in boys and girsl Low/Low (solid line) denotes low maternal anxiety at both timepoints, High/Low (triangles/semi-dashed line) denotes high prenatal anxiety only, Low/High (inverted triangles/dashed line) denotes high maternal anxiety at 33 months postpartum which High/High (diamond line) refers to children exposed to high levels of maternal anxiety at both assessments. Estimates are based on SDQ scores generated using growth curve analysis, controlling for birthweight, gestational age, substance use in pregnancy, maternal age, education, crowding as index of SES, parenting style, maternal depression at 8 weeks postnatal, maternal postnatal anxiety at 33 months, paternal prenatal anxiety, paternal postnatal depression at 8 weeks, and paternal postnatal anxiety at 33 months.

with mothers who were in the top 15% for anxiety prenatally but not postnatally, postnatally but not prenatally or both. The results are shown in Figure 17.1.

The curves show that the magnitude of the association between prenatal anxiety or postnatal anxiety and child outcomes were quite similar, and if the mother was in the top 15% for anxiety at both these times, the effects were additive. The curves using depression instead of anxiety were very similar. The magnitude of the associations between prenatal anxiety and child outcome were similar in boys and girls, although the trajectories of the curves were somewhat different for the three SDQ subscales and the two sexes.

Underlying mechanisms

A possible mediating factor is increased exposure of the fetus to cortisol. Glucocorticoids (cortisol in humans and primates, corticosterone in rodents) are known to have a range of effects on the developing fetus, including on the brain (Herbert *et al.* 2006; Buss *et al.* 2012). Whilst they are essential for fetal development and tissue maturation, overexposure of the fetus to glucocorticoids can have effects which predispose to ill health in later life (Harris and Seckl 2011). Fetal overexposure to glucocorticoids could occur through increases in maternal cortisol associated with anxiety and during periods of stress, which then crosses the placenta into the fetal environment. In animal models this has been shown to be one mechanism. Administration of adrenocorticotropic hormone (ACTH) to pregnant rhesus monkeys resulted in increased maternal cortisol production and adverse offspring neurodevelopmental outcomes, similar to those seen in response to prenatal stress (Schneider *et al.* 2002). The effects of prenatal stress in rats have been shown to be prevented by adrenalectomy and, at least for some outcomes, reinstated by corticosterone administration (Barbazanges *et al.* 1996). However, the human HPA axis functions differently in pregnancy from most animal models, because of the placental production of corticotrophin releasing hormone, which in turn causes an increase in maternal cortisol. The maternal HPA axis becomes gradually less responsive to stress as pregnancy progresses (Kammerer *et al.* 2002). And there is only a weak, if any, association between maternal mood and her cortisol level, especially later in pregnancy (Obel *et al.* 2005; Sarkar *et al.* 2006; O'Donnell *et al.* 2009). It thus seems unlikely that an increase in maternal cortisol is the primary mediating mechanism between prenatal maternal stress, anxiety, or depression in later pregnancy and altered fetal outcome.

However, fetal programming may be mediated by cortisol without increases in maternal levels. An alternative explanation is that stress or anxiety causes increased transplacental transfer of maternal cortisol to the fetal compartment. The placenta clearly plays a crucial role in moderating fetal exposure to maternal factors, and presumably in preparing the fetus for the environment in which it is going to find itself (O'Donnell *et al.* 2009). Thus, another mechanism by which the fetus could become overexposed to glucocorticoids is through changes in placental function, especially the enzyme 11β-hydroxysteroid dehydrogenase type II (11β-HSD2), the barrier enzyme that converts cortisol to the inactive cortisone. If there is less of this barrier enzyme then the fetus will be exposed to more maternal cortisol, independently of any change in the maternal cortisol level. There is some evidence in rat models that prenatal stress can affect placental 11β-HSD2. Restraining pregnant rats in a tube for short periods in the last week of pregnancy, a procedure they find stressful, has been shown to result in decreased placental 11β-HSD2 expression and activity (Mairesse *et al.* 2007). There is also evidence that reduced 11β-HSD2 causes an alteration in the behaviour of the offspring. (Welberg *et al.* 2000).

Indirect evidence in humans suggests that maternal anxiety may be associated with a decreased level of this enzyme. Glover and colleagues (Glover *et al.* 2009) reported that the correlation between maternal and amniotic fluid cortisol levels was greater in women with high anxiety compared to less anxious women, raising the possibility that prenatal anxiety in humans can increase the placental permeability to cortisol.

Our laboratory has recently found direct evidence that maternal prenatal anxiety and depression are associated with a downregulation of 11β-HSD2. Women were recruited the day before an elective caesarean and given self-rating psychometric questionnaires. The placentae were collected on delivery and the 11β-HSD2. mRNA expression and enzyme activity were measured. Higher levels of anxiety and depression were associated with less expression and enzyme activity (O'Donnell *et al.* 2012).

This provides direct evidence of an association between maternal mood in pregnancy and placental function. This adds further support to the fetal programming hypothesis, and that maternal mood in pregnancy may have a direct effect on fetal neurodevelopment.

Implications

These recent studies add to the evidence that there is a causal effect of prenatal anxiety or depression, which changes fetal neurodevelopment, in a way that persists into early adolescence, and is independent of the known effects of genetics and parenting. The implications are that improved emotional care of pregnant women should improve the emotional/behavioural outcome for their children to a clinically significant degree.

References

Afadlal, S., Polaboon, N., Surakul, P., Govitrapong, P., and Jutapakdeegul, N. (2010). Prenatal stress alters presynaptic marker proteins in the hippocampus of rat pups. Neuroscience Letters **470**(1): 24–7.

Austin, M. P., Hadzi-Pavlovic, D., Leader, L., Saint, K., and Parker, G. (2005). Maternal trait anxiety, depression and life event stress in pregnancy: relationships with infant temperament. Early Human Development **81**(2): 183–90.

Barbazanges, A., Piazza, P. V., Le Moal, M., and Maccari, S. (1996). Maternal glucocorticoid secretion mediates long-term effects of prenatal stress. Journal of Neuroscience **16**(12): 3943–9.

Barker, E.D., Jaffee, S.R., Uher, R., and Maughan, B. (2011). The contribution of prenatal and postnatal maternal anxiety and depression to child maladjustment. Depression and Anxiety **28**(8): 696–702.

Bergman, K., Sarkar, P., O'Connor, T. G., Modi, N., and Glover, V. (2007). Maternal stress during pregnancy predicts cognitive ability and fearfulness in infancy. Journal of the American Academy of Child and Adolescent Psychiatry **46**(11): 1454–1463.

Beversdorf, D.Q., Manning, S.E., Hillier, A., *et al.* (2005). Timing of prenatal stressors and autism. Journal of Autism and Developmental Disorders **35**(4): 471–8.

Buitelaar, J.K., Huizink, A.C., Mulder, E.J., de Medina, P.G., and Visser, G.H. (2003). Prenatal stress and cognitive development and temperament in infants. Neurobiology and Aging **24**(Suppl 1): S5360; discussion S67–58.

Buss, C., Davis, E.P., Muftuler, L.T., Head, K., and Sandman, C.A. (2010). High pregnancy anxiety during mid-gestation is associated with decreased gray matter density in 69-year-old children. Psychoneuroendocrinology **35**: 141–53

Buss, C., Davis, E.P., Shahbaba, B., *et al.* (2012). Maternal cortisol over the course of pregnancy and subsequent child amygdala and hippocampus volumes and affective problems Proceedings of the National Academy of Sciences of the U S A **109**(20): E1312–9.

Coe, C.L., Kramer, M., Czeh, B., *et al.* (2003). Prenatal stress diminishes neurogenesis in the dentate gyrus of juvenile rhesus monkeys. Biological Psychiatry **54**(10): 1025–34.

Coe, C.L., Lulbach, G.R., and Schneider, M.L. (2002). Prenatal disturbance alters the size of the corpus callosum in young monkeys. Developmental Psychobiology **41**(2): 178–85.

Del Cerro, M.C., Perez-Laso, C., Ortega, E., *et al.* (2010). Maternal care counteracts behavioral effects of prenatal environmental stress in female rats. Behavioral Brain Research **208**(2): 593–602.

Diego, M.A., Field, T., Hernandez-Reif, M., Cullen, C., Schanberg, S., and Kuhn, C. (2004). Prepartum, postpartum, and chronic depression effects on newborns. Psychiatry **67**(1): 63–80.

DiPietro, J.A., Novak, M.F., Costigan, K.A., Atella, L.D., and Reusing, S.P. (2006). Maternal psychological distress during pregnancy in relation to child development at age two. Childhod Development **77**(3): 573–87.

Entringer, S., Epel, E.S., Kumsta, R., *et al.* (2011). Stress exposure in intrauterine life is associated with shorter telomere length in young adulthood. Proceedings of the National Academy of Sciences of the U S A **108**(33): E513–8.

Field, T., Diego, M., Hernandez-Reif, M., *et al.* (2002). Prenatal anger effects on the fetus and neonate. J Obstetrics and Gynaecology **22**(3): 260–6.

Glover, V. (2011). Annual Research Review: Prenatal stress and the origins of psychopathology: an evolutionary perspective. Journal of Child Psychology and Psychiatry **52**(4): 356–67.

Glover, V., O'Connor, T.G., Heron, J., and Golding, J. (2004). Prenatal maternal anxiety is linked with atypical handedness in the child. Early Human Development **79**(2): 107–18.

Glover, V., Bergman, K., Sarkar, P., and O'Connor, T.G. (2009). Association between maternal and amniotic fluid cortisol is moderated by maternal anxiety. Psychoneuroendocrinology **34**(3): 430–5.

Glover, V., O'Connor, T.G., and O'Donnell, K. (2010). Prenatal stress and the programming of the HPA axis. Neuroscience and Biobehavioural Reviews **35**(1): 17–22.

Hansen, D., Lou, H. C., and Olsen, J. (2000). Serious life events and congenital malformations: a national study with complete follow-up. Lancet **356**(9233): 875–80.

Harris, A., and Seckl, J. (2011). Glucocorticoids, prenatal stress and the programming of disease. Hormones and Behavior **59**(3): 279–89.

Henry, C., Kabbaj, M., Simon, H., Le Moal, M., and Maccari, S. (1994). Prenatal stress increases the hypothalamo-pituitary-adrenal axis response in young and adult rats. Journal of Neuroendocrinology **6**(3): 341–45.

Herbert, J., Goodyer, I.M., Grossman, A.B., *et al.* (2006). Do corticosteroids damage the brain? Journal of Neuroendocrinology **18**(6): 393–411.

Huizink, A.C., Bartels, M., Rose, R.J., *et al.* (2008). Chernobyl exposure as stressor during pregnancy and hormone levels in adolescent offspring. Journal of Epidemiology and Community Health **62**(4): e5.

Huizink, A.C., de Medina, P.G., Mulder, E.J., Visser, G.H., and Buitelaar, J.K. (2002). Psychological measures of prenatal stress as predictors of infant temperament. Journal of the American Academy of Child and Adolescent Psychiatry **41**(9): 1078–85.

Huizink, A.C., Dick, D.M., Sihvola, E., *et al.* (2007). Chernobyl exposure as stressor during pregnancy and behaviour in adolescent offspring. Acta Psychiatrica Scandinavica **116**(6): 438–46.

Huizink, A.C., Robles de Medina, P.G., Mulder, E.J., Visser, G.H., and Buitelaar, J.K. (2003). Stress during pregnancy is associated with developmental outcome in infancy. Journal of Child Psychology and Psychiatry **44**(6): 810–18.

Kammerer, M., Adams, D., Castelberg Bv B., and Glover, V. (2002). Pregnant women become insensitive to cold stress. BMC Pregnancy and Childbirth **2**(1): 8.

Khashan, A.S., Abel, K.M., McNamee, R., *et al.* (2008). Higher risk of offspring schizophrenia following prenatal maternal exposure to severe adverse life events. Archives of General Psychiatry **65**(2): 146–52.

Kinney, D.K., Miller, A.M., Crowley, D.J., Huang, E., and Gerber, E. (2008). Autism prevalence following prenatal exposure to hurricanes and tropical storms in Louisiana. Journal of Autism and Developmental Disorders **38**(3): 481–88.

Laplante, D.P., Brunet, A., Schmitz, N., Ciampi, A., and King, S. (2008). Project Ice Storm: prenatal maternal stress affects cognitive and linguistic functioning in 5 1/2-year-old children. Journal of the American Academy of Child and Adolescent Psychiatry 47(9): 1063–72.

Li, J., Vestergaard, M., Obel, C., et al. (2009). A nationwide study on the risk of autism after prenatal stress exposure to maternal bereavement. Pediatrics 123(4): 1102–7.

Maccari, S., Piazza, P.V., Kabbaj, M., et al. (1995). Adoption reverses the long-term impairment in glucocorticoid feedback induced by prenatal stress. Journal of Neuroscience 15(1 Pt 1): 110–16.

Mairesse, J., Lesage, J., Breton, C., et al. (2007). Maternal stress alters endocrine function of the feto-placental unit in rats. American Journal of Physiology, Endocrinology and Metabolism 292(6): E1526–33.

Matthews, S.G. (2000). Prenatal glucocorticoids and programming of the developing CNS. Pediatrics Research 47(3): 291–300.

Mennes, M., Stiers, P., Lagae, L., and Van den Bergh, B. (2006). Long-term cognitive sequelae of prenatal maternal anxiety: involvement of the orbitofrontal cortex. Neuroscience and Biobehavioural Reviews 30(8): 1078–86.

O'Connor, T.G., Caprariello, P., Blackmore, E.R., et al. (2007). Prenatal mood disturbance predicts sleep problems in infancy and toddlerhood. Early Human Development 83(7): 451–458.

O'Connor, T.G., Heron, J., Golding, J., Beveridge, M., and Glover, V. (2002). Maternal prenatal anxiety and children's behavioural/emotional problems at 4 years. Report from the Avon Longitudinal Study of Parents and Children. British Journal of Psychiatry 180: 502–508.

O'Connor, T.G., Heron, J., Golding, J., and Glover, V. (2003). Maternal prenatal anxiety and behavioural/emotional problems in children: a test of a programming hypothesis. Journal of Child Psychology and Psychiatry 44(7): 1025–36.

O'Donnell, K., O'Connor, T.G., and Glover, V. (2009). Prenatal stress and neurodevelopment of the child: focus on the HPA axis and role of the placenta. Developmental Neuroscience 31(4): 285–92.

O'Donnell, K.J., Bugge Jensen, A., Freeman, L., et al. (2012). Maternal prenatal anxiety and downregulation of placental 11beta-HSD2. Psychoneuroendocrinology 37(6): 818–26.

O'Donnell, K.J., Glover, V., Barker, E.D., and OConnor, T.G. (in press). The persisting effect of maternal mood in pregnancy on childhood psychopathology. Development and Psychopathology, in press.

Obel, C., Hedegaard, M., Henriksen, T. B., Secher, N.J., and Olsen, J. (2003). Psychological factors in pregnancy and mixed-handedness in the offspring. Developmental Medicine and Child Neurology 45(8): 557–561.

Obel, C., Hedegaard, M., Henriksen, T.B., Secher, N.J., Olsen, J., and Levine, S. (2005). Stress and salivary cortisol during pregnancy. Psychoneuroendocrinology 30: 647–56

Pawlby, S., Hay, D., Sharp, D., Waters, C.S., and Pariante, C.M. (2011). Prenatal depression and offspring psychopathology: the influence of childhood maltreatment. British Journal of Psychiatry 199: 106–12.

Rice, F., Harold, G.T., Boivin, J., et al. (2010). The links between prenatal stress and offspring development and psychopathology: disentangling environmental and inherited influences. Psychological Medicine 40(2): 335–45.

Rodriguez, A., and Bohlin, G. (2005). Are maternal smoking and stress during pregnancy related to ADHD symptoms in children? Journal of Child Psychology and Psychiatry 46(3): 246–54.

Rodriguez, A., and Waldenstrom, U. (2008). Fetal origins of child non-right-handedness and mental health. Journal of Child Psychology and Psychiatry 49(9): 967–76.

Sarkar, P., Bergman, K., Fisk, N.M., and Glover, V. (2006). Maternal anxiety at amniocentesis and plasma cortisol. Prenatal Diagnosis 26(6): 505–9.

Schneider, M.L., Moore, C.F., Kraemer, G.W., Roberts, A.D., and DeJesus, O.T. (2002). The impact of prenatal stress, fetal alcohol exposure, or both on development: perspectives from a primate model. Psychoneuroendocrinology **27**(12): 285–98.

Talge, N.M., Neal, C., and Glover, V. (2007). Prenatal maternal stress and long-term effects on child neurodevelopment: how and why? Journal of Child Psychology and Psychiatry **48**(34): 245–61.

Van Den Bergh, B.R., and Marcoen, A. (2004). High prenatal maternal anxiety is related to ADHD symptoms, externalizing problems, and anxiety in 8- and 9-year-olds. Child Development **75**(4): 1085–97.

Van den Bergh, B.R., Mulder, E.J., Mennes, M., and Glover, V. (2005). Prenatal maternal anxiety and stress and the neurobehavioural development of the fetus and child: links and possible mechanisms. A review. Neuroscience and Biobehavioural Reviews **29**(2): 237–58.

van Os, J. and Selten, J. P. (1998). Prenatal exposure to maternal stress and subsequent schizophrenia. The May 1940 invasion of The Netherlands. British Journal of Psychiatry **172**: 324–6.

Wadhwa, P.D., Sandman, C.A., Porto, M., Dunkel-Schetter, C., and Garite, T.J. (1993). The association between prenatal stress and infant birth weight and gestational age at birth: a prospective investigation. American Journal of Obstetrics and Gynecology **169**(4): 858–65.

Weinstock, M. (2001). Alterations induced by gestational stress in brain morphology and behaviour of the offspring. Progress in Neurobiology **65**(5): 427–51.

Weinstock, M. (2008). The long-term behavioural consequences of prenatal stress. Neuroscience and Biobehavioural Reviews **32**(6): 1073–1086.

Welberg, L.A., Seckl, J.R., and Holmes, M.C. (2000). Inhibition of 11beta-hydroxysteroid dehydrogenase, the foeto-placental barrier to maternal glucocorticoids, permanently programs amygdala GR mRNA expression and anxiety-like behaviour in the offspring. European Journal of Neuroscience **12**(3): 1047–54.

Yehuda, R., Engel, S.M., Brand, S.R., *et al.* (2005). Transgenerational effects of posttraumatic stress disorder in babies of mothers exposed to the World Trade Center attacks during pregnancy. Journal of Clinical Endocrinology and Metabolism **90**(7): 4115–8.

Chapter 18

Postpartum psychosis—important clues to the aetiology of mood disorders

Ian Jones

Introduction

It is of great regret that although corresponding with him at the start of my research career, I never met Channi Kumar face to face. His work, however, as evidenced by this book, remains an important influence on our field. I share his belief in the 'maternal brain as a model for investigating mental illness' (Kumar 2001), and this conviction has underlined much of my research. In this chapter I will discuss the concept of postpartum psychosis (PP), explore what we know about the relationship of these episodes to other mood and psychotic disorders, and consider research strategies aimed at understanding the nature of the postpartum trigger. I will argue that the nosological confusion surrounding this condition has been unhelpful and that it is time, perhaps, to consider whether we should revive postpartum psychosis as a diagnostic concept.

What do we mean by the term 'postpartum psychosis'?

Episodes of mood disorder in relation to pregnancy and childbirth are very common. In our group we have recently examined the history of perinatal episodes in over 1,500 women with mood disorder who have participated in our genetic studies and find that approximately two thirds of parous women, with both bipolar and unipolar disorder, have experienced a significant mood episode in the perinatal period (Di Florio et al. 2013). PP refers to some of the most severe forms of postpartum psychiatric disorder. Although the boundaries of this condition are not easy to define, the core concept is the acute onset of a manic or affective psychosis in the immediate postpartum period. Depending on the definition employed, the incidence is approximately 1 in 1,000 deliveries (Jones et al. 2010).

Women may go from being very well to severely ill within hours. Affective (mood) symptoms, both elation and depression, are prominent, as is a disturbance of consciousness marked by an apparent confusion, bewilderment, or perplexity. As the name suggests, psychotic phenomena occur, with delusions and hallucinations prominent. Some women with severe manic episodes, but who do not show psychotic symptoms, may receive the diagnosis, although it is also possible to reserve the label for those women with frank psychotic presentations. Mixed episodes, in which manic and depressive symptoms occur simultaneously, are common, and the clinical picture often shows a constantly changing, 'kaleidoscopic', picture. The term refers to the new onset, although not necessarily the first episode, of a severe affective psychosis in the first couple of weeks following delivery. Accordingly, continuing symptoms of a chronic psychosis, such as schizophrenia, would not be appropriately labelled as PP.

PP should be considered a psychiatric emergency and, in the vast majority of cases, requires hospitalization. The latter point is particularly true because of the clinical picture often changing rapidly, with wide fluctuations in the intensity of symptoms and severe swings of mood. Women with PP can deteriorate very rapidly and services must respond quickly, factoring the fluctuating clinical picture into the assessment made.

Studies of PP are complicated by marked variations in inclusion criteria and definitions of the puerperal period. However, they demonstrate that the majority of PP episodes are affective, with mania particularly common in the 2 weeks following childbirth (Brockington 1996). An old, but interesting, study examined the symptoms experienced in 58 postpartum episodes compared to 52 episodes of non-puerperal psychotic illness occurring in women of childbearing age (Brockington *et al.* 1981). The study found that systematization of delusions, persecutory ideas, auditory hallucinations, odd affect, and social withdrawal were less common in the postpartum patients, whereas manic symptoms—elation, rambling speech, flight of ideas, lability of mood, distractibility, euphoria, and excessive activity—were all more frequent and severe. Similarly, studies from across the globe have consistently shown that the majority of cases of PP are within the bipolar spectrum, including bipolar I disorder, schizoaffective disorder, and major depressive disorder with psychotic features (Brockington *et al.* 1981; Dean and Kendell 1981; Katona 1982; Klompenhouwer and Van Hulst 1991; Meltzer and Kumar 1985; Kendell *et al.* 1987; Kumar *et al.* 1995; Robling *et al.* 2000).

Not all episodes, however, fit neatly into the mood disorder rubrics of the current diagnostic systems. There are clearly major issues with the classification of episodes that fit the classic concept of PP.

How are postpartum episodes treated by the classification systems?

In recent decades the concept of postpartum mood disorders has come under close scrutiny. It has been argued that: (i) episodes of non-psychotic depression are no more common following childbirth; (ii) the symptoms of postpartum depression are no different; and (iii) women with depression at this time respond to the same psychological and pharmacological treatments as do women with depression not related to childbirth. As we will see, these criticisms do not apply to the severe end of the postpartum mood disorder spectrum, but it is clear that for episodes of non-psychotic depression, childbirth is often considered a non-specific life event like any other. According to this view specific postpartum diagnostic categories are considered unnecessary and unhelpful. An approach which has led us to the unsatisfactory situation we face in both the International Classification of Diseases (ICD) and *Diagnostic and Statistical Manual* (DSM) classification systems, which many feel do not deal with the perinatal landscape in an optimal way.

Severe postpartum episodes of psychiatric disorder are subject to particular difficulties in the classification systems with a large number of diagnostic categories available to disorders that share more characteristics than for which they differ. PP was included in ICD-8, but its use was qualified by the instruction to only use this diagnosis when another category was not possible. The category disappeared in ICD-9 and -10, and was replaced by the ragbag category 'mental and behavioural disorders associated with the puerperium, not elsewhere classified'. This is available for episodes with onset within 6 weeks of delivery, and only if they do not meet the criteria for disorders classified elsewhere.

Turning to the DSM classification presents a similar picture. DSM-II included a category of PP but again carried the instruction to use only if 'all other possible diagnoses have been excluded'. By DSM-IV, although the category had disappeared, a 'postpartum onset specifier' was included in the mood disorders chapter for onsets within 4 weeks of delivery. In the DSM, therefore, episodes of PP are treated as mood disorders with a postpartum trigger. It is not possible, for example, to code a postpartum onset for a 'brief psychotic disorder'.

Despite the classification systems not recognizing PP as a separate nosological entity, the term postpartum or puerperal psychosis has remained in widespread clinical use and it is clear that the label has resonance with women who experience severe postpartum episodes—the key user group in the UK, for example, is known as Action on Postpartum Psychosis (www.app-network.org).

A woman with the abrupt onset of a severe postpartum psychiatric episode, with a mixture of affective and psychotic symptoms—the core concept of PP—may therefore receive (depending on the exact mix of her symptoms, the particular time she is assessed, or local diagnostic conventions) a range of diagnoses. This is clearly not the ideal situation and has undoubtedly led to difficulties in research on PP that relies on clinical diagnoses such as registry-based studies.

One issue is that the nature of PP, with prominent mood and psychotic symptoms, does not sit comfortably with the Kraeplinian dichotomy that has dominated psychiatric thinking for the last century. With research findings now suggesting a reappraisal of this dogma (Craddock and Owen 2005, 2010), this may have implications for the how PP is treated in future classification systems. I believe the nosological confusion causes problems in clinical practice and has hindered research into this important disorder, a theme I will return to later.

The link to childbirth

Although it has been argued that episodes of non-psychotic depression are not more common in the postpartum period, at the severe end of the spectrum there is little doubt that there is a greatly increased risk of episodes of postpartum psychosis. Clear evidence supports a specific relationship to childbirth for episodes of severe affective psychosis and for bipolar disorder, in particular (Jones and Craddock 2005).

In the 1980s, a landmark study of psychiatric admissions of women in Edinburgh showed that women are at a 23-fold increased risk of being admitted in the first postpartum month compared to other times in a woman's reproductive years (Kendell *et al.* 1987). More recently, great insights into the relationship of severe psychiatric episodes and childbirth have been gained by the studies of Trine Munk-Olsen and her colleagues in Denmark. In a large study of the Danish admission and birth registries that examined over 600,000 pregnancies and postpartum periods, women were over 23 times more likely to be admitted with an episode of bipolar disorder in the first postpartum month (relative risk (RR) 23.33, 95% confidence interval (CI) 11.52–47.24) (Munk-Olsen *et al.* 2006). A previous history of admission with bipolar disorder was associated with an even larger increased risk of admission following pregnancy (RR 37.22, 95% CI 13.58–102.4) (Munk-Olsen *et al.* 2009). Women with bipolar disorder have at least a 1 in 4 risk of suffering a severe recurrence following delivery (Di Florio *et al*, in press; Jones and Craddock 2001). Those with a previous history of a severe postpartum episode (postpartum/puerperal psychosis) and those with a family history of postpartum psychosis are at particularly high risk, with greater than 1 in 2 deliveries being affected (Jones and Craddock 2001; Robertson *et al.* 2005). Severe postpartum episodes have a close temporal relationship to childbirth. In a study from our group of 111 episodes of postpartum psychosis, 97% of women retrospectively reported the onset of symptoms within the first 2 weeks postpartum, with the majority being on days 1–3 (Heron *et al.* 2007).

The risk of admission in the postpartum period also appears to be raised in women with a history of schizophrenia, with Scandinavian register studies documenting increased postpartum admission rates (Munk-Olsen et al. 2006; Harlow *et al.* 2007). Indeed, one study from the Swedish register found 15% of women with a previous diagnosis of schizophrenia were admitted in the postpartum months (Harlow *et al.* 2007). However, the association with childbirth is not as dramatic as it is for bipolar disorder, neither does it have such a close temporal relationship to delivery. For bipolar disorder, the risk is for the new onset of an episode of severe affective psychosis. Women with schizophrenia may be admitted for other reasons, due to difficulties in parenting for example, or owing to the influence of more longstanding psychotic symptoms.

The Danish register studies have also found that women are at a higher risk of admission with a diagnosis of a unipolar major depression in the postpartum period (Munk-Olsen *et al.* 2006 *et al*, 2009), although again the increased risk is considerably lower than for bipolar disorder and extends over a longer period following childbirth. In addition, we have also recently demonstrated that an admission with unipolar major depression in the immediate postpartum is a marker of an increased risk for subsequent conversion to a bipolar disorder diagnosis (Munk-Olsen *et al.* 2011).

In summary, although the postpartum period may be a period of risk for women with a wide variety of psychiatric disorders, the data suggests that it is women with a history of bipolar disorder who are at a particularly high risk of a severe recurrence.

What causes postpartum psychosis?

Many episodes of PP may therefore represent an underlying bipolar disorder diathesis acted on by a specific puerperal trigger. An important goal of research is to understand the nature of this trigger, which will be of great benefit to women who become unwell at this time. It will enable us to target better existing treatments, allow for the development of novel treatments for PP based on an understanding of aetiology, and perhaps even enable the prevention of illness in those women at high risk. In addition, understanding the triggering of postpartum episodes may give important clues that will enable us to understand more about the aetiology of mood disorders in general. This is clearly and important question. What then, is currently known about the nature of the trigger?

Does PP result from changes in medication?

A plausible explanation of episodes occurring in relation to childbirth is that they result form the fact that, due to concerns over the reproductive safety of psychotropic medication, women often stop or change medication preconception or in early pregnancy. Although simple and intuitively appealing this explanation does not seem to stand up to close examination. Viguera and colleagues (2000) employed survival analysis to examine the course of illness in 42 women with previous bipolar episodes who stopped lithium due to pregnancy, compared to 59 age-matched non-pregnant lithium discontinuers. The study found that recurrence risks were very similar for both groups up to 40 weeks but following delivery the women who had delivered a baby were far more likely to experience an episode of illness (70% vs 24% recurrence). The increased risk of recurrence following childbirth for bipolar women is not, it appears, merely a result of women stopping mood stabilizing medication.

Are psychosocial or obstetric factors important?

Becoming a mother is a complex and often difficult psychosocial transition and this clearly plays a major role in many episodes of postnatal depression. It is a common belief, shared currently by the DSM and ICD classification systems, that childbirth acts as a general and non-specific psychosocial stressor like any other life event. However, psychosocial factors have not been shown to play a major role in determining vulnerability to *psychosis* in the puerperium. Four high risk studies that have examined this issue are consistent in finding no association between stressful life events and the occurrence of an episode following childbirth (McNeil 1988; Brockington *et al.* 1990; Dowlatshahi and Paykel 1990; Marks *et al.* 1991).

A further area that has received attention is the possibility that certain obstetric factors are associated with PP. Both obstetric complications and caesarean section rates have been found to be higher in some studies of women with PP. In a study from our group we compared affected and unaffected deliveries in over 50 women with PP and found that experiencing a complication during delivery more than doubled the risk of PP (Blackmore *et al.* 2006). Other factors which have been examined such as sex of the child, gestation of pregnancy have not been consistently supported as risk factors (McNeil and Blennow 1988; Videbech and Gouliaev 1995; Kirpinar *et al.* 1999).

What about hormones and sleep?

As we have seen, there is little evidence implicating psychosocial factors in the aetiology of PP. It is also clear that the majority of episodes have an abrupt onset in the first postpartum week, particularly on days 1 to 3 following delivery (Heron *et al.* 2007). This is a time of major physiological change and suggests that biological, possibly hormonal, factors may be of fundamental importance. The role of several hormones has been considered, but the sex steroids oestrogen and progesterone have perhaps received the greatest attention. It is also important to note that the peripartum is a time of major change in other hormonal systems such as the thyroid axis and the hypothalamus–pituitary–adrenal system.

One intriguing hormonal theory in the aetiology of postpartum psychosis comes from the work of Channi Kumar himself (Weick *et al.* 1991). The growth hormone response to the dopamine agonist apomorphine, was found to be enhanced 4 days following delivery in women at high risk who went on to experience a severe postpartum episode. These results suggest that the onset of affective psychosis after childbirth is associated with increased sensitivity of dopamine receptors in the hypothalamus, and possibly elsewhere in the brain, and that such changes may be triggered by the sharp fall in circulating oestrogen concentrations after delivery.

The studies that have examined a range of hormonal measures in women with postpartum affective episodes and controls have not demonstrated consistent hormonal differences (Hendrick *et al.* 1998; Bloch *et al.* 2003) and the evidence for the involvement of reproductive hormones in the aetiology of PP remains predominantly circumstantial. One study, however, provides more direct evidence for the involvement of oestrogen and progesterone in the puerperal triggering of affective symptoms. Bloch and colleagues (2000) simulated the very high gonadal steroid levels of pregnancy and the dramatic postpartum withdrawal in eight women with, and eight women without, a history of postpartum depression. They found that five of the eight women with a history of postpartum depression and none of the women in the comparison group developed significant mood symptoms during the withdrawal period.

It is unlikely, therefore, that women with postpartum mood disorders show gross abnormalities in endocrine physiology. The evidence more suggests that a vulnerability to postpartum triggering represents an abnormal response to the normal hormonal fluctuations of pregnancy and childbirth. As we will see below, it is likely that genetic factors play a role in determining this vulnerability.

Another plausible hypothesis that has remained surprisingly under-researched is that the sleep deprivation that is an almost universal feature of delivery and the immediate postpartum period is responsible for puerperal triggering of illness (Sharma and Mazmanian 2003; Sharma *et al.* 2004). More research in this area is clearly needed to differentiate sleep disturbance as an early symptom of an episode of illness from sleep disturbance as a trigger.

Parity

A potentially important clue to the aetiology of PP is the well-established effect of parity, with episodes being more common following first babies (Blackmore *et al.* 2006). In both register based (Kendell *et al.* 1981; Videbach and Gouliaev 1995) and clinical studies (Kirpinar *et al.* 1999; Thomas and Gordon 1959; Blackmore *et al.* 2006; Bergink *et al.* 2011) PP has been shown to be more common after first deliveries. An important bias is that women with a severe postpartum episode may be less likely to go on to have further children, but this is unlikely to be the main explanation (Kendell *et al.* 1987; McNeil 1988; Blackmore *et al.* 2006). Both biological and psychosocial factors may underpin the link between parity and severe mood disorders. First pregnancies are a greater psychosocial stressor than subsequent deliveries, but there are significant biological differences that may also play a role and which are candidates for further study.

The association with parity is an important clue to aetiology and points to links with other pregnancy related conditions such as pre-eclampsia (PE), which are also found more frequently in relationship to first pregnancies. There are a number of important overlaps in the clinical presentation and epidemiology of PP and PE. Associations between pre-eclampsia and mood episodes have been described (Cripe *et al.* 2011), and psychosis can be a dramatic feature of eclampsia (Brockington 2010). It is of interest that psychotic symptoms related to eclampsia are not merely sequelae of convulsions (i.e. post-ictal), but occur prior to this end-stage and are therefore thought to be part of the systemic effects of pre-eclampsia on the central nervous system. Whilst there are important differences between PE and PP (for example, PE is predominantly a condition of pregnancy while the onset of PP is usually in the first few postpartum days (Heron *et al.* 2007)), it is clear that PE is a heterogeneous condition—20% of women who develop eclampsia, for example, do not have proteinuria (Noraihan *et al.* 2005) and eclamptic seizures can infrequently occur 48 hours to 1 month postpartum, in which case the condition is described as late postpartum eclampsia (Santos *et al.* 2008). Interestingly, one-third or more of patients with postpartum eclampsia present without ever having manifested signs and symptoms of PE (Sibai *et al.* 2005). Studies of the potential overlap in aetiological factors between PE and PP is therefore a promising avenue for further research.

Do genetic factors play a role in vulnerability to the puerperal trigger?

A potentially fruitful avenue of research is the attempt to define genetic factors that influence risk of PP. The evidence from family studies suggests that vulnerability to affective disorders is increased in the relatives of women with puerperal psychosis (Jones and Craddock 2001). Moreover, studies have suggested that episodes of PP are a marker for a more familial form of bipolar disorder (Jones and Craddock 2002) and that a specific vulnerability to the puerperal triggering of bipolar illness is familial (Jones and Craddock 2001). Further support for the involvement of genetic factors comes from the report of familial clustering of puerperal psychotic episodes associated with consanguinity which raises the possibility of a recessive gene contributing to susceptibility (Craddock *et al.* 1994).

The relationship between genetic factors determining vulnerability to postpartum psychosis and those for bipolar disorder remain unclear. It is possible that one or more susceptibility genes for bipolar illness also lead to a vulnerability to puerperal triggering. Alternatively, the genetic factors influencing puerperal vulnerability may be completely distinct from those that determine the bipolar diathesis and act as course modifiers. It is likely that only when the genetic factors are found will the relationship be resolved.

Molecular genetic studies of PP are ongoing with linkage evidence pointing to a gene or genes for PP on the long arm of chromosome 16 (Jones *et al.* 2007). Although we have conducted a number of candidate gene studies of PP (Jones and Craddock; 2007) the main limitation of this approach is that our knowledge of the pathophysiology of psychiatric disorders remains limited and therefore potentially important biological pathways are unlikely to be tested. For psychiatric disorders, there are distinct advantages in approaches that are genome-wide and hypothesis free, and attention in the field has therefore turned to genome wide association studies (GWAS) as technological advances have made this approach tenable. It has also become clear that large samples are required in GWAS studies of psychiatric disorders to achieve the power required to identify genes of small to modest effect. In our group, we have been building up the sample of women with PP as part of the Bipolar Disorder Research Network study (www.bdrn.org), and in the coming years we will have samples making GWAS studies of PP realistic.

Conclusion—What is the status of postpartum psychosis?

As we have seen, the status of PP and its clinical boundaries remain subject to debate. There is a considerable amount of confusion in both clinical practice and research that I believe has been a significant impediment in understanding more about this condition.

There appears to be little reason to believe that PP is a condition in its own right separate from other diagnoses on the mood and psychosis spectrums. The literature pointing to a specific relationship to bipolar disorder is strong and compelling and it is clear that a majority of women experiencing episodes of PP will have a lifetime diagnosis of bipolar disorder or schizoaffective bipolar disorder. However, this is not the case for all women, and particularly for women who experience PP as a first episode of illness under the current diagnostic systems a variety of disorders may be diagnosed. This is clearly not optimal. Women with a severe postpartum episode—irrespective of lifetime diagnosis—are at considerable risk of recurrence following further pregnancies. An episode of postpartum psychosis therefore carries considerable prognostic implications. The introduction of a specific episode diagnosis of postpartum psychosis to ICD and DSM classification systems would go some way to address these issues. Despite decades of neglect postpartum psychosis as a diagnostic term refuses to go away, perhaps its time to bring it back.

References

Berginck, V., Lambregtse-van den Berg, M.P., Koorengevel, K.M., Kupka, R., and Kushner, S.A. (2011). First-onset psychosis occurring in the postpartum period: a prospective cohort study. Journal of Clinical Psychiatry **72**: 1531–7.

Blackmore, E., Jones, I., Doshi, M., *et al.* (2006). Obstetric factors associated with bipolar affective puerperal psychosis. British Journal of Psychiatry **188**: 32–6.

Bloch, M., Schmidt, P.J., Danaceau, M., *et al.* (2000). Effects of gonadal steroids in women with a history of postpartum depression. American Journal of Psychiatry **157**(6): 924–30.

Bloch, M., Daly, R.C., Rubinow, D.R. (2003). Endocrine factors in the etiology of postpartum depression. Comprehensive Psychiatry **44**(3): 234–46.

Brockington, I.F. (1996) Puerperal psychosis. In Motherhood and mental health. Oxford. Oxford University Press. pp. 200–84.

Brockington, I. (2010). *Eileithyia's Mischief.* Eyry Press, Bredenbury.

Brockington, I.F., Cernick, K.F., Schofield, E.M., *et al.* (1981). Puerperal psychosis: phenomena and diagnosis. Archives of General Psychiatry **38**: 829–33.

Brockington, I.F., Martin, C., Brown, G.W., Goldberg, D., and Margison, F. (1990). Stress and puerperal psychosis. British Journal of Psychiatry **157**: 331–4.

Craddock, N., Brockington, I., Mant, R., *et al.* (1994). Bipolar affective psychosis associated with consanguinity. British Journal of Psychiatry **164**: 359–64.

Craddock, N. and Owen, M.J. (2005). The beginning of the end for the Kraepelinian dichotomy. British Journal of Psychiatry **186**: 364–66.

Craddock, N. and Owen, M.J. (2010). The Kraepelinian dichotomy—going, going . . . but still not gone. British Journal of Psychiatry **196**(2): 92–5.

Cripe, S.M., Frederick, I.O., Qiu, C., and Williams, M.A. (2011) Risk of preterm delivery and hypertensive disorders of pregnancy in relation to maternal co-morbid mood and migraine disorders during pregnancy. Paediatrics and Perinatal Epidemiology **25**(2):116–23.

Dean, C. and Kendell, R.E. (1981). The symptomatology of puerperal illnesses. British Journal of Psychiatry **139**: 128–33.

Di Florio, A., Forty, L., Gordon-Smith, K., *et al.* (2012). Perinatal episodes across the mood disorder spectrum. JAMA Psychiatry **70**: 168–75.

Dowlatshahi, D. and Paykel, E.S. (1990). Life events and social stress in puerperal psychosis: absence of effect. Psychological Medicine **20**: 655–62.

Harlow, B.L., Vitonis, A.F., Sparen, P., *et al.* (2007). Incidence of hospitalization for postpartum psychotic and bipolar episodes in women with and without prior prepregnancy or prenatal psychiatric hospitalizations. Archives of General Psychiatry **64**: 42–8.

Hendrick, V., Altshuler, L.L., and Suri, R. (1998). Hormonal changes in the postpartum and implications for postpartum depression. Psychosomatics **39**(2): 93–101.

Heron, J., Robertson-Blackmore, E., McGuinness, M., Craddock, N., and Jones, I. (2007). No 'latent period' in the onset of bipolar affective puerperal psychosis. Archives of Womens Mental Health **10**: 79–81.

Jones, I. and Craddock, N. (2001). Familiality of the puerperal trigger in bipolar disorder: results of a family study. American Journal of Psychiatry **158**: 913–7.

Jones, I. and Craddock, N. (2002). Do puerperal psychotic episodes identify a more familial subtype of bipolar disorder? Results of a family history study. Psychiatric Genetics **12**: 177–80.

Jones, I. and Craddock, N. (2005).Bipolar disorder and childbirth: the importance of recognising risk. British Journal of Psychiatry **186**: 453–4.

Jones, I. and Craddock, N. (2007). Searching for the puerperal trigger: molecular genetic studies of bipolar affective puerperal psychosis. Psychopharmacology Bulletin **40**(2): 115–28.

Jones, I., Hamshere, M.L., Nangle, J.M., *et al.* (2007). Bipolar affective puerperal psychosis—genome-wide significant evidence for linkage to chromosome 16. American Journal of Psychiatry **164**(7): 1099–104.

Jones, I., Heron, J., and Robertson Blackmore, E. (2010). Puerperal psychosis. In The Oxford Text Book of Womens Mental Health, D. Kohen, editor. Oxford, Oxford University Press.

Katona, C.L. (1982). Puerperal mental illness: comparisons with non-puerperal controls. British Journal of Psychiatry **141**: 447–52.

Kendell, R.E., Rennie, D., Clarke, J.A., and Dean, C. (1981). The social and obstetric correlates of psychiatric admission in the puerperium. Psychological Medicine **11**(2): 341–50.

Kendell, R.E., Chalmers, J.C., and Platz, C. (1987). Epidemiology of puerperal psychoses. British Journal of Psychiatry **150**: 662–73.

Kirpinar, I., Coskun, I., Cayköylü, S., Anac, S., and Ozer, H. (1999). First-case postpartum psychosis in Eastern Turkey: a clinical case and follow-up study. Acta Psychiatrica Scandinavica **100**: 199–204.

Klompenhouwer, J.L. and van Hulst, A.M. (1991). Classification of postpartum psychosis: a study of 250 mother and baby admissions in The Netherlands. Acta Psychiatrica Scandinavica **84**(3): 255–61.

Kumar, R.C. (2001). The maternal brain as a model for investigating mental illness. Progress in Brain Research **133**: 333–8.

Kumar, R., Marks, M., Platz, C., and Yoshida, K. (1995). Clinical survey of a psychiatric mother and baby unit: characteristics of 100 consecutive admissions. Journal of Affective Disorders **33**(1): 11–22.

Marks, M.N., Wieck, A., Checkley, S.A., and Kumar, R. (1991). Life stress and postpartum psychosis: a preliminary report. British Journal of Psychiatry **158**: 45–9.

McNeil, T.F. and Blennow, G. (1988). A prospective study of postpartum psychoses in a high risk group. 6. Relationship to birth complications and neonatal abnormality. Acta Psychiatrica Scandinavica **78**: 478–84.

McNeil, T.F. (1988). A prospective study of postpartum psychoses in a high risk group. 4. Relationship to life situation and experience of pregnancy. Acta Psychiatrica Scandinavica **77**: 645–53.

Meltzer, E.S. and Kumar, R. (1985). Puerperal mental illness, clinical features and classification: a study of 142 mother-and-baby admissions. British Journal of Psychiatry **147**: 647–54.

Munk-Olsen, T., Laursen, T., Pedersen, C., Mors, O., and Mortensen, P. (2006). New parents and mental disorders: a population-based register study. JAMA **296**: 2582–9.

Munk-Olsen, T., Laursen, T.M., Mendelson, T., et al. (2009). Risks and predictors of readmission for a mental disorder during the postpartum period. Archives of General Psychiatry **66**(2): 189–95.

Munk-Olsen, T., Laursen, T.M., Meltzer-Brody, S., Mortensen, P.B., and Jones, I. (2011). Psychiatric disorders with postpartum onset: possible early manifestations of bipolar affective disorders. Archives of General Psychiatry **69**: 428–34.

Noraihan, M.N., Sharda, P., and Jammal, A.B. (2005). Report of 50 cases of eclampsia. Journal of Obstetrics and Gynaecology Research **31**: 302–9.

Robertson, E., Jones, I., Haque, S., Holder, R., and Craddock, N. (2005). Risk of puerperal and non-puerperal recurrence of illness following bipolar affective puerperal (post-partum) psychosis. British Journal of Psychiatry **186**: 258–9.

Robling, S.A., Paykel, E.S., Dunn, V.J., Abbott, R., and Katona, C. (2000). Long-term outcome of severe puerperal psychiatric illness: a 23 year follow-up study. Psychological Medicine **30**(6): 1263–71.

Santos, V.M., Correa F.G., Modesto, F.R., Moutella, P.R. (2008). Late-onset postpartum eclampsia: still a diagnostic dilemma? Hong Kong Medical Journal **14**(1): 60–3.

Sharma, V., Smith, A., and Khan, M. (2004). The relationship between duration of labour, time of delivery, and puerperal psychosis. Journal of Affective Disorders **83**(2–3): 215–20.

Sharma, V. and Mazmanian, D. (2003). Sleep loss and postpartum psychosis. Bipolar Disorders **5**(2): 98–105.

Sibai, B.M. (2005). Diagnosis, prevention, and management of eclampsia. Obstetrics and Gynecology **105**: 402–10.

Thomas, C.L. and Gordon, J.E. (1959). Psychosis after childbirth: ecological aspects of a single impact stress. American Journal of Medical Science **238**: 363–88.

Videbech, P. and Gouliaev, G. (1995). First admission with puerperal psychosis: 7–14 years of follow-up. Acta Psychiatrica Scandinavica **91**(3): 167–73.

Viguera, A.C., Nonacs, R., Cohen, L.S., *et al.* (2000). Risk of recurrence of bipolar disorder in pregnant and nonpregnant women after discontinuing lithium maintenance. American Journal of Psychiatry **157**: 179–84.

Wieck, A., Kumar, R., Hirst, A.D., *et al.* (1991). Increased sensitivity of dopamine receptors and recurrence of affective psychosis after childbirth. BMJ **303**(6803): 613–6.

Chapter 19

The biology of postpartum psychosis
A hypothetical model

Paola Dazzan

Introduction

I had the pleasure of meeting Channi Kumar as a junior psychiatry trainee at the Maudsley Hospital, when I elected to work in his clinical service as part of my rotation. It is therefore for me an honour to contribute to a book that celebrates his legacy. While working with him, I had the opportunity to seeing him in both the clinical and the academic settings. I came to know Channi as a gentle and charismatic clinician with patients, and an inspiring scientist. Channi was fascinated by the predictability of postpartum psychosis, which he used to discuss extensively with his patients, and he led seminal work on the biology of this disorder. I have been stimulated by this work and motivated to advance what remains a largely unexplored area of psychiatry. This chapter will discuss evidence on how biological factors relevant to the pathophysiology of psychoses and the perinatal period could interact in explaining the vulnerability and onset of postpartum psychosis. The role of genetic factors is extensively covered in Chapter 18, and will therefore not be discussed here.

The importance of postpartum psychosis

Psychiatric disorders contribute to 12% of all maternal deaths (UK Confidential Enquiry into Maternal Deaths; RCPG 2002), and puerperal (or postpartum) psychosis is the most severe psychiatric disorder associated with childbirth, with an estimated suicide rate of 2 per 1,000 sufferers (Oates 2003), and an incidence of 1–2/1,000 deliveries (Munk-Olsen et al. 2006). Although the last few decades have seen a fall in mortality and morbidity from childbirth, this has not been paralleled by a fall in the incidence of postpartum psychosis, which has remained remarkably stable at 0.5–1.0 per 1,000 deliveries (Munk-Olsen et al. 2006). Postpartum psychosis can have dramatic clinical and social consequences: child separation from the mother; lack of emotional bonding between mother and child; impaired child cognitive, physical, and psychological development; and, in some cases, suicide, infanticide, or both. This devastating impact is remarkable, especially considering that postpartum psychosis is highly predictable: in fact, between 30 and 50% of women with a history of bipolar affective disorder, or of schizoaffective disorder, will suffer postpartum psychosis after giving birth (Jones and Cradock 2001); and up to 50–70% of women with a previous history of postpartum psychosis (Jones and Craddock 2001).

Although postpartum psychosis occurs in concomitance with the biological changes of childbirth (most often within 6 weeks), there has been little research on the pathophysiology of this disorder, and its underlying neurobiology remains poorly understood. Therefore, studies evaluating gonadal and stress hormonal states, neurotransmitter activity, and functional imaging of frontal and mesolimbic areas in relation to the risk of postpartum psychosis, have been warranted in recent literature. For example, the 2007 perinatal mental health NICE guidelines highlighted the paucity of evidence available in this area. Moreover, a recent editorial by K. Wisner published in the *American Journal of Psychiatry* (;The last therapeutic orphan: the pregnant woman;) highlighted how:

> further advancement of the care for pregnant women with serious mental illness involves identification of the clinical, biological, and/or genetic characteristics of women who are at higher (and lower) risk for recurrence during pregnancy, to allow targeting of prophylactic treatment for the most vulnerable candidates (Wisner 1994).

The neurobiological basis of postpartum psychosis

Several clinical features make postpartum psychosis atypical compared to classical mania and other psychoses, including the rapid onset, the mood lability, and the unusual psychotic symptoms, often mood incongruent. Furthermore, compared to other psychotic disorders, women who suffer from postpartum psychosis usually have higher premorbid functioning and a lack of long-term impairment (Sit *et al.* 2006). In addition, the confusion, the cognitive disorganization, and the olfactory, visual and tactile hallucinations, that often accompany postpartum psychosis, make it more similar to an organic syndrome (Sit *et al.* 2006; Wisner *et al.* 1994). Therefore, identifying the biological mechanisms by which psychotic symptoms emerge after childbirth would help us understand which women are more at risk and could benefit from preventative interventions, and guide these interventions.

The role of reproductive hormones

Because of the chronological proximity to childbirth, the rapid decline of reproductive (estrogen and progesterone) steroid hormones concentrations that occurs after childbirth has long been thought to play a role in postpartum psychosis onset (Kumar *et al.* 1993). Steroid hormones enter the brain easily, and the concentrations of these hormones in the brain and the cerebrospinal fluid are highly correlated. Among reproductive hormones, estrogen may be particularly relevant. For example, at central level oestrogen seems to modulate the function of dopamine, a neurotransmitter thought to be crucial in the development of psychotic symptoms. Elevated oestrogen has been suggested to decrease the activity of tyrosine hydroxylase, a rate-limiting enzyme involved in dopamine synthesis (Blum *et al.* 1987). The reduction in synaptic dopamine could for example lead to a supersensitivity of dopamine (DA) 2 receptors, which could then be involved in the production of psychotic symptoms after delivery (Blum *et al.* 1987).

Although the hypothesis that levels of reproductive hormones may be lower after delivery in those women who develop postpartum psychosis has been an attractive one, studies that have evaluated the absolute levels of reproductive hormones in women with postpartum psychosis indicate that the levels of these hormones are similar to those of well-women (Wisner and Stowe 1997). On the basis of the oestrogen hypothesis, Channi conducted crucial experimental work, exploring the potential benefit that could derive from administering oestrogen to women at high risk of developing postpartum psychosis. However, his work suggests that oestrogen administration in the postpartum does not prevent postpartum psychosis (Kumar *et al.* 2003). On the basis of this evidence, it is reasonable to conclude that rapid changes in these hormones alone are not sufficient to explain the precipitous onset of this psychosis. Instead, it is possible that physiological changes in reproductive hormones act on an existing vulnerability in systems relevant to the pathogenesis of psychosis, such as the dopaminergic ones described above. To explore this model, Channi conducted an important study using apomorphine, a dopamine agonist (Wieck *et al.* 1991). The secretion of growth hormone following a small dose of this agonist has been considered an index of responsiveness of dopamine-sensitive neurons in the hypothalamus or elsewhere in the brain, possibly via stimulation of postsynaptic D2 receptors. In this study, women at risk of postpartum psychosis because of a history of bipolar or schizoaffective psychosis were given a subcutaneous injection of apomorphine on the fourth day postpartum, and the subsequent growth hormone secretion was measured. The results showed that the women who went on to develop an episode of postpartum psychosis were the ones who had shown greater growth hormone response to apomorphine. These findings further point to the presence of an increased sensitivity to dopaminergic stimulation in women who develop the disorder.

The role of stress hormones

Interestingly, gonadal steroids are also important regulators of the main stress response system, the hypothalamic–pituitary–adrenal (HPA) axis. The HPA axis is one of the main physiological systems involved in the neuroendocrine response to stress. In humans, the HPA axis follows a circadian rhythm with a peak in the secretion of the main hormone, cortisol, in the first hour after awakening (*awakening response*, considered a natural stressor), followed by a gradual decline during the course of the day. Changes in this rhythm have been described in several psychiatric conditions, including affective disorders and psychoses (Mondelli *et al.* 2010).

Changes in the HPA axis are also present in relation to inter-individual differences in response to stress, as well as in physiological conditions like pregnancy and the postpartum, when the HPA axis undergoes major changes. High levels of adrenocorticotropin (ACTH) and cortisol are seen in gestation, in response to rising levels of placental corticotropin-releasing hormone (CRH) (Magiakou *et al.* 1996). The abrupt withdrawal of placental CRH at birth then results in lower cortisol levels, with a re-equilibration of the maternal HPA axis in the days post-delivery (Magiakou *et al.* 1996). These major shifts in the regulation of the stress response have been thought to contribute to perinatal psychiatric disorders. For example, depression during pregnancy is associated with HPA axis hyperactivity, with cortisol hypersecretion in the evening, in a diurnal pattern similar to that of major depression (O'Keane *et al.* 2011). This is consistent with evidence that HPA hyperactivity is also present in psychoses independent from gestation. We have also shown that individuals at their very first episode of any psychosis have a blunted cortisol response to awakening, as well as higher levels of diurnal cortisol, indicating the presence of a hyperactivation of the HPA axis in psychosis (Mondelli *et al.* 2010). What is particularly interesting, when considering the HPA response in relation to risk for psychosis, is that subjects who experience attenuated psychotic symptoms show increased cortisol levels as well as increased pituitary and reduced hippocampal volumes (Aiello *et al.* 2012). Moreover, this HPA axis hyperactivity seems to be even greater among those individuals who subsequently develop frank psychosis. Relatives of individuals with psychosis also show increased sensitivity to stress, as suggested by increased emotional reactivity to daily life stress, increased ACTH in response to stress, increased pituitary volume, and reduced hippocampal volume. An enhanced HPA axis response to stress thus appears to be part of the biological vulnerability to psychosis, present prior to the onset of psychosis.

Studies that have evaluated the HPA axis in relation to pregnancy and childbirth have not focused on women at risk of postpartum psychosis, but rather on stress responsivity in the postpartum. One of these studies has found that the maternal awakening cortisol response in late pregnancy is negatively predictive of cortisol response and ACTH to an acute psychosocial stress in the 8th week postpartum (Meinlschmidt *et al.* 2010). These data suggest that differences in HPA activity in pregnancy are indicative of responsiveness to stress in the postpartum, leaving open the question of whether processes related to this response may be related to the onset of postpartum psychiatric disorders. Although what underlies differences in HPA activation in pregnancy remains unclear, the experience of early trauma is a strong candidate factor (Mondelli *et al.* 2010). For example, Brand and colleagues (2010) found that women with a history of early life trauma had altered HPA response to stress at 6 month postpartum. Maternal stress maladaptations may therefore represent factors relevant to the pathophysiology of not only affective disorders, but also of psychoses starting soon after childbirth.

Increased peripheral inflammation is associated with psychoses

Other important biological factors that play a role in the postpartum period are inflammatory biomarkers, such as pro-inflammatory cytokines. These are crucially involved in the mechanisms of parturition, and tend to be higher during pregnancy (Curry *et al.* 2008). Interestingly, the stress response discussed in the previous section is typically associated with an activation of the immune system, at least acutely, with increases of circulating markers such as pro-inflammatory cytokines. The postpartum period is in fact a time of immune activation, as indicated also by evidence that inflammatory diseases like rheumatoid arthritis or multiple sclerosis may have re-exacerbation or even first onset at this time (Haupl *et al.* 2008; Hellwig *et al.* 2009; Bergink *et al.* 2011).

More specifically to psychiatric disorders, there is evidence that depressive symptoms in the context of chronic psychosocial stress increase inflammation during pregnancy (Coussons-Read *et al.* 2007). This is of note, since an increase in inflammatory markers has long been implicated in both affective and non-affective psychoses. For example, patients with a first episode of any psychosis have higher interleukin (IL)-1α, IL-1β, IL-8, tumour necrosis factor-α, and IL-6, paralleling the increase in cortisol levels (Mondelli *et al.* 2011). Recent data also provide evidence of immune activation in women with postpartum psychosis (Bergink *et al.* 2012; Weigelt *et al.* 2013). For example, women with postpartum psychosis have been found to lack the normal postpartum T cell elevation, but to have a significant elevation of monocyte levels and a significant upregulation of several immune-related monocyte genes, when compared with control subjects postpartum and non-postpartum. More specifically, microRNAs which regulate immune activation genes have been found to be differentially expressed in monocytes of postpartum patients and healthy women. This evidence converges in suggesting the presence of an inflammatory state in postpartum psychosis, similarly to what seen in other psychoses.

Among factors potentially responsible for the hyperactivation of the stress and immune response discussed in the previous sections, good candidates would be personal adversity and trauma (Mondelli *et al.* 2010). Severe trauma, like childhood sexual and physical abuse, separation from parents and domestic violence in adulthood (Howard *et al.* 2010) may all shape response to stress. Furthermore, these factors have been suggested to increase the risk of psychoses non related to childbirth, with a particularly strong link in women (Howard *et al.* 2010; Fisher *et al.* 2009). Surprisingly, while these factors have been extensively studied in the context of postpartum depression (Fisher *et al.* 2009), the same cannot be said for postpartum psychosis (Trevillion *et al.* 2012).

Brain vulnerability and neuroplasticity

Although the number of neuroimaging studies conducted in psychoses not related to childbirth has grown enormously over the last few decades, there is no neuroimaging study in women with postpartum psychosis. Therefore, to study brain vulnerability to this condition, one has to look at evidence derived from other at-risk and psychotic groups. Studies conducted in these other groups suggest two non-mutually exclusive pathways that may lead to structural and functional brain alterations in psychosis: an existing brain structural vulnerability to developing the illness, and a decreased neuroplasticity due to the cortisol and inflammatory hyperactivity associated with psychosis.

Neuroimaging studies in affective and non-affective psychoses have consistently shown that, even at first episode, psychoses are associated with abnormalities of brain structure (Mourao-Miranda *et al.* 2012). Interestingly, psychoses in the affective spectrum—that is, with a clinical picture more similar to that seen in postpartum psychosis—have been particularly associated with changes in areas involved in emotional regulation, such as the amygdala and the subgenual cingulate cortex (Morgan *et al.* 2007). These changes have been considered to represent vulnerability markers, and as such they precede the onset of psychosis (Dazzan *et al.* 2011; McDonald *et al.* 2004). For example, both individuals at-risk who subsequently develop schizophrenia or an affective type of psychosis, show smaller cortical volumes than at-risk subjects who do not develop psychosis (Dazzan *et al.* 2011). In addition, these subjects seem to have further reductions, depending on the type of psychosis they subsequently develop. For example, the subgroup that goes on to develop an affective psychosis has significantly smaller subgenual cingulate volumes. This suggests that there are volumetric abnormalities in high-risk individuals, and that some of these may be specific to the nature of the subsequent disorder (Dazzan *et al.* 2011).

On the wave of evidence that psychosis is associated with an increase in peripheral inflammatory markers, attention has moved to estimating *in-vivo* the role of inflammatory processes as potentially involved in the brain structural and functional changes seen in psychosis. In fact, both proinflammatory cytokines and HPA axis have been reported to affect neurotrophic factors, such as brain-derived neurotrophic factor (BDNF), and to influence neurogenesis in areas relevant to psychosis such as the hippocampus (Zunszain *et al.* 2011). Consistently with this model, in patients with first episode psychosis, higher IL-6 and cortisol levels, together with low levels of BDNF, explain more than 70% of the smaller hippocampal volume found with magnetic resonance imaging at psychosis onset (Mondelli *et al.* 2011). Also, experimentally-induced inflammation has been associated with changes in brain function, including increased activity of amygdala and anterior cingulate cortex, especially in response to emotionally-salient faces in functional MRI experiments (Harrison *et al.* 2009). These changes correlate with changes in peripheral IL-6, suggesting that concomitant central and peripheral processes occur when the immune response is activated (Harrsion *et al.* 2009). This is interesting since the same neural changes during emotion recognition have been found in individuals at risk of affective and non-affective psychoses (Modinos *et al.* 2012), and with postpartum depression (Moses-Kolko *et al.* 2010).

Finally, as well as grey matter structure and neural function, inflammatory processes can affect white matter, as a consequence of microglia activation. Abnormalities in myelin, the main white matter constituent, are often found in neurological diseases with evidence of inflammatory infiltration and microglial activations that lead to aberrant cell development, cytotoxicity and oligodendrocytes loss (Schmitz and Chew 2008). Consistently with this, two studies have shown evidence of microglia activation in patients with schizophrenia (van Berckel *et al.* 2008; Doorduin *et al.* 2009). This is particularly important since demyelinating diseases may present with affective and psychotic symptoms, and since white matter disconnectivity has been proposed as one of the main alteration of both affective and non-affective psychotic disorders, and of risk for these disorders (Carletti *et al.* 2012; Walterfang *et al.* 2008).

Understanding the neurobiology of postpartum psychosis

Current evidence on biological factors that increase the risk for other psychiatric disorders can be very informative for our understanding of the pathophysiology of postpartum psychosis. There is enough evidence that genetic factors, reproductive and stress hormones, together with an underlying brain vulnerability, play an important role in the onset of postpartum psychosis. However, as for other psychiatric disorders, it is clear that studying a single biological system will not be sufficient to characterize the neurobiological substrate of this disorder. Instead, studying multiple biological systems and integrating knowledge from both postpartum physiology and the pathophysiology of psychoses, can truly advance our understanding of this devastating, yet highly predictable, perinatal disorder and move forward to more individualized intervention strategies.

References

Aiello, G., Horowitz, M., Hepgul, N., Pariante, C.M and Mondelli, V. (2012). Stress abnormalities in individuals at risk for psychosis: A review of studies in subjects with familial risk or with 'at risk' mental state. Psychoneuroendocrinology 37: 1600–13.

Bergink, V., Burgerhout, K.M., Weigelt, K., *et al.* (2012). Immune system dysregulation in first-onset postpartum psychosis. Biological Psychiatry 73: 1000–7.

Bergink, V., Kushner, S.A., Pop, V., *et al.* (2011). Prevalence of autoimmune thyroid dysfunction in postpartum psychosis. The British Journal of Psychiatry 198: 264–8.

Blum, M., McEwen, B.S., and Roberts, J.L. (1987). Transcriptional analysis of tyrosine hydroxylase gene expression in the tuberoinfundibular dopaminergic neurons of the rat arcuate nucleus after estrogen treatment. The Journal of Biological Chemistry 262: 817–1.

Brand, S.R., Brennan, P.A., Newport, D.J., *et al.* (2010). The impact of maternal childhood abuse on maternal and infant HPA axis function in the postpartum period. Psychoneuroendocrinology 35: 686–93.

Carletti, F., Woolley, J.B., Bhattacharyya, S., *et al.* (2012). Alterations in white matter evident before the onset of psychosis. Schizophrenia Bulletin 38: 1170–9.

Coussons-Read, M.E., Okun, M.L., and Nettles, C.D. (2007). Psychosocial stress increases inflammatory markers and alters cytokine production across pregnancy. Brain Behavior and Immunity 21: 343–50.

Curry, A.E., Vogel, I., Skogstrand, K., *et al.* (2008). Maternal plasma cytokines in early- and mid-gestation of normal human pregnancy and their association with maternal factors. Journal of Reproductive Immunology 77: 152–60.

Dazzan, P., Soulsby, B., Mechelli, A., *et al.* (2011). Volumetric abnormalities predating the onset of schizophrenia and affective psychoses: An MRI study in subjects at ultrahigh risk of psychosis. Schizophrenia Bulletin 38: 1083–91.

Doorduin, J., de Vries, E.F., Willemsen, A.T., *et al.* (2009). Neuroinflammation in schizophrenia-related psychosis: a PET study. Journal of Nuclear Medicine 50: 1801–7.

Fisher, H., Morgan, C., Dazzan, P., *et al.* (2009). Gender differences in the association between childhood abuse and psychosis. British Journal of Psychiatry 194: 319–25.

Harrison, N.A., Brydon, L., Walker, C., *et al.* (2009). Inflammation causes mood changes through alterations in subgenual cingulate activity and mesolimbic connectivity. Biological Psychiatry 66: 407–14.

Haupl, T., Ostensen, M., Grutzkau, A., *et al.* (2008). Reactivation of rheumatoid arthritis after pregnancy: increased phagocyte and recurring lymphocyte gene activity. Arthritis and Rheumatism 58: 2981–92.

Hellwig, K., Beste, C., Schimrigk, S., and Chan, A. (2009). Immunomodulation and postpartum relapses in patients with multiple sclerosis. Advances in Neurological Disorders 2: 7–11.

Howard, L.M., Trevillion, K., Khalifeh, H., *et al.* (2010). Domestic violence and severe psychiatric disorders: prevalence and interventions. Psychological Medicine **40**: 881–93.

Jones, I. and Craddock, N. (2001). Familiality of the puerperal trigger in bipolar disorder: results of a family study. American Journal of Psychiatry **158**: 913–17.

Kumar, R., Marks, M., Wieck, A., *et al.* (1993). Neuroendocrine and psychosocial mechanisms in postpartum psychosis. Progress in Neuropsychopharmacology and Biological Psychiatry **17**: 571–9.

Kumar, C., McIvor, R.J., Davies, T., *et al.* (2003). Estrogen administration does not reduce the rate of recurrence of affective psychosis after childbirth. Journal of Clinical Psychiatry **64**: 112–18.

Magiakou, M.A., Mastorakos, G., Rabin, D., *et al.* Hypothalamic corticotropin-releasing hormone suppression during the postpartum period: implications for the increase in psychiatric manifestations at this time. Journal of Clinical Endocrinology and Metabolism **81**: 1912 1 –17.

McDonald, C., Bullmore, E.T., Sham, P.C., *et al.* (2004). Association of genetic risks for schizophrenia and bipolar disorder with specific and generic brain structural endophenotypes. Archives of General Psychiatry **61**: 974–84.

Meinlschmidt, G., Martin, C., Neumann, I.D., and Heinrichs, M. (2010). Maternal cortisol in late pregnancy and hypothalamic-pituitary-adrenal reactivity to psychosocial stress postpartum in women. Stress **13**: 163–71.

Modinos, G., Pettersson-Yeo, W., Allen, P., *et al.* (2012). Multivariate pattern classification reveals differential brain activation during emotional processing in individuals with psychosis proneness. Neuroimage **59**: 3033–41.

Mondelli, V., Dazzan, P., Hepgul, N., *et al.* (2010). Abnormal cortisol levels during the day and cortisol awakening response in first-episode psychosis: the role of stress and of antipsychotic treatment. Schizophrenia Research **116**: 234–42.

Mondelli, V., Cattaneo, A., Murri, M.B., *et al.* (2011). Stress and inflammation reduce brain-derived neurotrophic factor expression in first-episode psychosis: a pathway to smaller hippocampal volume. Journal of Clinical Psychiatry **72**: 1677–84.

Morgan, K.D., Dazzan, P., Orr, K.G., *et al.* (2007). Grey matter abnormalities in first-episode schizophrenia and affective psychosis. British Journal of Psychiatry Supplement **51**: s111–s116.

Moses-Kolko, E.L., Perlman, S.B., Wisner, K.L., *et al.* (2010). Abnormally reduced dorsomedial prefrontal cortical activity and effective connectivity with amygdala in response to negative emotional faces in postpartum depression. American Journal of Psychiatry **167**: 1373–80.

Mourao-Miranda, J., Reinders, A.A.T.S. Rocha-Rego, V., *et al.* (2012). Individualized prediction of illness course at the first psychotic episode: a support vector machine MRI study. Psychological Medicine **42**: 1037–47.

Munk-Olsen, T., Laursen, T.M., Pedersen, C.B., Mors, O., and Mortensen, P.B. (2006). New parents and mental disorders: a population-based register study. JAMA **296**: 2582–9.

Oates, M. (2003). Suicide: the leading cause of maternal death. British Journal of Psychiatry **183**: 279–81.

O'Keane, V., Lightman, S., Marsh, M., *et al.* (2011). Increased pituitary-adrenal activation and shortened gestation in a sample of depressed pregnant women: a pilot study. Journal of Affective Disorders **130**: 300–5.

Plaza, A., Garcia-Esteve, L., Torres, A., *et al.* (2012). Childhood physical abuse as a common risk factor for depression and thyroid dysfunction in the earlier postpartum. Psychiatry Research **200**: 329–35.

RCOG (2002).The Confidential Enquiries into Maternal Deaths in the United Kingdom. Why mothers die: 2000–2002 report. London, royal College of Obstetricians and Gynaecologists Press.

Schmitz, T. and Chew, L.J. (2008). Cytokines and myelination in the central nervous system. ScientificWorldJournal **8**: 1119–47.

Sit, D., Rothschild, A.J., and Wisner, K.L. (2006). A review of postpartum psychosis. Journal of Womens Health (Larchmt) **15**: 352–68.

Trevillion, K., Oram, S., Feder, G., and Howard, L.M. (2012). Experiences of domestic violence and mental disorders: a systematic review and meta-analysis. PLoS One 7: e51740.

van Berckel, B.N., Bossong, M.G., Boellaard, R., *et al.* (2008). Microglia activation in recent-onset schizophrenia: a quantitative (R)-[11C]PK11195 positron emission tomography study. Biologocal Psychiatry **64**: 820–22.

Walterfang, M., McGuire, P.K., Yung, A.R., *et al.* (2008). White matter volume changes in people who develop psychosis. British Journal of Psychiatry **193**: 210–15.

Weigelt, K., Bergink, V., Burgerhout, K.M., *et al.* (2013). Down-regulation of inflammation-protective microRNAs 146a and 212 in monocytes of patients with postpartum psychosis. Brain Behavior and Immunology **29**: 147–55.

Wieck A, Kumar R, Hirst A D, Marks M N, Campbell I C, Checkley S A. Increased sensitivity of dopamine receptors and recurrence of affective psychosis after childbirth. BMJ, 1991; **303**: 613–616.

Wisner K L, Peindl K, Hanusa B H. Symptomatology of affective and psychotic illnesses related to childbearing. J Affect Disord, 1994; **30**: 77–87

Wisner K L, Stowe Z N. Psychobiology of postpartum mood disorders. Semin Reprod Endocrinol, 1997; **15**: 77–89.

Wisner K L. The last therapeutic orphan: the pregnant woman. The American journal of psychiatry, 2012; **169**: 554–556.

Zunszain P A, Anacker C, Cattaneo A, Carvalho L A, Pariante C M. Glucocorticoids, cytokines and brain abnormalities in depression. Prog Neuropsychopharmacol Bol Psychiatry, 2011; **35**: 722–729.

Safeguarding mothers and children: the ongoing debate

Chapter 20

Psychiatric causes of maternal deaths

Lessons from the Confidential Enquiries into Maternal Deaths

Margaret R. Oates

Introduction

The UK Confidential Enquiries into Maternal Deaths, published triennially, are over 50 years old (see Figure 20.1). Its forebears are even older; enquiries into maternal deaths began early in the 19th century in Scotland. In the 20th century the numbers of women dying from childbirth has steadily declined, influenced by many factors, including improved public health and maternity care, smaller family size, blood transfusions, and antibiotics, to name but a few. The introduction of the Abortion Act in 1967 was followed by a marked reduction of deaths in pregnancy from the consequences of illegal abortion. The rate and causes of maternal death have always been influenced by changes in reproductive epidemiology and technology, and continue to be so.

Maternal deaths in pregnancy and in the 6 weeks following delivery are required to be reported to the Coroner, if directly related to childbirth. However, there are other causes of maternal death due to conditions exacerbated by pregnancy: for example, diabetes, cardiac disease, epilepsy. These are referred to as indirect deaths. Women who die from conditions unrelated to pregnancy or childbirth are counted and described as coincidental deaths.

Over the years as the direct causes of maternal death have fallen, the indirect causes of maternal death have achieved more prominence and case ascertainment has improved.

Improvements in medical care and in particular intensive care have resulted in some women developing their fatal condition within 6 weeks of childbirth, only to die beyond it. For this reason, the UK Enquiry extended their period of surveillance beyond 6 weeks to include late maternal deaths, both a small number of late direct deaths and a larger number of late indirect deaths.

Suicide in pregnancy and following delivery has always been included in the Enquiries. However, prior to 1994 the cases were not separately analysed and were included in the group of late Coincidental Deaths (i.e. not thought to be related to pregnancy or childbirth).

The 1994–1996 Enquiry, under the Directorship and Editorship of Dr Gwyneth Lewis and Professor James O'Drife, heralded a change in presentation of the Enquiry. The

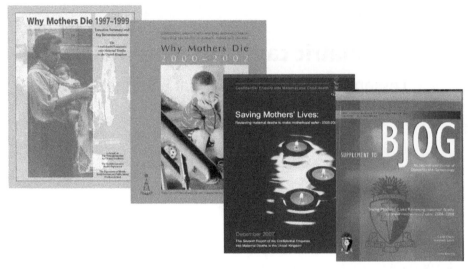

Fig. 20.1 UK Maternal Death Enquiries publications 1997–2008.

Directors realized that a significant number of maternal deaths were due to suicide and other psychiatric causes. They felt that childbirth was a significant aetiological factor in the deaths of the majority of women who killed themselves and that maternal suicide should be more properly classified as an indirect cause of maternal death. These cases were sufficiently numerous to be separately analysed and described. A perinatal psychiatrist joined the panel of assessors of maternal deaths. Psychiatric causes of maternal deaths from that time have been separately analysed and described in Chapter 11, Psychiatric Causes of Maternal Death, of the triennial publication of the Enquiry. Channi Kumar was the first perinatal psychiatrist to be involved in the Enquiry from 1994–1996. Margaret Oates took over this role for the 1997–1999, and subsequent, Enquiries.

Case ascertainment relies upon the reporting of maternal deaths to regional offices and regional assessors by midwives, obstetricians, primary care professionals, and coroners. Since the 1997–1999 Enquiry, this case ascertainment has been augmented in England by an Office of National Statistics Linkage Study, which links all deaths of women with all births. This has resulted in an increase in the numbers of maternal deaths detected mostly of indirect deaths and in particular deaths from psychiatric causes. This led to the finding that maternal suicide is commoner than previously thought and that the majority of deaths from psychiatric causes occur after 42 days (i.e. are late indirect rather than early indirect deaths).

The UK Maternal Deaths Enquiry combines both maternal deaths surveillance and Enquiry into individual deaths. The maternal mortality statistics including quantitative variables such as maternal social class, age, cause of death and other obstetric variables together. The quantitative aspect of the Maternal Deaths Enquiry is internationally distinctive because of the very high levels of case ascertainment and the inclusion and scrutiny of indirect causes of maternal death as well as late causes of maternal death.

It is, however, the qualitative component of the Enquiry that makes the UK study truly distinctive. To quote the World Health Organization (WHO) it goes 'beyond the numbers'. It is sentinel event reporting. Maternal death is mercifully rare, and within this rare event psychiatric causes of maternal death rarer still. The observation and description of individual cases with the publication of illustrative case vignettes tells stories from which clinicians learn. The findings of the Maternal Deaths Enquiries have a major impact on clinical practice. Individual providers of maternity care have an obligation to implement the findings and recommendations. The Enquiry generates hypotheses and future research and has resulted in a number of clinical guidelines produced by the Royal College of Obstetricians and Gynaecologists, with demonstrable effect on both mortality and morbidity from individual causes. Anonymity of the women, professionals, and services involved is maintained throughout the assessment and publication process, which promotes free reporting of deaths and acceptance of findings.

There are, however, limitations to the methodology, and therefore the findings of the Maternal Deaths Enquiry, which has attracted criticism. These include generalizing the findings of very small numbers of deaths. We know little about the women who share the same characteristics, but who survive. We also suffer from a lack of accurate denominator data. Judgements about the quality of care that the woman who died are made knowing the outcome, which may influence the opinion of the assessor. Criticisms of the Enquiry have been made about the undue harshness of the views of assessors and the lack of standardized criteria against which they make their judgements.

The maternal mortality rate uses the number of deaths from 22 weeks of pregnancy to 42 days postpartum. The maternal mortality ratio uses the number of deaths following delivery of more than 24 weeks of gestation to 42 days postpartum. The International Classification of Diseases-10 (ICD-10), 'pregnancy related death' includes all deaths in pregnancy up to 1 year postpartum. Care needs to be taken when making international comparisons that the appropriate expression of maternal mortality is used.

In the UK Maternal Deaths Enquiry, maternal deaths are classified both by cause and timing. Deaths from conditions directly related to maternity—e.g. pre-eclampsia, haemorrhage, sepsis, etc.—are classified as *indirect* if they occur after 22 weeks of pregnancy but before 42 days after delivery. If they are later they are classified as *late direct*. Deaths from conditions not thought to be directly caused by the maternity, but exacerbated by it, are classified as *indirect* if they occur after 22 weeks of pregnancy but before 42 days of delivery. Examples include deaths from pre-existing medical conditions: cardiac disease, epilepsy, some cancers, etc. All suicides are classified as indirect. If the death occurs after 42 days it is classified as *late indirect*.

Figure 20.2 shows the change in the maternal death rate since 1985 both from direct and indirect causes. It can be seen that more women have died from indirect than from direct causes since 1994. Part of this increase is due to improved case ascertainment but other factors are also likely to have played a part. There have been changes in reproductive epidemiology with childbearing women becoming older, increased rates of obesity, and more women with pre-existing medical and psychiatric conditions becoming pregnant.

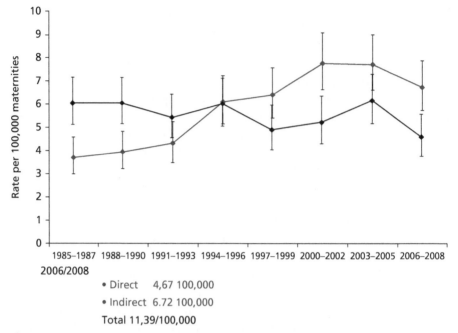

Fig. 20.2 Direct and indirect maternal mortality rates, UK 1984–2008.

The increased number of asylum seekers and refugees has also played a part recently. In general, causes of maternal mortality that directly relate to childbirth are within the influence of changed practice by maternity services. Indirect causes of maternal death that require wider changes in society or the actions of other branches of medicine may be more difficult to influence.

Table 20.1 shows the categories of psychiatric death.

Findings of the Enquiries 1997–2008

In the last Enquiry 2006–2008 there were 67 deaths from psychiatric causes, 29 of which were suicides.

Timing and cause of death

Table 20.2 shows the timing of deaths from, or associated with, psychiatric causes in the UK 2006–2008. There has been no significant change in either the numbers of deaths overall, or the numbers from suicide, since 1997.

Table 20.3 shows the number of maternal deaths during pregnancy and up to 6 months postpartum during the last three Enquiries. There has been no significant change in the numbers of suicide since 1997. From Table 20.3 it can be seen that only considering suicide in pregnancy and up to 6 weeks following delivery gives a misleading picture, as the number doubles if the period is extended to 6 months. The majority of women who died

Table 20.1 Definition of terms

Suicide	Pregnancy to 42 days after delivery	Indirect*
	43–182 days	Late indirect
Psychiatric associated deaths		
	Substance misuse—accidental overdoses	Coincidental**
	Medical conditions caused by/mistaken for psychiatric disorder**	
	Accidents due to maternal psychiatric disorder	Coincidental**

*Contributes to maternal mortality rates.

** Counted elsewhere but described in Chapter 11 Psychiatric Causes of Maternal Death of the Confidential Enquiry.

Table 20.2 Timing of maternal deaths from, or associated with, psychiatric causes in the UK 2006–2008

Cause	Pregnancy undelivered	Up to 42 days after end of pregnancy	*Late* deaths 43–182 days after end of pregnancy	Total
Suicide	4	9	16	29
Accidental overdose from drugs misuse	2	3	5	10
Medical conditions, including those associated with substance misuse	4	16	5	25
Accidents	2	1	0	3
Total	**12**	**29**	**26**	**67**

Table 20.3 Number of maternal deaths during pregnancy and up to 6 months postpartum during the last three Enquiries

Timing of death	2000–2002 *n* (Rate)	2003–2005 *n* (Rate)	2006–2008 *n* (Rate)
In pregnancy			
Before 28 weeks	1(0.10)	5(0.24)	2(0.09)
28–41 weeks undelivered	4(0.05)	3(0.14)	2(0.09)
Postnatal *indirect*			
Up to and including 42 days after delivery	5(0.25)	4(0.19)	9(0.39)
All indirect	10(0.50)	12(0.57)	13(0.57)
Over 6 weeks after delivery late indirect			
43–90 days	5(0.25)	2(0.19)	4(0.17)
91 days to 26 weeks after delivery	7(0.35)	6(0.57)	12(0.52)
All late indirect deaths	12(0.60)	8(0.38)	16(0.70)
All suicides during pregnancy and up to and including 6 postnatal months	22(1.10)	20(0.95)	29(1.27)

after 42 days but before 6 months had the onset of their illness within the first 6 weeks following delivery.

Method of suicide

Table 20.4 demonstrates the method of maternal suicide before 6 months since 1997.

It can be seen that there has been a consistent finding, since 1997, of women dying violently, with only 20% dying from an overdose of prescribed drugs. This stands in contrast to the method of suicide amongst women in the general population.

The psychiatric diagnosis

Since 1997 over half of the women who committed suicide were suffering from a serious mental illness following childbirth predominantly a serious affective disorder including bipolar illness. Table 20.5 shows the psychiatric diagnosis of women who died in the 2006–2008 triennium. There was evidence from the documentation that 59% of these suicides were suffering from a serious illness, consistent with the findings since 1997.

Table 20.4 Method of maternal suicide before 6 months since 1997

Method of suicide	1997–1999 n	2000–2002 n	2003–2005 n	2006–2008 n	All n
Hanging	10	8	14	9	41
Jumping from a height	5	4	4	9	22
Cut throat	4	1	0	1	6
Intentional road accident	1	2	0	0	3
Self-immolation	1	1	2	3	7
Drowning	1	1	2	2	6
Gunshot	1	0	0	0	1
Railway track	0	0	1	0	1
Carbon monoxide/bleach	0	0	0	2	2
Overdose of prescribed drugs	3	0	9	3	24
Total stated	**26**	**26**	**32**	**29**	**113**
Not stated	0	0	1		

Table 20.5 Psychiatric diagnosis of deaths 2006–2008

Diagnosis	n	%
Psychosis	11	38
Severe depressive illness	6	21
Adjustment/grief reaction	3	10
Drug dependency	9	31
Total	**29**	**100**

In this triennium, as previously since 1997, approximately one third of the suicides occurred in women who were drug dependent, the majority on heroin. In this, as in previous reports, small numbers of suicides were known to be suffering from a variety of non-psychotic disorders.

Of those women who died with serious mental illness, approximately half were suffering from a first onset postpartum psychosis, or very severe depressive illness, and one half were suffering from a recurrence of a bipolar or schizo-affective disorder. In the last three triennia very few women were suffering from a recurrence of a previous puerperal psychosis.

Of the women suffering from a severe mental illness, in many cases the initial diagnosis made on first contact with Psychiatric Services was of anxiety and depression, or postnatal depression, despite documented evidence of symptoms that would lead to a more serious diagnosis.

Previous illness and risk of recurrence

Since 1997 the Enquiries have consistently found that half of the suicides had a psychiatric history that could have been identified at early pregnancy assessment. One of the recommendations of the 1997–1999 Enquiry was that all women should be asked at 'booking clinic' about their psychiatric history, and those with a previous serious mental illness should be referred for assessment during pregnancy. These findings confirmed previous research that women with a past history of serious affective disorder faced a 50% risk of recurrence following delivery. Despite these recommendations, repeated in subsequent reports, the 2006–2008 Enquiry found that half of the women who died from suicide (all diagnoses) had a previous psychiatric history, but of these less than half were identified, and in very few cases was this risk managed (see Table 20.6). Unfortunately this finding too is consistent with previous Enquiries.

Psychiatric care received

All the women suffering from serious mental illness were receiving psychiatric care. However, only one of the nine substance misuse suicides were receiving the appropriate treatment from Drug and Alcohol Treatment Services.

Table 20.6 Past psychiatric history of suicides 2006–2008

Past psychiatric history	n	%
No history, first illness	10	34
Past psychiatric history	19	66
Past psychiatric history identified	9	47
Past history appropriately managed	4	21
Total	**29**	**100**

Table 20.7 Level of psychiatric care of mothers who committed suicide 2006–2008

Level of care	n	%
Mother and baby unit	2	7
General psychiatric inpatient	6	21
Perinatal psychiatric team	0	0
General psychiatric team	9	31
Drug and alcohol team	1	3
GP only	4	14
None	7	24
Total	**29**	**100**

All those with serious illness received care from general adult psychiatric teams, either as an inpatient or in the community. This included two suicides who had been in mother and baby units. These two women had received general adult care both as outpatients and inpatients in a non-specialized service prior to, and subsequent to, their admission on a mother and baby unit. In previous Enquiries only one of the suicides since 1997 had been admitted to a mother and baby unit.

Table 20.7 shows the highest level of psychiatric care of mothers who committed suicide in 2006 to 2008.

All of the seriously mentally ill suicides had received care during their short illnesses from multiple psychiatric teams, a new finding in the 2006–2008 Enquiry. Eleven out of the 17 women who were seriously mentally ill and receiving psychiatric care were judged by the assessors to have received substandard care. The characteristics of this care, including misdiagnosis, were that despite documented symptoms of a severe or psychotic illness, a diagnosis of postnatal depression or anxiety and depression was made. They had received a standard response and threshold of intervention with delays in accessing treatment and lower levels of intervention, including admission, than were judged to have been needed with hindsight. Risk assessments were particularly poor, with previous histories of suicide attempts not being taken into consideration and documented evidence of suicidal thinking and preoccupation judged to have been ameliorated by 'good social support'. In general, this substandard care was also hallmarked by an apparent failure to recognize the severity of the unfolding, and often rapidly deteriorating, condition. This latter finding has also been frequently mentioned in the analysis of other causes of maternal death.

Illustrative cases

Case examples have always been an integral and distinctive feature of the UK Maternal Deaths Enquiry. They provide graphic examples of the key findings of the last four Enquiries.

Case example 1

A woman died from self-immolation within 42 days of delivery of her second child. She had a history of schizoaffective psychosis, including one postpartum episode, and had made a near fatal violent suicide attempt following the birth of her older child 5 years previously. Despite this, she had been well on medication for the previous 5 years and had been functioning normally. She remained in close contact with psychiatric services during her pregnancy and following delivery. However, the maternity services seemed to be unaware of the severity of her past illness. After delivery she was initially well, but within 4 weeks there was the sudden onset and rapid deterioration of an episode of affective psychosis. She was preoccupied with her previous suicide attempt and the notes describe her as suspicious, guilty, and with suicidal thoughts. The aim of her management was 'to keep her at home', and three more psychiatric teams were involved. She died one week after the onset of her illness by setting fire to herself.

This case demonstrates the abrupt onset and rapid deterioration of a postpartum psychosis, and the apparent difficulties the psychiatric team had in recognizing the additional risks of this illness. There seems to have been a preoccupation with home treatment. Multiple psychiatric teams were involved in her care with numerous healthcare professionals.

Case example 2

A young, single mother, recently separated, with significant social problems died from injuries sustained on a railway track 10 weeks after the birth of her second child. She had a long history of recurrent episodes of bipolar illness, but was last admitted to a psychiatric unit 5 years previously. She had remained well on sodium valproate, but this was withdrawn and she was discharged from psychiatric care at the beginning of her pregnancy. Her previous psychiatric history was not elicited in her antenatal care, although the general practitioner knew and had told the obstetrician. No psychiatric referral was made during pregnancy. On the third postpartum day the onset of unusual behaviour resulted in a referral to the duty psychiatrist. He did not find that she was mentally ill and took no action. Two weeks following delivery she went to see her GP complaining of depression. He did not think she was ill and attributed her distress to her social problems. Some weeks later her family became worried about her and telephoned the health visitor. However, she died the following day.

This case demonstrates the risk of recurrence of severe affective disorder following childbirth. This remains a risk even if there was no recurrence following the birth of a previous child. It also demonstrates the importance of preconception counselling and of continuing psychiatric care in high risk women when it is likely that they will have further children. She should have been re-referred during pregnancy. Both the duty psychiatrist and the general practitioner should have been alerted to the early manifestations of a recurrence of her illness. At the very least, this woman should have had regular contact with psychiatric services following delivery, and her family should have known what to do if they became concerned.

Case example 3

An older professional woman in comfortable social circumstances, with no previous psychiatric history, died by jumping from a height within 8 weeks of delivery of her first baby. In late pregnancy there was documentation that she had increasing morbid anxiety, leading to antenatal admission to a maternity unit, but not to psychiatric referral, or to any alert to the community midwife or GP that all was not well. Six weeks after delivery she presented to Accident and Emergency agitated and with bizarre hypochondriacal beliefs. She was seen by a duty psychiatrist who diagnosed an anxiety state, despite describing abnormal thinking. He referred her to the community mental health team. She presented again the following day.

The community mental health team rejected her referral with a letter to the GP saying that they only assessed those with serious mental illness. The GP referred her to a private psychiatrist. The letter describing severe depression with suicidal ideas arrived the day after her death.

This case demonstrates the findings of misdiagnosing serious mental illness as anxiety and depression, and the rapid deterioration of postpartum conditions. It also demonstrates the difficulties with a standard service response to a postpartum condition in someone with no prior psychiatric history. Presentation of such a condition shortly after delivery should prompt an early assessment.

Overall characteristics of maternal suicide

Between 1997 and 2008 the numbers, rates and characteristics of women committing suicide in pregnancy and up to six months postpartum have not changed significantly.

- 76% of suicides took place after delivery.
- 83% were well during pregnancy.
- 87% died violently.
- 60% were seriously ill; half were suffering from a first onset condition and half a recurrence of a previous condition.

The serious illnesses were characterized by acute onset and rapid deterioration. There was a median of 9 days between first contact with psychiatric services and death.

- 66% of al women who died from suicide (all diagnoses) had previous psychiatric illness but less than half were identified at booking and few were managed.
- 30% of those who died from suicide were substance misusers.
- 90% were white.

The median age of the women who died by suicide was 30 years (range 16–43); 76% were married or in stable cohabitation, and 76% were employed; 41% were educated to A level or above, and 28% university educated.

Of those suffering from serious mental illness, 80% were aged 30 or older, were married, educated, and employed. In contrast, those substance misusers who committed suicide were in the main single, unemployed, young, and the majority were socially excluded.

In this triennium there were no infanticides, and since 1997 only 2 out of 114 women who died from suicide were associated with infanticide.

Psychiatric associated causes of maternal death

Suicide was not the only psychiatric cause of maternal death. Women died from accidental overdose of drugs of misuse. Women also died from medical conditions, including those associated with substance misuse that were either caused by a psychiatric disorder, or mistaken for one, and a small number from accidents attributable to substance misuse.

Table 20.5 shows the causes of death in women known to be substance misusers in the 2006–2008 Enquiry. These findings are consistent with the previous two Enquiries. The majority of these women died shortly after a child protection case conference and the decision to remove their child into care. This finding too is consistent with those of the last two Enquiries.

Three women died from gastrointestinal complications of alcoholism. The remaining substance misuse deaths were characterized by heroin abuse combined with poly-drug use, including cocaine, amphetamines, painkillers, and the inappropriate and erratic use of antidepressants. The focus of attention was, in the majority of cases, only on heroin and methadone substitution. The majority of the women were young, single, deprived and socially excluded. All were involved with child safeguarding. Very few of the women were receiving any specialized care from drug and alcohol treatment teams. The management was often naïve, with no routine checking of drug consumption, and a ready acceptance of the woman's declaration that she was not taking drugs. Attempts were often made to reduce methadone consumption, accompanied by an undeclared increase in the use of street drugs. The substance-misusing women were characterized by an avoidance of antenatal care. Child safeguarding case conferences were, in general, followed by a disengagement from maternity care and involvement of both maternity services and social services appeared to stop once the baby had been removed.

In the last as in previous Enquiries, a group of women died from medical conditions either attributable to their psychiatric disorder, as in the case of substance misusers, or mistaken for a psychiatric disorder. Examples of these include a woman with no psychiatric history who died from a ruptured aortic aneurysm and pulmonary embolus. Her distress and pain had been diagnosed as anxiety and depression. Numerous cases of acute confusional states, which have been misdiagnosed as postnatal depression, and of tachycardia attributed to anxiety have been noted. In one notable case where death occurred shortly after admission to a psychiatric unit, the post mortem revealed gangrene of the uterus. Deaths from malignancy and milliary tuberculosis were seen in women whose weight loss and loss of appetite had been attributed to anorexia nervosa.

Case example 4

An older professional woman with no prior psychiatric history died from pneumonia and encephalopathy within 42 days of the birth of her first baby. Eighteen months previously she had been diagnosed with systemic lupus erythematosus. Her presenting symptoms had been weight loss and malaise. She withdrew her medication in early pregnancy. In mid-pregnancy she complained of malaise, weight loss, and loss of appetite. She became agitated. This was attributed, without further investigation, to depression, and she was referred many times to a liaison psychiatrist. No psychiatric disorder was found. She collapsed on the second postpartum day whilst waiting to see a psychiatrist and died some weeks later in intensive care.

International comparison

Suicide is classified as an indirect cause of maternal death. The WHO supports this classification internationally. However, international comparison of maternal suicide is difficult as many countries do not include indirect causes of maternal death in their national statistics. However, those that do, including Finland, Denmark, and New Zealand, have similar findings to the UK, in that suicide accounts for at least 15% of all maternal deaths and is a leading cause of maternal death.

Discussion

In common with many other indirect causes of maternal death (for example cardiac causes, neurological causes, etc.) the rate is not falling. In common with the recommendations made by the assessors of other indirect causes of maternal death the importance of preconception counselling for those women who have medical or psychiatric conditions likely to be affected by pregnancy is underlined. Also, in common with other indirect causes of death, the importance of recurrence of the pathoplastic effects of pregnancy on illness is underlined, with a tendency to rapid deterioration and severity. It is not only amongst the psychiatric causes of maternal death, but also other causes of maternal death, that there is a problem with misattribution of serious mental illness, either to problems with pregnancy itself or to psychiatric disorder. Other assessors responsible for the assessment of indirect causes of maternal death have commented on the need for specialist cardiologists, diabetologists, neurologists, and psychiatrists who have special expertise in maternal conditions and who can work closely with maternity services. They all comment on the importance of an altered service response to women who are pregnant or postpartum, with medical and psychiatric conditions, and of a need for a lowered threshold of concern and intervention.

There have been numerous changes in the National Health Service and the way it delivers its services. A triennial report is able to see the impact of these changes. In psychiatric causes of maternal death the introduction of functional psychiatric teams was evident in the multiple psychiatric teams involved in the short illness in the women who died. Also evident was the impact of the exclusion of the GP from maternity care, and the fact that midwives are increasingly not located within GP surgeries. The responsibility of disclosing a previous psychiatric history therefore rested entirely on the woman's shoulders.

In the last Enquiry all of the women who died from suicide died whilst under the care of general adult psychiatrists, even though in two cases they had been admitted to a mother and baby unit. In addition, since 1997, only one woman has died on a mother and baby unit. In none of these deaths was there a specialized perinatal community psychiatric team available, and in the three deaths that have occurred since 1997 the admission to a mother and baby unit was to a remote, out of area unit, after considerable delay.

The findings of the last four Enquires would suggest that, not only should direct admission of mother and infant together to a mother and baby unit take place if admission is necessary, but also that specialist community perinatal community psychiatric teams are as important as mother and baby units. They have specialized understanding of the distinctive clinical features of early onset postpartum conditions, the additional risks faced to both mother and infant, and the need for lowered thresholds for concern and interventions.

The findings of the last four Enquiries contain lessons for psychiatry:

- The importance for preconception counselling for women with serious mental illness, particularly serious affective disorder.
- The predictable risk of recurrence of serious affective disorder after delivery.

- That serious illness deteriorates quickly and requires prompt referral to specialized care.
- That general adult psychiatric services should alter their response to women presenting with mental illness after delivery.
- The risk of suicide is not related to socioeconomic deprivation.
- That medical conditions can present as or complicate a psychiatric disorder and that substance misuse is dangerous to mothers and infants, and requires expert specialized care.

Conclusion

Psychiatric disorder increases the risk of maternal death. Late pregnancy and the early puerperium increases the risk of suicide. The risks are reducible.

Further reading

Oates, M.R. (2001) Chapter 11. Deaths from psychiatric causes in Why Mothers Die 1997–1999. Fifth Report of the Confidential Enquiries into Maternal Deaths in the United Kingdom. London, RCOG Press.

Oates, M.R. (2004). Chapter 11. Deaths from psychiatric causes in Why Mothers Die 2000–2002. Sixth Report of the Confidential Enquiry into Maternal and Child Health (CEMACH). London, The Royal College of Obstetricians and Gynaecologists.

Oates, M.R (2007). Chapter 12, Deaths from psychiatric causes in Saving Mothers' Lives Reviewing maternal deaths to make motherhood safer 2003–2005. In Seventh Report of the Confidential Enquiry into Maternal Deaths in the United Kingdom. Lewis, G., editor. London, CEMACH.

Oates, M. and Cantwell, R. (2011). Chapter 11: Deaths from psychiatric causes in Saving Mothers' Lives: Reviewing maternal deaths to make motherhood safer: 2006–2008. Eighth Report of the Confidential Enquiries into maternal deaths in the United Kingdom (CMACE). Supp to BJOG: An International Journal of Obstetrics and Gynaecology Vol **118**, Supp 1.

Chapter 21

The Children Act 1989

Success or failure

Simonetta Agnello Hornby

The Children Act of 1989

Heralded as the most progressive legislation of the world, the Children Act of 1989 revolutionized children's law in England and Wales. It is underpinned by six principles: (1) the supremacy of the child's interest in all decisions concerning their upbringing and education; (2) the recognition that it is best for any chid to be brought up by their blood family, that his religious and ethnic background must be respected,and that siblings should not be separated; (3) the abolition of the stigma of illegitimacy and its replacement with the attribution at birth of paternal responsibility to the child's father; (4) the unification of public and private law, and the creation of the 'menu' of Residence, Contact, Prohibition, and Specific Issue orders available to the court; (5) the establisment of the new principle that time is of the essence in all cases relating to children; and (6) the creation of the presumption that 'no order is better than an order' thus the ingerence of the court must be minimal.

I believed in those principles and in the benefits that the Children Act would bring to my clients—children and parents alike. I had some reservations: the system was expensive to implement on two counts: first, it gave the child a 'guardian' (a qualified social worker appointed by the court through CAFCASS, a governmental agency), as well as their own solicitor paid for by Legal Aid, as was the representative of the parents, who had the right to instruct independent experts; second, because its requirements of social services and other agencies involved further training and increased resources, as well as further involvement of the judiciary, and increased court time. Hornby and Levy were at the forefront of its implementation: our entire staff received in-house training that was open to other disciplines, within the spirit of cooperation between agencies that permeated the Act and its implementation. I also lectured in Britain and abroad and was proud to tell others that social services were under a duty to keep families united, rather than removing children from parents, and make efforts to return to the family the child removed from it, or if this failed, to place the child within the extended family, or with adoptive parents, within a year. Parental responsibility did not cease on the making of a Care Order, and cooperation and consultation between parents and social services was to continue beyond the making of that order. I told them that while a child was separated from their family, contact with the parents and siblings and relevant adults continued unless it was demonstrated to the court's satisfaction that it was not beneficial to the child. Last but not least, I told foreign lawyers, judges, and social workers that the the voice of the child (their wishes and feelings) was heard in court though the 'guardian', and the specialist solicitor, instructed by the 'guardian', who had the added duty to decide if the child had the capacity to give instructions directly, in which case the solicitor was bound to take istructions from the child only and not from the 'guardian'. Without doubt, the Children Act greatly improved the lot of the 60,000 children in care or accommodated, and of the 4,000 refuges looked after in England and Wales. Cases were dealt with swftly, the child's 'guardian', social workers, and parents collaborated directly and though their respective lawyers, and the court's decisions were implemented without delay.

However, this is no longer the case. The life of the child in care is, in many cases, more miserable than before the intervention of social services. Seventy-three per cent of children in care live some distance from their home, in foster families no longer recruited and trained by social services, but by private companies that manage them and the children on behalf of social services; more often than not such placements necessitate change of schools and create difficulties in keeping contact with families and friends. These arrangements have no stability. The average child in care has four foster placements. Of the other children in care, 10% are placed in children's homes and 17% avait adoption, or live in residential homes or specialist insititutions.

The profile of children in care is chilling: 60% have been abused or neglected, 20% come from dysfunctional families, and 4% are looked after by social services because of their carers' incapacity or illness. Fortyfive per cent of those between the age of 5 and 17 years suffer from mental illness, 10% have learning difficulties, and 5% have drug addcition.

Compared to ther children of the same age, they are twicemore likely to have been involved in criminal proceedings, four times more likely to be unemployed at the age of 16, five times more likely to be expelled from school, and only 14% (against the 65% of other children) achieve GCSEs or similar grades. There has been no improvement in these figures over the years.

WHY has the system failed?

There are seven most compelling reasons.

1 Scarcity, low quality of social workers, and their organization. Unfilled vacancies, scarcity, discontinuity of allocated social workers, overall lack of experience, and an increasing self protective burocratic culture, paralyse the process and do not create space for effective and meaningful social work. Furthermore, unlike all the other professions, social workers who advance in their career become managers and no longer practise social work; they do not meet the family and the child, and concentrate on supervising the junior staff.

2 Poor legal work. Lack of resources in local authorities affects care proceedings at all the stages, including the running of the case: statements and legal documents are drafted by

social workers and not lawyers; there is no continuity in legal representation; and low fees mean less experienced and able barristers; assessments are not carried out speedily or comprehensively. Social workers feel unable to give opinions and their lawyers rely on experts' reports.

3 High turnover of social workers. Lack of consistent social work means that in too many cases the child, placed with a foster family outside the borough, is literally forgotten, leaving the foster family—who receive scanty information on the child from the liaison officer, who in turn knows the little that his or her employers have been told by social services—to deal with his emotional problems, his educational needs in a new school, and contact or the lack of it. In most cases contact is made difficult by logistics and by the requests that the parents do visit social services to receive travel warrants; it is not supported by the social worker of the child; there is little or no preparation at all of both child and parents about contact, and no discussion after the visit with the parents to improve the quality of contact and reaffirm its purpose. Social workers often forget (or discourage outright) to arrange contact with grandparents and the extended family.

4 Lengthy court proceedings and lack of resurces in lawyers and CAFCASS. Children's and parents' lawyers are paid at lower rates than before. Fewer people, and of lower calibre, choose to work under the conditions imposed by legal aid. CAFCASS suffers forn chronic shortage of staff, and cases last longer waiting for the appointment of a 'guardian'. Delays are the norm. Cases, that in the intention of the legislators shouldhave been completed in 3 months, (rather optimistically) take over 2 years. There is a pervasive culture of despondency. Advocates meetings are useless because the lawyers do not have instructions, and pleadings have not been filed as ordered by the court. Agreed 'threshold criteria' documents are not filed when due. Parents forget to come to court and solicitors send barristers with scanty instructions

5 Delegation of professional responsibilities and the proliferation of experts' reports. Social workers are afraid of being blamed by the press and society for the mistakes that they feel are not only their fault. They have a point, but the result is that they no longer feel competent or wish to make in-depth assessments of children's needs and of their families. They rely on the reports and the assessments of overworked, and thus slow, independent experts, such as other social workers, child psychiatrists, and psychologists. Many of these are retired and have chosen the lucrative career of court experts. The quality of these reports often leaves much to be desired.

6 Incompetence, self protection, and antagonism among professionals and between them and parents in the context of the proceedings. The antagonism between social services and parents has increased and can also exisit between them and 'guardians'. There is no longer a social worker who works with the family. The social worker of the child—the subject of the proceedings—is seen by the parents as the enemy. Cooperation is but a word. In my experience, opportunities for dialogue are missed at court, where social workers and their team leaders hardly acknowledge the presence of the parents. They are told not to take their files for fear of being asked to give evidence on them, and not to

engage in conversation with other than their own representative to protect themselves. Even contact arrangements are not made at court: the parent will be requested to make a special visit to the social worker's office after the hearing.

7   The role of the judiciary. The written evidence, intended to be less voluminous that in the past, has, on the contrary, increased substantially; through 'cut and paste' it is repeated in the documentation. It has decreased in quality because of lack of clear thinking, inaccurate reporting, and use and abuse of jargon. The 'guardian's report' is now an analysis that follows a template that no longer contains a chronology and cannot give a complete and coherent account of the facts. The judiciary sought to remedy this disarray in the proceedings establishing procedures, protocols, and memoranda of good practice that should have set out the procedures to follow and speed up the case. Each of these has failed to achieve its purpose because of lack of manpower and the laissez-faire culture that unites dispirited and overworked social services and lawyers. The judge may give directions that set out timetables, request reports and information to be given by a specific date, but is, in practice, powerless when these are not complied with. At the final hearing, due to the pressures on judicial time and for the avoidance of further delays, often the parties have no option but to reach an agreement both on the facts and on the disposal of the case without a hearing to test the evidence, leaving the implementation of the agreement to parents and social workers who do not trust each other. In the end, it is the child who suffers.

Where is the child?

He or she is not to be seen nor heard. The guardian's evidence is filed weeks before the hearing and often the guardian has not seen the child since. Similarly the solicitor rarely visits in the week before the hearing. The child's presence in court is discouraged by the judiciary, even in respect of teenaged children, on the bais that their wishes and feelings have been reported to the court adequately by the 'guardian' and is the child will be kept informed of the proceedings by the 'guardian' and by the solicitor. There are no practice directions that regulate how the child can have access to the documentation filed in their case, and the full judgement at the time of the final hearing or later, and on reaching majority. The child is not told that they have the right to have sight of the documentation, and to receive copies of the evidence, even when they are adult.

The chid has no right to meet the judge; this depends on the discretion of the judge. Those of my child clients, who have kept in contact as adults, tell me that they have no real undestanding of what was decided at court and why. Some of them, who had the courage to speak about their abuse and neglect, regret having done so. They say that life after the care order was worst than before—the true failure of the hopes pinned on the Children Act.

Chapter 22

Child abuse in the United States

Margaret Spinelli

Introduction

Child abuse is a major cause of morbidity and mortality in the United States and other countries. It is the second leading cause of death among children in the US. All 50 States, the District of Columbia, and the US Territories have mandatory child abuse and neglect reporting laws that require certain professionals and institutions to report suspected mal-treatment to a child protective services (CPS) agency. Four major types of maltreatment are considered: neglect, physical abuse, psychological maltreatment, and sexual abuse (Centers for Disease Control and Prevention 2010).

Once an allegation or referral of child abuse is received by a CPS agency, the majority of reports receive investigations to establish whether or not an intervention is needed. Some reports receive an alternative response in which safety and risk assessments are conducted, but the focus is on working with the family to address issues. Investigations involve gathering evidence to substantiate the alleged maltreatment.

National Child Abuse and Neglect Data System

Data from reports on child abuse is derived from the National Child Abuse and Neglect Data System (NCANDS), which aggregates and publishes statistics from state child protection agencies. The first report from NCANDS was based on data for 1990. Case-level data include information about the characteristics of reports of abuse and neglect that are made to CPS agencies, the children involved, the types of maltreatment that are alleged, the dispositions of the CPS responses, the risk factors of the child and the caregivers, the services that are provided, and the perpetrators (Centers for Disease Control and Prevention 2010).

During 2010, the NCANSDS reported that an estimated 3.3 million referrals estimated to include 5.9 million children were received by CPS agencies. Of the nearly 2 million reports that were screened and received a CPS response, 90.3% received an investigation response and 9.7% received an alternative response (Centers for Disease Control and Prevention 2010).

Of the 1,793,724 reports that received an investigation in 2010, 436,321 were substantiated; 24,976 were found to be indicated (likely but unsubstantiated); and 1,262,118 were found to be unsubstantiated. Three-fifths of reports of alleged child abuse and neglect were made by professionals. The four largest percentages of report sources were from such professionals as teachers (16.4%), law enforcement and legal personnel (16.7%), social services staff (11.5%), and medical personnel (8.2%) (Centers for Disease Control and Prevention 2010). More than 80% of perpetrators of child maltreatment are parents (Asnes and Leventhal 2010); two-fifths of victims were maltreated by their mothers; one-fifth were maltreated by their fathers; one-fifth were maltreated by both parents.

The duplicate count of child victims counts a child each time he or she was found to be a victim. The unique count of child victims counts a child only once regardless of the number of times he or she was found to be a victim during the reporting year. More than 3.6 million (duplicate) children were the subjects of at least one report. One-fifth of these children were found to be victims with dispositions of substantiated (19.5%), indicated (1.0%), and alternative response (0.5%). The remaining four-fifths of the children were found to be nonvictims of maltreatment.

Repeat victimization

The duplicate victim rate in the US (includes children who were victims more than once) was 10.0 victims per 1,000 children in the population. For 2010, an estimated 754,000 duplicate and 695,000 unique children were victims of maltreatment. The rate of victimization for the past 5 years has decreased, and most states reported a decreased number of victims, when compared to 2009. However, if duplicate children are reported more than once because they have been re-victimized, what prophylactic measures are taken after the initial evaluation to prevent repeat abuse of the child? What happens to the investigated cases over time? The problem of repeat victimization speaks to the action taken by CPS after the investigation, adjustment of modifiable risk factors, and prevention over time.

Demographics

The youngest children are the most vulnerable to maltreatment. 39.2% of victims were younger than 4 years; 9.5% of victims were in the age group 4–7 years of age (NCANDS)). Children younger than 1 year had the highest rate of victimization at 42.4%. Data collected through the NCANDS shows children younger than 1 year had the highest rate of neglect at 20.6 per 10,000 children in the population of the same age. Victimization is equal between the sexes. The rate and percentage of 88% of unique victims were comprised of three races or ethnicities—African-American (21.9%), Hispanic (21.4%), and White (44.8%), a rate that has remained stable for years. Four-fifths (78.3%) of unique victims were neglected, 17.6% were physically abused, 9.2% were sexually abused, 8.1% were psychologically maltreated, and 2.4% were medically neglected.

Risk factors

Several risk factors make children more vulnerable to abuse. They include children with a disability: mental retardation, emotional disturbance, visual or hearing impairment, learning disability, physical disability, behavioural problems, or other medical problems. Sixteen percent of unique victims were reported as having a disability.

Children may also be victims of the alcohol abuse, drug abuse, and domestic violence caregiver risk factors. With respect to domestic violence, the caregiver could have been either the perpetrator or the victim of the domestic violence. More than 25.7% of victims were exposed to this behaviour. The current national standard for the absence of maltreatment recurrence is 94.6% after 6 months. The question to ask is what happens after that?

Consequences of abuse

In addition to the obvious physical harm experienced by the abused child, there are also long-term sequelae. Traumatized children are at risk for chronic forms of post-traumatic stress disorder. Physical health consequences include damage to the spinal cord or brain from shaken baby syndrome (National Institute of Neurological Disorders and Stroke 2007), impaired cognitive, language and academic abilities (Watts-English *et al.* 2006) and increased physical ailments as adults (Springer *et al.* 2007). Psychological consequences include toddler depression and withdrawal (Dubowitz *et al.* 2002). As many as 80 percent of young adults who had been abused met diagnostic criteria for at least one psychiatric disorder (Silverman *et al.* 1996) in addition to antisocial traits, behavioural problems, delinquency, adult criminality, teen pregnancy, and drug use (Kelley *et al.* 1997).

Child fatalities

Almost five children die each day as a consequence of child abuse (National Child Abuse Statistics 2010). Of 23,976 children and adolescents who died in the US in 2007, the leading cause of death was unintentional injuries, which accounted for 42.1% of all deaths. The second leading cause of death was homicide, which accounted for 11.5% of deaths (Heron *et al.* 2010). The weighted mean age of victims depicted in most filicide studies is 5.5 years (West *et al.* 2009).

The NCANDS reports fluctuating rates in the past 5 years. The rate rose substantially from 2006–2007 (to 2.35 from 2.05 per 100,000), a 15% rise in one year. In its data on child maltreatment fatalities, the latest NCANDS shows little change for fatalities for 2008 (Finkelhor *et al.* 2009). However, the most recent reported rate from NCANDS was 2.07 per 100,000 in 2010 from 2.32 in 2009.

The true incidence of fatal child abuse in the US is unknown because of an absence of accurate data. This is caused by restrictions and inaccuracies in coding, causes of death, incomplete or inaccurate information on death certificates and police reports, varying case definitions and lack of perpetrator information (Herman-Giddens *et al.* 1999). From 1985 through 1996, 9,467 homicides among US children younger than 11 years were estimated to be due to abuse rather than the 2,973 reported. The International Classification of Diseases-9 (ICD-9) cause of death coding under-ascertained abuse homicides by an estimated 61.6%.

When reviewing 259 cases of child fatality in North Carolina, West *et al.* (2009) found that the state vital records system under-recorded the coding of those deaths due to battering or abuse by 58.7%. Black children were killed at three times the rate of white children.

Males made up 65.5% of assailants. Biological parents accounted for 63% of the perpetrators of fatal child abuse.

Decrease in reports of child abuse

After nearly two decades of increase, reports of child maltreatment have decreased each year since 1994. The decline is attributed to passage of laws for mandated reporting of child maltreatment and increased recognition of maltreatment. Several other theories have been proposed to explain the decrease (Johnson 2002); improved economy and less stress on caretakers, day care for vulnerable children, treatment of victims to prevent reactive abuse, imprisonment of offenders, decreased use of corporal punishment, earlier recognition and reporting, and prevention programmes, including home visitors and less corporal punishment in school (Asnes and Leventhal 2010). Other possible factors that may account for the dramatic downward trend in physical and sexual abuse are increases in the numbers of law enforcement and child protection personnel, more aggressive prosecution and incarceration policies, growing public awareness, and dissemination of new treatment options for families with mental health problems.

During the 1990s there was a remarkable 39% decline in US cases of sexual abuse substantiated by child protective agencies from an estimated 150,000 cases in 1992 to 92,000 cases in 1999 (Jones and Finkelhor 2003). One explanation for this trend is the investment by the US in public awareness campaigns, prevention programs, criminal justice interventions and treatment. Overall from 1992 to 2009 sexual abuse declined 61%. Overall from 1992 to 2009 physical abuse declined 55% and neglect declined 10% (Finkelhor *et al.* 2009).

Inconsistencies and barriers in reporting child abuse

Even when there are high levels of suspicion, only one in four children is reported to CPS. Current barriers to reporting child abuse include failure to identify maltreatment and refusing to report abuse to the state authorities (Sege and Flaherty 2008). Other concerns include fears that the child may be separated from the parents. Only a fraction of CPS reports results in removal of a child from the home and most likely in cases of suspected serious injury or serious neglect. Even when removal occurs, reunification is always the goal and is considered in every case. Families do not necessarily lose custody of their children; instead they receive services through the auspices of CPS. Removal is an option of last resort, and is used only when a child's safety cannot be assured.

Recent surveys describe a large majority of child abuse reporting physicians have suffered adverse personal consequences after reporting child maltreatment. Physicians have been sued for reporting despite laws protecting physicians who report suspected abuse. In addition, internet and social networks have been used to destroy the reputations of reporting physicians. Other reasons for not reporting include lack of certainty that the injury was caused by child abuse and the belief that the practitioner can intervene more effectively than child services.

Steps needed to improve outcomes include broad education of all providers to the common patterns of child abuse, supporting front line physicians by providing use of abuse physicians, process oriented education, and improved CPS assessments and interventions.

Role of the practitioner

Forty years after implementing a mandatory child reporting system in the United States, we continue to fall short when protecting young and vulnerable victims. The management of child maltreatment is never easy, but considering and reporting suspected cases of child abuse and neglect are important clinical skills and obligations of a clinician. The use of a stepwise approach has been outlined by Asnes and Lenenthal (2010). The mandatory reporting laws state that once a practitioner has reasonable cause to suspect that a child has been abused or neglected, he or she is obligated by state law to make a report to CPS (Tilden *et al.* 1994). Risk factors associated with child maltreatment should be part of the medical record including poverty, family violence, social isolation, disabled children, and a household that has many children younger than 5 years of age. Also included is a parental history of maltreatment as children. Another worrisome parental behavior, which can be monitored by the practitioner, is failure of empathy between a parent and child and the assignment of inherent value to the use of physical punishment.

The practitioner should ask if the history obtained includes a reasonable mechanism to explain the injury? Does the history make sense in terms of the severity of the injury? Does the history adequately explain the injury with respect to timing?

The practitioner should know when and how to get help and consider if siblings are also involved. There should be no delay telling parents about the report then continue to advocate and care for the child and family after making a CPS report.

Recurrence rates

Although we have witnessed a decrease in the rates of physical and sexual abuse, tragedies continue to occur. The rates of neglect and fatalities have not exhibited such consistent decline. Furthermore, repeated maltreatment is not uncommon, which may indicate that there are risk factors that have not been addressed.

CPS investigations should be associated with subsequent improvements, but CPS investigation may also be disruptive to a household and associated with worsening risk factors. Interventions such as family preservation and family support are not associated with reductions in repeat maltreatment or foster care placement. While targeted interventions such as parent training programmes after physical abuse, cognitive behavioural treatment after sexual abuse, and therapeutic peer intervention after neglect, are promising, they are not implemented on a wide basis and modifiable risk factors are frequently not addressed.

Analysis of NCANDS data on 1.4 million children from nine states found that one-third of abused children were re-reported within 5 years (Waldfogel 2009). Children who received post-investigation services were more likely to be re-reported than those who did not receive services. One explanation may be that many families receive few services beyond periodic visits by usually overburdened caseworkers. Another explanation may be that services such as respite care, parenting education, housing assistance, substance abuse treatment, day care, home visits, individual and family counselling, and home help are poor in quality and insufficient in quantity.

Modifiable risk factors

Studies have found that families in which parents have modifiable risk factors such as substance abuse, mental health problems and domestic violence (Marcenko *et al.* 2011) are more likely than others to be re-reported, suggesting that developing and delivering more effective treatment services for such parents could help prevent maltreatment. When researchers examined cases of investigated child abuse 4 years after reports to CPS and compared them to those who were not investigated, they found that investigated households continued to be at increased risk for family violence and parental dysfunction, for child medical and behavioural problems and for future incidents of maltreatment (Marcenko *et al.* 2010).

When household, family and child risk factors were examined, the investigated subjects were not perceptibly different from non-investigated subjects in social support, family functioning, poverty, maternal education and child behaviour problems. Mothers of investigated subjects had more depressive symptoms than non-investigated subjects (Campbell *et al.* 2010).

A lack of improvement in described modifiable risk factors suggests that we may be missing an opportunity for secondary prevention of maltreatment and maltreatment consequences (Campbell *et al.* 2010). Only 38% of children receive post investigation services and only 28% receive mental health services within 12 months of report. Forty percent of caregivers report ongoing intimate partner violence after 18 months, and 22% to 62% of children will be referred back for new concerns of maltreatment.

Low-income, unmarried women with low levels of educational achievement are at highest risk of mood disorders, which often co-exist with anxiety and substance abuse. An estimated 5.5% of women living with children under the age of 18 have abused or been dependent on alcohol and/or illicit drugs. Substance abuse is associated with higher rates of child maltreatment. Poverty and attendant hardships are also risk factors for child abuse. Children in low socioeconomic households are five times more likely to experience maltreatment than other children.

The following case example describes a case of severe mental illness in a mother who killed her five children. The case was never reported to child services by the hospital personnel, neighbours, or friends.

Case example 1

In 2001, the United States was riveted when Andrea Yates drowned her five children in the bathtub of her Houston, Texas home (http://crime.about.com/od/current/p/andreayates.htm?r=et). Perhaps no other case of infanticide or filicide demonstrates the danger of postpartum psychosis and associated infanticide. Andréa Yates was a devoted mother who home-schooled her children. She had remained pregnant and/or breast feeding over the previous 7 years and had recurrences of postpartum depression and psychosis. Two suicide attempts after her fourth pregnancy were driven by attempts to resist satanic voices commanding her to kill her infant (Spinelli 2002).

Six months after her fifth child, Andrea Yates appeared 'catatonic.' Her neighbour described her walking around the house like a 'caged animal.' After two psychiatric hospitalizations, she continued to deteriorate. Upon discharge from the hospital there were no child services referrals by staff. She was left alone on the morning of June 21, 2001 when she drowned her five children. She stated that Satan directed her to kill her children to save them from the fires and turmoil of hell.

Intimate partner violence is another modifiable risk factor with negative consequences for exposed children with a lifetime prevalence of 20% in women. In a sample of female caregivers who were reported for child maltreatment, 45% experienced domestic violence in their lifetime. Almost 70% of women who had co-occurring substance abuse, mental health problems, and interpersonal trauma were separated from their children against their will and 26% had their rights to one or more children terminated.

Case example 2

One of the most notorious cases of child abuse and filicide was the case of Lisa Steinberg, a 6-year-old illegally adopted daughter of Joel Steinberg and Hedda Nussbaum. On November 2, 1987 the police came to their Greenwich Village home to find Joel Steinberg carrying his pale and still naked daughter whose body was mottled with bruises. The child was unconscious and cyanotic, with bruising and welts on her back. Lisa died from a subdural haematoma after a beating that occurred 11 hours before help was called. This tragedy occurred despite the fact that neighbours, relatives, teachers, and social workers had witnessed the signs of neglect and abuse that had gone on for years.

Hedda Nussbaum had endured years of abuse before Lisa was killed. Like most battered women, she hoped he would change or the beatings would stop. She was fired from her job because of frequent absences. A friend at work described that she saw her walking with her baby in a stroller. The baby had a cut lip and Hedda had on sunglasses and a bandage. Over the years she had sustained black eyes, broken cheekbones, nose, and ribs. She had burns, and ulcers on her legs so widespread that they were life threatening. Her face was bruised, mangled, and swollen. Over a period of 6 years, neighbours watched the sad, anguished life of a little girl who never had a chance against the two people whose callousness and parental abdication became symbolic of child abuse in America (Gado 1987; Ehlich 1989). Despite availability of child services, cases like these frequently go unnoticed and unreported. Homicides of infants and young children are most often committed in the home by parents and caregivers using 'weapons of opportunity' (Bennett *et al.* 2006).

In general, investigated households continue to be at increased risk for family violence and parental dysfunction, for child medical and behavioural problems, and for future incidents of maltreatment compared to households not investigated by CPS. Therefore, CPS intervention may represent a missed opportunity to improve outcomes for children at high risk for future maltreatment, medical problems and behaviour problems.

Role of caseworkers

There is scarce empirical evidence about how CPA management affects children over time (Wells 2006). Management by the caseworker includes specific judgements when investigating allegations of abuse or neglect; deciding whether children need to be placed outside the home; developing treatment plans to prevent further mistreatment and/or risky behaviours by the child; referring children and caregivers to appropriate services; and monitoring cases. The caseworkers pursue these goals with limited resources, balancing information about needs of and challenges facing vulnerable families with awareness of service availability and competing demands on their own time. Often referrals needed include those that have shortages in services such as physical and mental health care, substance abuse treatment, and housing. Not only abused and neglected children, but also the caregivers who struggle to raise them have risk factors that may be modified to prevent recurrence and adverse long-term outcomes.

One important variable which determines outcome of a mental health referral is the strategy used by the caseworker (Bunger *et al.* 2012). There is strength of available evidence about the benefits of participatory management techniques about what child welfare managers ought to be doing to manage change. The question may really be how they can involve caseworkers on the frontline to effectively change initiatives, given frequent skill deficiencies among both caseworkers and the managers themselves, scarce training budgets, inadequate time to meet, and structural and cultural constraints endemic to child welfare services (Wells 2006).

A limitation of the system is the caseworker referral strategy. Caregivers often have many persistent mental health needs. Over one half of child welfare reported caregivers meet diagnostic criteria for major depression. Mental illness can impair parenting skills and child development and increase the risk of maltreatment. Connecting community based mental health services can increase the likelihood of family reunification. Yet only one quarter to one third of caregivers with behavioural health needs received services. Caregivers who belong to a minority, or more skeptical caregivers, are less likely to utilize mental health services. Other issues include lack of health insurance or transportation money. Caseworker referral strategists may be either 'informational' or 'social'. Informational strategies include providing the caretaker with information on available services, but responsibility of seeking out and utilizing services belongs to the caregiver. Social referral strategies provide assistance in obtaining appointment, filling out paperwork, or accompanying clients to the appointments. Encouraging caseworkers to play a more active role in obtaining services may enhance safety, permanency and well-being for children and families (Bunger *et al.* 2012).

Prevention programmes

Reduction of physical abuse and neglect is a combined focus in many prevention programmes. The Nurse Family Partnership has undergone the most rigorous and extensive evaluation of child maltreatment outcomes (Krugman *et al.* 2007). Home visitation is provided by nurses to low-income first-time mothers beginning prenatally and during infancy. The first and second Nurse–Family Partnership trials included a condition of prenatal visitation without the intensive postpartum component. The phrase 'nurse-visited' refers here to the group receiving prenatal and intensive postnatal intervention, because it showed the most positive outcomes (MacMillan *et al.* 2009). The intervention reduced child physical abuse and neglect, as measured by official child protection reports, and associated outcomes, such as injuries in children of first-time disadvantaged mothers.

The Early Start programme is an intensive home-visiting programme targeted to families facing stress and difficulties (Fergusson *et al.* 2005). At age 3 years, children in Early Start had significantly lower attendance rates at hospital for childhood injuries than controls and fewer admissions to hospital for severe abuse and neglect. Early Start children have about one third of the rate of parent-reported physical abuse.

The TripleP-Positive Parenting Program involved the dissemination of Triple P professional training to the existing workforce alongside universal media and communication strategies across 18 randomly assigned counties in one US states (Prinz *et al.* 2009). Compared with the services as usual control condition, there were positive effects in the Triple P-Positive Parenting Program counties for rates of substantiated cases of child maltreatment, child out-of home placements, and child maltreatment injuries.

The most widely adopted prevention strategy in US hospitals aims to prevent abusive head traumas (shaken impact syndrome). Dias and colleagues (2004) assessed an educational intervention (leaflet, video, posters) in 16 hospitals about the dangers of infant shaking and ways to handle persistent crying provided to parents in 16 hospitals in New York State. The incidence of abusive head trauma was substantially reduced during the 66 months after introduction of the programme compared with the 66 months before the study.

Although the field of child maltreatment is changing, it needs rigorous designs applied to the assessment of programmes across the range of interventions, and a commitment across disciplines to apply evidence based principles to link science with policy.

Has CPS outlived its usefulness? While there has been considerable decline in both physical and sexual abuse, the number of cases of child neglect has not changed, and remains responsible for the higher volume of reports to CPS (Bergman 2010). Bergman suggests reallocation of responsibilities of the programs so that investigations of physical and sexual abuse are the responsibility of law enforcement, and public health nurses are first-time responders to concerns about child neglect. About 15% of child welfare staff holds a bachelor's degree and 13% hold a master's degree in social work. The average tenure for the workers is less than 2 years. Improving staff education would be beneficial.

Still child abuse cases remain unreported. Professional education must continue and be incorporated into the curriculum of undergraduate and graduate education. Societies should emulate other societies where corporal punishment has been outlawed. There should be clearly defined laws that describe abuse with consequences for failure to report.

Research priorities should include consensus about definition, better diagnostic and research instruments, epidemiological studies of incidence and prevalence, risk consequences research, determination of cultural variables and role of media, a national research plan, adequate budgeting, and ethical research designs. If children belong to the world community, then these international issues must be discussed and resolved by agencies in all countries working together under the guidance of an international maltreatment agency. A liaison with domestic violence services is necessary due to the association with it and child maltreatment (Johnson 2002).

The Department of Health and Human Services has been implementing major initiatives aimed at bringing down the rate of child abuse and neglect such as the recently funded Family Violence Prevention and Services Act (2010), grants geared towards domestic violence victims and organizations, as well as grants to reduce long-term foster care, and development of innovative intervention strategies to help our children into permanent homes.

President Obama's 2011 budget reflects a further commitment to reducing child maltreatment, by requesting child abuse state grants for child abuse prevention programmes, community-based child abuse prevention, and child abuse discretionary activities. The budget also requests additional grants for family violence prevention and service programs (Child and Family Alliance 2011).

The lowest rates of child abuse are found in countries that invest in families and prevention (Gregoire and Hornby 2011). There is good evidence that parent–child interaction therapy reduces recurrence of physical abuse. The nurse family partnership has demonstrated robust evidence for effectiveness (Spinelli and Howard 2011).

Although we have seen a dramatic decline in child abuse in the USA, it is clear that the system is in need of improvement by encouraging reports by society and practitioners, increased education, improved guidelines and better staffing for caseworkers who must be accountable for better assessment and improvement in long-term outcomes with attention to modifiable risk factors. It is essential that society and the medical profession continue to develop and refine prevention and intervention strategies aimed at curtailing the incidence and prevalence of child abuse and homicide (Bennett *et al.* 2006).

References

Asnes, A.G. and Leventhal, J.M. (2010). Managing child abuse: general principles. Pediatrics Review **31**: 47–55.

Bennett, Jr., M.D., Hall, J., Frazier, L., Jr., *et al.* (2006). Homicide of children aged 0–4 years, 2003–2004: results from the National Violent Death Reporting System. Injury Prevention. **12** (suppl II), ii39–ii43.

Bergman, A.B. (2010). Child protective services has outlived its usefulness. Archives of Pediatric Adolescent Medicine **164**(10): 978–79.

Bunger, A.C., Chuang, E., and McBeath, B. (2012). Facilitating mental health service use for caregivers: referral strategies among child welfare caseworkers. Child and Youth Services Review 1, **34**(4): 696–703.

Campbell, K.A., Cook, L.J., LaFleur, B.J., and Keenan, H.T. (2010). Household, family, and child risk factors after an investigation for suspected child maltreatment: a missed opportunity for prevention. Archives of Pediatric Adolescent Medicine **164**(10): 943–49.

Child Abuse and Neglect Fatalities 2011: Statistics and Interventions. retrieved October, 2013 https://www.childwelfare.gov

Centers for Disease Control and Prevention. National Center for Injury Prevention and Control (2010). Child Maltreatment. retrieved October, 2013 at http://www.cdc.gov/violenceprevention/childmaltreatment/

Dias, M.S., Smith, K., DeGuehery K., *et al.* (2004). Preventing abusive head trauma among infants and young children: a hospital-based, parent education program. Pediatrics **115**: e470–471.

Dubowitz, H., Papas, M.A., Black, M.M., and Starr, R.H. Jr. (2002). Child neglect: outcomes in high-risk urban preschoolers. Pediatrics **109**(6): 1100.

Ehrlich, S. (1989). Lisa, Hedda & Joel: The Steinberg Murder Case. New York, St. Martin's Press.

Family Violence Prevention and Services Act (2010). retrieved October 2013 http://www.nnedv.org/policy/issues/fvpsa.html

Fergusson, D.M., Grant, H., Horwood, L.J., and Ridder, E.M. (2005). Randomized trial of the Early Start program of home visitation. Pediatrics **16**(6): e803–9.

Finkelhor, D., Jones, L., and ShattuckA. (2009). Updated Trends in Child Maltreatment. retrieved October 2013 http://www.cola.unh.edu/ccrc/trends-child-victimization

Gado, M. (1987). The killing of Lisa Steinberg. retrieved October, 2013. http://www.trutv.com/library/crime/notorious_murders/family/lisa_steinberg/1.html

Gregoire, A. and Hornby, S.A. (2011). Has child protection become a form of madness? Yes. BMJ. **342**: d3040.

Herman-Giddens, M.E., Brown, G., Verbiest, S., *et al.* (1999). Underascertainment of child abuse mortality in the United States. JAMA **282**(5): 463–9.

Heron, M., Sutton, P.D., Xu, J., and Ventura, S.J. (2010). Annual Summary of Vital Statistics: 2007. Pediatrics **125**(1): 4–15.

Johnson, C.F. (2002). Child maltreatment 2002: recognition, reporting and risk. Pediatrics International **44**(5): 554–60.

Jones, L.M. and Finkelhor, D. (2003). Putting together evidence on declining trends in sexual abuse: a complex puzzle. Child Abuse and Neglect **27**: 133–35.

Kelley, S.J., Yorker, B.C., and Whitley, D. (1997). To grandmother's house we go . . . and stay. Children raised in intergenerational families. Journal of Gerontological Nursing **23**(9): 12–20.

Krugman, S.D., Lane, W.G., and Walsh, C.M. (2007). Update on child abuse prevention. Current Opinion in Pediatrics **19**(6): 711–18.

Macmillan, H.L., Nadine Walthan, C., Barlow, J., and Fergusson, D.M. (2009). Child maltreatment 3. Interventions to prevent child malreatment and associated impairment. Lancet **373**: 250–66.

Marcenko, M.O., Lyons, S.J., and Courtney, M. (2011). Mothers experiences, resources and needs: the context for reunification. Children and Youth Services Review **33**: 431–8.

National Child Abuse Statistics (2010). National Child Abuse Hotline: 1–800–4-A-CHILD. Child Abuse in America. Available from http://www.childhelp.org/pages/statistics (accessed 20 September 2013).

National Institute of Neurological Disorders and Stroke (2007). Shaken baby syndrome. retrieved October, 2013 http://www.ninds.nih.gov/disorders/shakenbaby/shakenbaby.htm,

Prinz, R.J., Sanders, M.R., Shapiro, C.J., and Whitaker, D.J., (2009). Population-based prevention of child maltreatment: The US triple P system population trial. Prevention Science **10**, 1–12.

Profile of Andrea Yates. retrieved October, 2013 at http://crime.about.com/od/current/p/andreayates.htm?r=et

Sege, R.D. and Flaherty, E. G. (20081). Forty years later: inconsistencies in reporting of child abuse. Archives of Disease in Childhood **93**: 822–4. Alliance for Children and families. retrieved October, 2013 http://alliance1.org/policy/briefs-analyses/child-welfare/capta

Silverman, A.B., Reinherz, H.Z., and Giaconia, R.M. (1996). The long-term sequelae of child and adolescent abuse: a longitudinal community study. Child Abuse and Neglect **20**(8): 709–23.

Spinelli, M. (2002). Infanticide: Psychosocial and legal perspectives on mothers who kill. Washington DC, American Psychiatric Press.

Spinelli, M. and Howard, L.M. (2011). Has child protection become a form of madness? No. BMJ. **342**: d3063.

Springer, K.W., Sheridan, J., Kuo D., and Carnes, M. (2007). Long-term physical and mental health consequences of childhood physical abuse: results from a large population-based sample of men and women. Child Abuse and Neglect **31**(5): 517–30.

Tilden, V.P., Schmidt, T.A., Limandri, B.J., and Chiodo, G.T. (1994). Factors that influence clinicians' assessment and management of family violence. American Journal of Public Health **84**: 628–33.

Waldfogel, J. (2009). Prevention and the child protection system. Future Child **19**(2): 195–210.

Watts-English, T., Fortson, B.L., Gibler, N., *et al.* (2006). The psychobiology of maltreatment in childhood. Journal of Social Sciences **62**(4): 717–36.

Wells, R. (2006). Managing child welfare agencies: what do we know about what works? Children and Youth Services Review **28**: 1181–94.

West, S.G., Friedman, S., and Resnick, P. (2009). Fathers who kill their children: an analysis of the literature. Journal of Forensic Science **54**(2): 463–8.

Chapter 23

Not a native son

Remi Kapo

Introduction

In the summer of 1953, aged 7, I arrived with my father at the port of Southampton from the colony of Nigeria. We were making for Ledsham Court School, a boarding school in St Leonards-on-Sea, Sussex. It was a stately building sitting among many green acres. After about an hour with the headmistress, Mrs Redfarn, my father said goodbye, turned and returned to Nigeria. I did not know then that I would not see or hear from him for 10 years, by which time I had forgotten what he looked like.

Ledsham's only black pupil began his academic life speaking no English. I was duly placed in the kindergarten with daily lessons in the native tongue. After catching up with my age group, in addition to the core subjects I was thereafter given instruction in Latin, ancient Greek, poetry, and nature study. To eradicate 'that funny African accent' I was solely accorded a daily class of elocution for a year—one hour a day with a speech therapist, held in a long, oak-panelled gallery with a book on my head to improve my deportment. Although in receipt of the beginnings of a good classical education, I was also given what I came to understand was a prototypical quantity of punishment for a 'darkie'—for most of that first year I was caned daily and frequently 'sent to Coventry' for the slightest indiscretion, usually for not understanding the customs and traditions of an alien white culture. Thus, for refusing to eat salad on my first day, I received 'three of the best'. The staff were undoubtedly ignorant of the eggs that parasites can lay on raw vegetables in a tropical climate like Nigeria, where all vegetables were cooked and salad was unheard of. Perhaps, I thought with a child's naivety, that with all the mosquitoes and eating of salad, no wonder West Africa was called the white man's grave in my books and comics. I woke up—for I had clearly landed in the mother country in the wrong skin colour. It hurt.

I had arrived knowing myself to be Yoruba. Suddenly, I was called 'coloured' and 'darkie'. Plainly vexed by my presence, several teachers and pupils resorted to belittling taunts and name-calling. It was made worse by there being nobody to whom I could appeal. Despite the daily onslaught on my race, I found first one white friend and then two more. Because of those friends, I am also able to recall good times during my time there.

Regrettably, after 5 years, my father could not sustain the fees. I had to leave Ledsham Court School. Even now I can see the carriage drive at the moment of departure. The headmistress tearfully removed the crucifix from her neck and placed it around mine, before the car driven by her husband took me away. It was the kindest act I had received from an adult in my time there. I was utterly distraught. Leaving behind the few people I knew and cared for, I belonged to nowhere, again. I felt an outcast, again.

Entering care

In the Empire mentality of the 1950s, when the ethic of white superiority was axiomatic, when class division seemed a hierarchical pillar of the populace, and when there were no rights legislation on the Statute Books, anything and everything happened to children of colour, especially to children who had further transgressed by apparently belonging to nobody.

On the long, scary, downwards skid from one middling school to another, from foster home to foster home, the London County Council was my arrester wire. My temporary home for the next 6 months was Earlsfield House Reception Centre in Wandsworth. Beechholme Children's Home in Banstead, Surrey was to be permanent. At first sight, an onlooker would perceive a sought-after suburban estate, befitting its Surrey surroundings. Established either side of a long salubrious avenue lined by mature trees, it possessed substantial properties and lawns sitting in pacific order. In truth, it felt like a place for outcasts; a State boarding school without the trimmings of private education. Had I broken some law to be sent there? Nobody would tell me what I had done. A curse like the mark of Cain settled upon me.

Beechholme

Managed by the London County Council, Beechholme comprised 24 houses named after trees, housing boys and girls in dormitories, constructed on an isthmus of land between the railway line and Fir Tree Road. Halfway down the avenue was the administration block, opposite the junior school and the war memorial. At one end of the leafy thoroughfare was a gymnasium and at the other end, a 30-bed sick bay in the charge of Sister 'Killer' Thompson, SRN. There were some 33 buildings in all on the site, including a covered swimming pool and the Chapel of the Good Shepherd, destroyed by a fire in 1968, a laundry, press shop, shoe repairer, clothes shop, and scout and guide huts.

These facilities enabled Beechholme to be more or less self-sufficient. The cottages were each run semi-independently by houseparents with Superintendent G.A. Banner, his deputy 'Taffy' Evans and the matron, Miss Hoare, overseeing the whole. Given such a large number of houses 'managed' by a motley collection of often untrained and sometimes despotic houseparents gifted with unfettered power, there were many Beechholmes, each with its own precarious ecosystem.

I was placed, aged 13, in Acacia with a housemother and three other female members of staff. There were about 14 to 16 boys and girls, each displaying shifting shades of despondency—from parental desertions and neglect, orphan fatigue, bullying, or some other sort of abuse. I think there was one other black child who was much younger. Feeling numbed and humiliated by my whirlwind ejection and downfall from boarding school, I attempted to make a new set of friends. Shunned by the majority of the white children, I got by with the few who befriended me.

Gale Parsons was one such friend. Noting the spurning on my arrival, she appointed herself to 'look after' me and show me the ropes. Younger than I and being the product of rejection and discrimination, she displayed no bigotry towards me and called me by my given name. Momentarily, she became my anchor, with no cost attached. Yet on that first encounter, I felt she was stricken by an emotional frailty I had not the maturity to understand. She had odd habits seemingly borne from the stress of deep unhappiness. Several years after leaving Beechholme, my friend Gale died alone, a beggarly heroin addict, off the Thames Embankment. Her lasting epitaph is the BBC2 Man Alive series documentary *Gale is Dead*. Directed by Jenny Barraclough in 1970 it tells of Gale's 19 difficult years on this earth. In the span of a lifetime, my time with Gale was a brief encounter, but one that had an enduring effect on me.

I saw no evidence that the powers that be in Beechholme manifestly tried to comprehend 'odd behaviour'. You were either all right or you were not. Those who were not all right were said to be 'overactive', 'underactive', or 'round the bend'. It was that clear-cut. Whilst some may say that mental health is a discipline inching towards adolescence, at Beechholme, there were no signs that it was even in its infancy. Then there was the other major institution in our neighbourhood. A few miles from Beechholme stood Belmont Hospital, specializing in psychiatric medicine. With blood-curdling gossip swirling about escaped patients, credited with all manner of crazed deeds, we regarded our institutional neighbour with great trepidation. In our unfettered imaginations, Belmont was a terrifying Bedlam. Yet some of us were living beside those with 'problems', labelled by uninformed staff as 'introverted', 'bonkers', and 'loonies', etc. And as children, we replicated what we heard. For children like my friend Gale, those fears became a later reality.

Acacia held two dormitories and staff bedrooms on the first floor and a sitting room, dining room, and kitchen on the ground floor. The large detached 'cottage' had a tarmac yard at the rear. Vested with absolute power, members of staff dispensed justice. By turns fair-minded and capricious, they determined right and wrong and their word was law. When I asked for a comb, a staffer retorted:

'Coloureds don't need combs.'

That was that and there was no appeal—my hair remained uncomfortably and unsightly knotted.

If they deemed a wrongdoing justified severe punishment, such as the cane, the sinner was sent to 'Old Banner', the Superintendent and final arbiter, who seldom resorted to corporal punishment. In my view, G.A. Banner was a misunderstood social revolutionary, a gentle, kindly man who was seen by many children as comfortably off and stuck-up, his refined accent setting him yet further apart. Arriving at Beechholme just a few years before me, he had heralded a mistral of change. However, tolerance, compassion, and a readiness to listen were not qualities shared by all the staff at the institution he had inherited. Furthermore, the sobering truth was that many children had long ceased to have any relationship with the consideration and liberal sympathy he manifested, and clung to their suspicions like a much-loved comforter.

In contrast to my regimented early education, I now lived alongside children who preferred comics to books, and for whom homework was definitely optional. Poetry for many went no further than the oft-recited Beechholme ditty:

There is a mouldy dump down Beechholme way,
Where we get lousy food three times a day.
Egg and bacon we don't see,
We get sawdust in our tea,
That's why we're gradually
Fading away.

On balance, it was defiant contempt. Although the houses were well-built and the food was adequate, hunger always lurked. It was a powerless way of articulating that we did not want to be 'in care'. Having previously been exposed at boarding school to Tennyson's 'The Lady of Shalott' and the broader domain of literature, I felt uncomfortably incongruous. Attempting to integrate into a sea of cockney accents, I tried unsuccessfully to mask both my elocution and education. Indignant at having plummeted in educational standards in a society where knowing one's place was an omnipresent despot, my colour put me bottom of the class pile. Anticipation and circumvention became constant companions.

Secondary school

Being of secondary school age, I was sent to Alvering Secondary School in Wandsworth, which held a handful of black pupils. Leaving the house every morning at seven, I would make the 20-minute walk along the lane to Banstead Station, to take the 39 bus via Sutton or the 84 directly to Clapham Junction, and then bus to St Anne's Hill, to arrive just before 9am. I would seek out my only school friend, Arthur Lum, a Chinese student, and proceed to our classes.

Ashamed of being from a children's home and in an attempt to avoid the disparagement that had been accorded those who had been too honest, like everyone else, I quickly concocted a fantasy about the home life that cosily bracketed my school day.

The daily routine of attending school was intimately coupled with staying clear of the bullies stalking the grounds. Many merely vilified my colour and delighted in telling me about the superiority of their race—'nigger', 'sambo', 'wog', 'darkie', and 'coloured'. However, some bullies went further, physically articulating the sentiments of the majority.

For two tormenters in particular, with everything of the night about them, I was their arrant bête noire. Passing by one during a metalwork class, he thrust a quarter-inch chisel into my lower right calf muscle; stabbing what I later learned was the posterior tibial artery. Blood spurted. Turning ashen, the horrified teacher screamed for the ambulance. Had I provoked the attack? No. Truly? I did not have to.

While having a tourniquet tied around my leg and waiting for the ambulance, I witnessed the feeble grilling:

'Why?' asked the teacher of my tormenter.
'Chisel slipped, sir,' the bully replied, curtly.

The bully's mates giggled.

'What?' the teacher sputtered. 'Your chisel slipped over five feet and into his leg?'
'Floor's slippery, sir,' said the bully, cockily.

Rolling his eyes in utter futility at the response, the teacher spat:

'In my class, you stay away from him.'
'Yes, sir.'

Shrugging off the feather-like scolding, the bully made a face at his sniggering mates, who were ready to serve as his 'blind' witnesses. In those wild days, there were some teachers who did not want to be observed siding with a 'coloured'—'nigger lover' was a taunt too far.

That was then. To this day I sometimes see my former antagonists, still glued together, chugging around Wandsworth in a flatbed truck collecting rag and bone, as they did all those years ago with dray horse and cart after leaving school.

To circumvent the playground assassins at lunchtime, I went hungry and retreated to the usually empty school library, my haven, where I immersed myself in history books. At the end of the school day, I would walk a gauntlet of jeers from some white pupils. But terror kicked in fully at the school gates. My two waiting antagonists would give chase the whole way to Clapham Junction Station and even onto the platform where, with abject fear, I would beg the protection of railway staff until the train arrived.

Unluckily, the welfare and child care officers were cold and indifferent individuals who, unwittingly or not, were likely to provoke new problems. Reporting a white pupil invited retaliation. Instead, I became accustomed to accepting the blame for things I had not done to lessen the cataclysm, and learned to console myself afterwards. These officials therefore learned nothing inconvenient from me. With blame for many things being frequently laid at my door, I learned to make myself invisible—to be in a room and be barely noticed.

Only the annual Sports Day in Beechholme rendered me appreciably visible. My membership of the team suddenly became imperative—'you coloureds are fast runners!' But once the great day of 'friendship' was over, I resumed being an outcast. The cold shouldering had the curious benefit of keeping me out of trouble, mischief-making tending to be a group activity.

Instead, I retreated to books and running, encircling Beechholme's broad playing fields every night. My isolation was finally breached on the great day I was invited to audition for the Beechholme choir by G.A. Banner, who was also its choirmaster. It had been almost 8 years since being invited to join anything in my host country. Desperate to 'belong' to something, I practised constantly before my audition and was ecstatic when I was accepted. Each Sunday now found me in the deep sanctum of the Church of England, trilling the praises of a god I thought had long forgotten me.

'The sun will never set on the British Empire.' I had had this pumped into me since arriving in Britain. When colonial independence was clearly underway, however, a new and chagrined cry surfaced:

'We don't need them anyway. They cost too much.'

Now here was Britain out on the daunting slopes of 1960s liberation, slipping, sliding and squealing into introspection, losing an empire and searching for a role. Suddenly, immigration crashed onto the agenda. The effect at Beechholme of this new reality and its consequent edicts was immediate. My normally high anxiety quotient shot up further. Now I was really scared.

'Wouldn't you feel better being among your own people?' asked a Beechholme housefather.

'When I qualify as a barrister,' I replied, weakly. 'Then I'm going home.'

'Barrister?' the housefather exclaimed, laughing out loud. 'No one from here has ever gone to university. Not clever enough. An' what is a coloured lad going to look like in a white wig? A black and white minstrel—that's what! A trade would suit you better—carpentry and plumbing. They will need carpenters in Nigeria,' he added, confidently.

His words and judgement hurt. My skin colour and my presence here had truly become a serious political issue. Providing I did not call Britain *home*, and that I was not trying to aspire to anything much or intending to settle here, I was safe from further assault, verbal and otherwise. I gained the distinct adolescent impression that decolonization aroused the populace, while the issue of immigration united them. Promulgated by mischievous politicians and disseminated by the baying press of the day, the issue of immigration inflamed the staff and fostered resentment. In the prickly aftermath of Independence celebrations, I represented Africa in the eyes of many in Beechholme. Disparaging remarks repeatedly scorched my ears:

> 'They can't govern.'
> 'You know they can't manage.'
> 'They'll fall apart without us.'
> 'Soon they'll be begging us to take them back.'

Saying goodbye to world power takes a particular grace. And I saw little of it.

'Ignore them,' said my welfare officer, chummily, as if he was my friend. 'What do they know about Nigeria? Half of them don't even know their own fathers. Now what's this I hear about you wanting to be a barrister? Why would you want to go bothering your head with all that bookwork? The other kids will only think you're trying to act big. Blend in with them. Lower your sights. Know your place.'

Intellectual and educational aspirations were scorned. Blue collar enterprise was encouraged with enthusiasm. I felt a captive in a padded compound with bodily needs guaranteed, but no prospect of setting a self-determined scholarly course considered counter to an in-care boy's station in life. No one seemed to notice the number of books I read.

Leisure time

Left to our own devices after school, boredom was the constant whinge. Indeed, weekends at Beechholme would have been most instructive to an onlooker. Many resorted to larking about in the back yards around Beechholme. Some built go-karts, bicycles and crystal radio sets from bits found on the local dump, trips to which were neither encouraged nor prevented. Others played endless card games and board games. Reflecting the disinterest in our education, homework was the rarest activity. School reports were furnished, and good reports eagerly flourished, but otherwise neither sought nor commented on by houseparents. However, homework was a habit I could not break and thus always completed. Besides, I enjoyed it.

Without homework to be concerned about, different routines came into play, in part guided by the temperament and encouragement of houseparents. Leisure in Beechholme's little galaxy ranged from those who sought the scout and guide packs' structured activities, to the defiantly errant, who gained notoriety by pinching sweets and cigarettes from The Chocolate Box in Nork and shops in Banstead Village. The local woods rustled as small bands pursued a brand of independence beyond Beechholme's perimeters, making fires, drifting around climbing trees, and sometimes crossing more private boundaries. Others played along the railway line, staged cricket and football tournaments in the yard, and teased our neighbours by playing knock-down-ginger on the doors of the houses along the avenue. During the fruit-picking season, scrumping in local orchards was both exhilarating and stomach-filling.

It was also at the weekends an onlooker would have seen the malaise of the angry, the introverted, the depressed and the excluded, for whom loneliness ruled. My weekends invariably comprised a five mile run, followed by homework, reading or listening to the Home Service and *Journey into Space*. My spirits rose when occasionally I was invited to listen to the Hit Parade on Radio Luxembourg before bed. It was usually a short-lived experience.

In many ways, Beechholme was an isolated, insulated and insular establishment where the *Lord of the Flies* could have been scripted in everything but gore. Between the children the hierarchy may well have tumbled from Darwin's theory of evolution. The bullies, who were generally the eldest and longest institutionalized, determined the state of play for all, frequently with the tacit agreement of the houseparents. Unfettered and unthinking prejudices abounded. Fear was a ubiquitous travelling companion.

Despite having a couple of tentative friendships in Acacia, I grew downhearted, a condition to which I became accustomed. Continuing rebuffs had normalised rejection. I withdrew. Worse still, I had lost the self-assurance needed for seeking out new interests, without disapproving comments and looks. Alarmed by my inner turmoil, an instinct said I must save myself. A chance encounter furnished me with a way out. On the train returning to Beechholme from Clapham Junction, I had met a resident of Kerria who invited me to tea. I was dumbfounded.

'You're allowed to invite someone to tea?' I asked, astonished.
'Sure. Uncle Bob won't mind. You'd like him.'

Weighed against the Spartan environs of Acacia, Kerria was positively abloom. Warming to the more homely atmosphere on repeated visits and hearing that there was a bed available, I tentatively asked them to accept me, which they did without hesitation—swapping houses was permitted provided you were accepted by the receiving house parents. Thus emboldened, I officially requested a move to Kerria House, convinced I would be happier in its more functional environment. A date was soon set.

Kerria House

Kerria House was the province of Bob and Beryl Green, a kind-hearted, middle-aged couple from Yorkshire. I know not how they came to join the social services. He was a moral, upright ex-serviceman who believed in the northern ethics of hard work. She had been a conventional housewife. Though I was now happier, I still felt deprived of affection, academic encouragement, personal guidance and advice—the friendly Uncle Bob was educationally ambivalent. In place of scholarship, he was a champion of blue-collar action, a virtuoso of the trades and an outstanding carpenter. Given his familiarity with service ablutions, Kerria was maintained by the children, shipshape and Bristol fashion. Drawing up a weekly rota, he had us peeling potatoes for 20, scrubbing and polishing floors, shoes, brass work, and even cooking under the supervision of Aunt Beryl. Punishment in Kerria favoured no one. Extra chores, loss of pocket money, and being confined to the house and yard were meted out irrespectively. Strangely, I was glad for that. Moreover, I never saw Uncle Bob lift his hand to a child. Thankfully, at a time when there were no race laws on the statute books, overt racial bigotry was prohibited. Gender bigotry, however, went unchecked, reflecting the chauvinism that extended beyond Beechholme.

Learning a trade took precedence over all other interests. Plumbing, carpentry and metalwork were his areas of expertise, together with caring for his beloved Ford Zodiac. Under his expert supervision we built an inspection pit and a portable garage, an enterprise that absorbed some of us after school over several months. Under Bob Green's tutelage I developed an unusual skill-set: carpentry, construction, metalwork, decorating, car mechanics, and mix and matching bits from a dump to build a bicycle from scratch.

In Kerria's lively environment, I felt more settled and my insecurities, anxieties and unresolved problems since leaving boarding school began to dissipate. But despite their efforts, Kerria also could not provide what we most lacked—a loving family, educational encouragement, and belief in a future. To a young Yoruba boy who knew he had been brought to Britain to receive an education, I felt I had failed before I had even had a chance to begin.

Despite my improved circumstances, I continued to harbour unease as to what would happen when the time came for me to leave Beechholme. What would I do? Where would I go? Where would I live? With what would I feed myself? The future looked bleak, and every child held that dread in common. Armageddon began on our 16th birthday, the date set for you to leave Beechholme. We often spoke gloomily about it among ourselves, pondering our unknown and fearful future. The professionals were unwilling or unable to grasp our scary reality, instead talking only of apprenticeships, our deeper apprehensions remaining unaddressed and untamed.

In theory, Beechholme was a laudable idea. *In loco parentis* was the role of the London County Council. As such, every child was provided with food, clothes, shelter, schooling and weekly pocket money according to age. For summer holidays, each house was given two weeks in resorts like Bournemouth, Paignton, Goodrington Sands, Torquay, Dawlish, Margate, and other resorts. There were senior and junior club activities, scouts, guides, and the choir. Every child received presents and cakes for birthdays and Christmas. This was far from the workhouse, which loomed in the recent past.

Nevertheless, there were systemic failures in the care at Beechholme. The word of a child carried little or no weight with the staff or child care professionals. Interest and support in academic achievement of any child was never shown. Personal problems deriving from disrupted and disfigured histories or from bullying were rarely resolved. Houseparents and assistants seemed mostly untrained in child care. I learned that many, not all, had previously worked in offices and factories before joining Beechholme. Sometimes they came from broken homes themselves. With unadulterated power over their vulnerable charges, the condescension of the day appeared to afflict them as well—thus disparagement tended to be their methodology with children. Child care professionals generally asked very few pertinent questions and always sided with the staff. 'Them against us' appeared to steer their behaviour. It certainly steered ours.

By the same token, what seems to have been missing in the management of Beechholme was tangible concern for reducing the often all-too-visible effects of the resentment, disorientation, psychological woes, and educational poverty that afflicted us all. Furthermore, we had all been taken into care at different ages with varying degrees of deprivation, both emotional and physical. During my time I witnessed browbeating and bullying as a daily occurrence and occasionally, other types of abuse. Naturally, sex was one.

Discussions about sex almost always resulted in embarrassed giggles. Sex education and loving relationships were a mystery. Sexual intercourse between a few children was an inevitable by-product, covertly sampled behind the many outhouses in Beechholme, in the out-of-sight hollows of Banstead Downs, in Nork woods, and other secluded places. The lack of developmental interest or educational guidance was akin to waving temptation at angry, wounded spirits. Sometimes girls would suddenly leave, to reappear 6 months later, inexplicably changed.

Sexual misconduct was not the special preserve of the children. A seriously inappropriate liaison crumbled when a married housemother was impregnated by a teenager. If an inquiry was conducted, the outcome was not for our ears, and as usual, a veil of secrecy was drawn over the scandal. Murky rumours from certain houses hinted that particular housefathers were acting suspiciously around girls or boys in their charge, or how certain assistant housemothers had been seen in compromising positions. They should have been reported. But to whom? Who would believe it? They must be caught red-handed. In an establishment the size of Beechholme? Unlikely. Had whistle-blowing been established in the homes for the children and staff, then maybe what we experienced may never have occurred.

The patent lack of comprehension and even compassion often exacerbated behavioural problems, which would later result in life-changing events.

'Stop doing that!' was the cure for anyone affected by a tic. 'You can stop if you want to, you're just not trying hard enough.'

The indignation and offensive retort from the chastized said everything and ultimately landed them in trouble. That chastizing mind-set was endemic, virtually guaranteeing that whatever dilemmas you arrived with, you left Beechholme with, with compound interest. That interest included an unerring suspicion of authority, and foreshortened horizons.

With child protection appearing to be guided by class attitudes, it was clear that we were the underclass in a deeply stratified society where joining the 'working class' was considered a laudable achievement in itself. Those who were deemed our protectors indeed inhabited a different world, speaking a language that had no vocabulary for our pain and fear. Thus we, too, remained inarticulate.

Legacy

It could be said that Beechholme was the consequence of a flawed and evolving system. Its overt defects could be characterized by a comprehensive disregard of children's rights and the silencing of our voices. Without apparent checks and balances behind the official façade, inexperienced individuals were allowed to interpret child care responsibilities according to their backgrounds and tendencies, covered by the ubiquitous mantle of silence. Anything can happen out of sight—an outlook that had sufficed in the colonies appeared to sufficed at home too. Statutes concerning children, race, gender, and the homeless have comprehensively altered the field, with broader definitions of human rights woven tightly into the tapestry of our legal system. Child welfare organizations comb the streets and operate phone lines, and psychologists and social workers are ever more alert. These belated laws, bodies, and sciences were but notions when I was at Beechholme. Could the unrestrained behaviour I experienced happen today? It seems so. As I write these words, the Oxford sex grooming case (Operation Bullfinch, 2013) is being heard at the Old Bailey court in London. Press revelations about the maltreatment of children under the noses of parents, care professionals, teachers, friends, and neighbours should tell us misjudgement is never far away—Haut de la Garenne, Bryn Estyn, Kincora Boys, Home, to name but a few.

What have we learned? Child psychologists and care professionals frequently complain of feeling overwhelmed by impossible caseloads. Of course they are, there is much to do. Like their charges, they too are unsupported by a complex and flawed system, open to political manipulation and short-sightedness. Like their forebears, there are the lingering mutterings of fecklessness and deprivation that few want to take responsibility for, but are quick to pontificate on.

Cottage homes like Beechholme were the transition between the workhouse and the current state care system. But what will this current system transform into? Beechholme typified the dilemma that continues to exist now. The 'problem' remains self-evident, but the solution to providing an alternative reality and future for children who are unloved and sometimes unlovely, or at least perceive themselves to be so, continues to present a formidable edifice. How does society love the forgotten and dispossessed, with their guileless pain all too evidently manifest?

Conclusion

At the conference that honoured the memory of Professor Channi Kumar, we debated whether child protection had become a form of madness. I think not. Channi Kumar's special gift to child psychology was his articulacy. We emerged from care with no words to express the loneliness, despair and hopelessness, depression, trauma, and lack of belonging. We were not listened to then, and are not listened to now. Perhaps it was because we couldn't articulate it. Channi Kumar had also experienced that intense loneliness as a child, and added a layer, that of empathizing with the voiceless. He represented the subaltern voice of the vulnerable.

Beechholme was an experience that I accidentally benefited from; in so much my antagonist was my benefactor. It taught me what I did not want. I was not a native son. I also found my voice.

Index

Note: 'n.' after a page number indicates the number of a note on that page

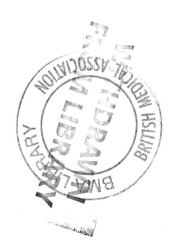